ATTACHMENT THEORY IN PRACTICE

Also from Susan M. Johnson

Attachment Processes in Couple and Family Therapy
Edited by Susan M. Johnson and Valerie E. Whiffen

Emotionally Focused Couple Therapy with Trauma Survivors: Strengthening Attachment Bonds
Susan M. Johnson

Emotionally Focused Therapy for Couples
Leslie S. Greenberg and Susan M. Johnson

ATTACHMENT THEORY IN PRACTICE

Emotionally Focused Therapy (EFT)
with Individuals, Couples, and Families

SUSAN M. JOHNSON

THE GUILFORD PRESS
New York   London

Library of Congress Cataloging-in-Publication Data

Names: Johnson, Susan M., author.
Title: Attachment theory in practice : emotionally focused therapy (EFT) with
    individuals, couples, and families / Susan M. Johnson.
Description: New York, NY : The Guilford Press, 2018. | Includes
    bibliographical references and index.
Identifiers: LCCN 2018045405 | ISBN 9781462538249 (hardback)
Subjects: LCSH: Family psychotherapy. | Marital psychotherapy. |
    Psychotherapy. | BISAC: PSYCHOLOGY / Psychotherapy / General. |
MEDICAL /
    Psychiatry / General. | SOCIAL SCIENCE / Social Work. | RELIGION /
    Counseling. | PSYCHOLOGY / Psychotherapy / Couples & Family.
Classification: LCC RC488.5 .J64 2018 | DDC 616.89/156--dc23
LC record available at *https://lccn.loc.gov/2018045405*

To my partner, John, the great miracle in my life,
who, every day, offers me a safe adventure that
lights up my heart and my soul
and makes me strong.

And to my colleagues—groundbreaking pioneers
in the science of adult bonding Mario Mikulincer
and Phil Shaver, and the outstanding clinicians
and trainers who are part of my EFT family.
Together we grow.

About the Author

Susan M. Johnson, EdD, is the leading developer of emotionally focused therapy (EFT). She is Professor Emeritus of Clinical Psychology at the University of Ottawa, Ontario, Canada; Distinguished Research Professor in the Marriage and Family Therapy Program at Alliant International University in San Diego; and Director of the International Centre for Excellence in Emotionally Focused Therapy. Dr. Johnson has been appointed to the Order of Canada, one of the country's highest civilian honors. She is a recipient of the Family Psychologist of the Year Award from Division 43 of the American Psychological Association and the Outstanding Contribution to Marriage and Family Therapy Award from the American Association for Marriage and Family Therapy, among other awards. Dr. Johnson is the author of acclaimed books for professionals, including *Emotionally Focused Therapy for Couples* and *Emotionally Focused Couple Therapy with Trauma Survivors*, as well as bestselling books for general readers, including *Hold Me Tight* and *Love Sense*.

Preface

> O body swayed to music, O brightening glance,
> How can we know the dancer from the dance?
> —WILLIAM BUTLER YEATS

I have to write. I write to try to tie down the chaos of life's moving kaleidoscope and to hold it still for a moment. I write notes while I am working in therapy. I write when I am unclear as to how to make sense of an experience or when I find something particularly significant or beautiful. I have to write about what my clients teach me in my sessions—and they always teach me something. Amazingly, I find that every session and every written reflection is still an adventure, a chance to clamber into this territory called being human. What will I find there? Always something I do not yet really understand.

As a psychologist, I also have the chance to be a perpetual student, listening to all the great names in psychology and psychotherapy share their insights and their conclusions and offer their suggestions for how our field should proceed into the 21st century. I teach therapists around the world and listen to their longings, their frustrations, and their dilemmas. So it is natural that over the last decade I have formed my own vision about the great endeavor called psychotherapy, about what our problems are and what is the best way forward, and it is natural that I must now write about this vision.

I am filled with hope for our profession; we are learning so much, and so fast, especially about intimate relationships and the role they play in who we are and how our lives unfold—for better and for worse. I am also filled with dismay, and some of the reasons I am sure will be clear in Chapter 1.

The world needs good therapists more than ever. And good therapists need a clear way of seeing human beings, a map of their struggles, and a clear route for guiding their clients toward wholeness and health. When we are safe and sound, confident and clear, then we can help our clients come home to the same place.

This book offers a synopsis of attachment theory as a comprehensive developmental perspective on personality and affect regulation and presents the implications of this theory for the general practice of psychotherapy. It delineates the clear links between attachment theory and the experiential humanistic model of intervention (using emotionally focused therapy [EFT] as a guide to following these links). It also offers an integrative approach to assessment and an outline of how the insights of attachment translate into effective intervention in individual, couple, and family therapy. Individual chapters on each modality expand this discussion, which is illuminated by clinical chapters showing interventions in action. In the first and, more briefly, in the last chapter, I summarize the promise of attachment theory and science for the practice of psychotherapy. In this book, the focus of intervention is on depression and anxiety—also referred to as "emotional disorders."

Those of you who know my work will not be surprised by my arguments or conclusions. The way forward is to honor both the relational heart of the practice of psychotherapy and the wisdom of our emotions and to tune in to attachment science as a guide to our craft. Attachment science is about biology, but it is also about common sense—what our deepest intuitions have always told us. It is, above all, about what makes us human—our relationships. Having a positive sense of connection with others is the best, and perhaps the only viable, way of helping human beings find a place called "safe and sound."

Contents

Chapter 1

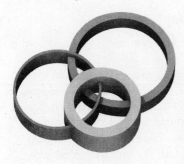

Attachment

An Essential Guide for Science-Based Practice

The most exciting breakthroughs of the 21st century
will not occur because of technology but because of an
expanding concept of what it means to be human.
       —JOHN NAISBITT

Proximity to social resources decreases the cost of climbing
both the literal and figurative hills we face, because the
brain construes *social* resources as *bioenergetic* resources,
much like oxygen or glucose.
       —JAMES A. COAN AND DAVID A. SBARRA (2015, p. 87)

There are now over a thousand different names for approaches to psychotherapy and 400 specifically outlined methods of intervention (Garfield, 2006; Corsini & Wedding, 2008). There are also numerous therapy "tribes" each with its own view of reality. Approaches and methods vary widely in the extent of their specification, the depth of theory they are based on, and the level of empirical support they have accrued. In addition, there are literally hundreds of specific in-session interventions for any problem a client can come up with. These interventions are often portrayed as fast cures for complex disorders, the focus being on symptom reduction rather than on considering the person and context in which this symptom arises. Having all these methods and techniques out

1

there, purportedly with at least some level of rigor behind them, strikes me as a perfect recipe for chaos in our field.

FOUR ROUTES OUT OF CHAOS

In the face of escalating numbers of "disorders" (which proliferate with every version of classification systems, such as the DSM), models, and interventions, the need to find clear, general, and parsimonious routes to training and intervention is obvious. Four routes seem to offer promise. The first is the path of dedicated empiricism. Conscientious therapists are exhorted to take the path of science, read all the empirical research, and then choose the best perspective, model, and intervention for each client's presenting problem at a particular time. Even for the most dedicated therapist, this seems like a daunting, if not impossible, task, especially since manualized treatment protocols are becoming more numerous, complex, and arduous to master. Under dedicated empiricism, the practice of therapy becomes one of following a set cognitive outline, and the therapist becomes primarily a technician.

The second path involves focusing on the process of change in therapy. The most concrete attempt at parsimony here seems to be the suggestion that therapists simply focus on common factors in the therapy change process, whatever and whoever they are trying to change. The justification for this orientation is that all treatments in large outcome studies seem to be equally effective, so specific models and interventions are interchangeable. In fact, this generalization is unfounded and is based on placing many different studies of varying quality into a soup called meta-analysis, and coming up with mean results that are often meaningless. In fact the whole idea of interchangeable effects across therapies would seem to be an artifact of evaluation methodology (Budd & Hughes, 2009); different manualized therapies often share a large number of active ingredients. There are also some areas in which specific treatments have been found to be more appropriate and more effective for specific disorders (Chambless & Ollendick, 2001; Johnson & Greenberg, 1985), although it is not clear if such differences are maintained at follow-up (Marcus, O'Connell, Norris, & Sawaqdeh, 2014).

Perhaps the most considered variables in the study of general change factors seem to be the quality of the alliance with the therapist and client engagement in the therapy process. The promise is that, if we get these general factors right, then suddenly the task of therapy—to create change—will become simple and manageable. A positive alliance and attention to the quality of client engagement are probably necessary for any kind of change; they are certainly key variables that potentiate the process of change. But they are hardly the whole story when it comes to intervention. The amount of variance in outcome accounted for by the alliance with the therapist has been calculated at around 10% (Horvath & Symonds, 1991; Horvath & Bedi, 2002). Furthermore, general factors become less general in the therapy room. Is alliance as operationalized by an experiential humanistic therapist the same as that shaped by a cognitive behavioral therapist? The concept of client engagement seems more promising. In the National Institute of Mental Health (NIMH) study of depression, Castonguay and colleagues found that more emotional engagement/experience on the part of clients predicted positive change across therapy models (Castonguay, Goldfried, Wiser, Raue, & Hayes, 1996), whereas a focus on distorted thoughts as they link to negative emotions (as exemplified by classic cognitive-behavioral therapy [CBT]) actually predicted more depressive symptoms after therapy. Of course, the level of engagement that is deemed sufficient for change will surely vary depending on the goals of a particular model of therapy.

A third proposed route to achieving clarity and efficiency in our field is to focus on commonalities in the problems clients bring to us. The promise here is that we can integrate areas of intervention focused on the so-called latent structure of, for example, emotional disorders (such as panic disorder, generalized anxiety disorder, and depression), viewing all these problems as a more general *negative affect syndrome*. Therapists then might work on modifying a small number of empirically outlined key symptoms of such general malaise. Negative affect syndrome, for example, can be defined as an overactive sensitivity to threat, a habitual avoidance of fearful situations, and automatic negative ways of responding or acting when triggered (Barlow, Allen, & Choate, 2004). Change is all about helping clients to reevaluate such threats and reduce catastrophizing, which makes it possible for them to then modify their habitual avoidance of fearful situations (which has prevented new learning and paradoxically maintained their anxiety). It should then be possible to persuade the client to actually respond in a different way when exposed to a negative trigger. Of course, the best ways to "persuade" and "reevaluate" are still unclear.

A fourth route is to focus on underlying processes, not just in the development of a disorder, but in the way people function when thriving and when dysfunctional. This equates to a broad orientation to how human beings continually construct a sense of self, make choices, and engage with others. From this vantage point, we understand why psychotherapy has evolved, not just in terms of following specific evidence-based interventions, grasping general common elements in therapy, and cataloging descriptions of client problems, all of which are useful, but also from general models of human functioning, that is, from attempts to depict and understand just what kind of creature a human being is. Such models offer therapists general definitions of health and positive functioning, and dysfunction and distress that go way beyond the disorders delineated in the formal classification systems (such as the DSM or ICD). The most current and most robust of these models call for therapy to focus on the whole person in his or her life-operating context. They call for the agenda of therapy to broaden in order to embrace growth and the optimal development of the personality, rather than focusing strictly on the relief of one or more specific symptoms. A broad conceptual model allows us to place descriptions of disorders and of core elements of change into an integrated explanatory framework. From this framework, we can assess clients' strengths and weaknesses and decide how best to engage with them. We can also make judgments about what changes really matter and are likely to last. All models of therapy are based on some kind of implicit model of human functioning, but these are often left vague or unexamined. The cognitive behavioral model of couple therapy, for example, is based on a rational economic model of close relationships, wherein skilled negotiation predicts relationship satisfaction. Emotionally focused couple therapy, on the other hand, is based on a model of relationships that prioritizes emotion and bonding processes and views emotional responsiveness as the key ingredient in satisfaction and stability.

No single perspective or model can capture the richness and complexity of a human life; as Einstein said, "Alas, our theory is too poor for experience." However, in order for clinicians to operate in an optimally efficient and effective fashion, we need a cohesive science-based theory of the essentials of human functioning that is capable of addressing emotional, cognitive, behavioral, and interpersonal dysfunction. This theory must apply across the modalities of individual, couple, and family therapies, and it must offer the three basics of any scientific endeavor: Systematic description based on observation and the outlining of patterns; predictions linking one factor to another; and a general explanatory framework, which must be supported by a large corroborating body of research. It must be convincing and falsifiable in its portrayal of optimal functioning and resilience, of the development and growth of a person over time, of dysfunction and how it is perpetuated, and of the necessary and sufficient conditions for meaningful lasting change.

Specifically, psychotherapy needs a theory (or a pathway or map) that guides us to help people to change on the level of core organizing variables, such as how emotion is habitually regulated, how core orienting cognitions about the self and other are structured and processed, and how pivotal behaviors and relationships with others are shaped. This theory has to step beyond the intrapsychic; it has to link self and system, intrapsychic individual realities, and interactional patterns in a parsimonious and systematic way. It has to correspond with the new cutting-edge research on neuroscience and the evidence that we are, more than anything else, social animals fixated on our connection with others.

ATTACHMENT THEORY: WHO WE ARE AND HOW WE LIVE

I submit that there is only one candidate that comes anywhere near fulfilling these criteria, and that is the developmental theory of personality termed attachment theory, as outlined by John Bowlby (1969, 1988). While initially attachment theory was presented in terms of early childhood development, it has been extended, particularly in the last few years, to adults and adult relationships. As Rholes and Simpson point out (2015, p. 1), "Few theories and areas of research have been more prolific during the past decade than the attachment field. . . . The ensuing flood of research that now supports the major principles of attachment theory rank among the most important achievements in the psychological sciences today." In addition, attachment science is consonant with current research from the fields of neuroscience, social psychology, health psychology, and clinical psychology, the central message of which is that we are first and foremost a social, relational, and bonding species. Over the lifespan, the need for connection with others shapes our neural architecture, our responses to stress, our everyday emotional lives, and the interpersonal dramas and dilemmas that are at the heart of those lives.

Recently attachment theory has been explicitly proposed by Magnavita and Anchin (2014) as the basis for a unified approach to psychotherapy. These authors suggest that this theory constitutes the long-sought-after "holy grail" that finally allows for a cohesive approach to a wide array of psychological disorders and addresses character change and permanent symptom alleviation. Others have recently suggested that attachment theory offers a substantive basis for intervention in a number of specific modalities, such as individual psychotherapy (Costello, 2013; Fosha, 2000; Wallin, 2007), couple therapy (Johnson & Whiffen, 2003; Johnson, 2002, 2004), and family therapy (Johnson, 2004; Furrow, Palmer, Johnson, Faller, & Palmer-Olson, in press; Hughes, 2007). All these authors stress the essentially integrative nature of attachment science and theory, and that this perspective allows us to move beyond compartmentalization and fragmentation into what E. O. Wilson terms "consilience" (1998). This term arises from the ancient Greek belief that the cosmos is orderly, and that this order can be discovered and systematically laid out in a series of interacting rules and processes. These rules emerge from the convergence of evidence drawn from different sets of phenomena and come together to give us viable blueprints for our world and ourselves.

PRINCIPLES OF ATTACHMENT THEORY

So what are the basic tenets of modern attachment theory that have evolved from the first model so brilliantly outlined by John Bowlby (Bowlby, 1969, 1973, 1980, 1988) and developed further by social psychologists in more recent years (Cassidy & Shaver, 2008; Mikulincer & Shaver, 2016)? I'll set forth 10. But first, note three general facts about this perspective. Attachment is fundamentally an interpersonal theory that places the individual in the context of his or her closest relationships with others; it views mankind as not only essentially social but also as *Homo vinculum*—the one who bonds. Bonding with others is viewed as the most intrinsic essential survival strategy for human beings. Second, this theory is essentially concerned with emotion and the regulation of emotion, and it particularly privileges the significance of fear. Fear is viewed not only in terms of everyday anxieties, but also on an existential level, as reflecting core issues of helplessness and vulnerability; that is, as reflecting survival concerns regarding death, isolation, loneliness, and loss. A key factor in mental health and well-being is whether these factors can be dealt with in a manner that enhances vitality and resilience. Third, it is a developmental theory; that is, it is concerned with growth and flexible adaptiveness and the factors that block or enhance this adaptiveness. Bonding theory assumes that the close connection with trusted others is the ecological niche in which the human brain, nervous system, and key behavioral patterns evolved and is the context in which we can evolve into our best selves.

In simple terms, the 10 core tenets of attachment theory and science are:

1. From the cradle to the grave, human beings are hardwired to seek not just social contact, but also physical and emotional proximity to special others who are deemed irreplaceable. The longing for a "felt sense" of connection to key others is primary in terms of the hierarchy of human goals and needs. Humans are most acutely aware of this innate need for connection at times of threat, risk, pain, or uncertainty. Threats that trigger the attachment system may be from the outside or the inside, for example, troubling construals of rejection by loved ones, negative images or concrete reminders of one's own mortality (Mikulincer, Birnbaum, Woddis, & Nachmias, 2000; Mikulincer & Florian, 2000). In relationships, shared vulnerability builds bonds, precisely because it brings attachment needs for a felt sense of connection and comfort to the fore and encourages reaching for others.

2. Predictable physical and/or emotional connection with an attachment figure, often a parent, sibling, longtime close friend, mate, or spiritual figure, calms the nervous system and shapes a physical and mental sense of a *safe haven* where comfort and reassurance can be reliably obtained and emotional balance can be restored or enhanced. The responsiveness of others, especially when we are young, tunes the nervous system to be less sensitive to threat and creates expectations of a relatively safe and manageable world.

3. This emotional balance promotes the development of a grounded, positive, and integrated sense of self and the ability to organize inner experience into a coherent whole. This grounded sense of self also facilitates the congruent expression of needs to attachment figures; such expressions are likely to result in more successful bids for connection, which then continue to build positive models of close others as accessible sources of support.

4. A felt sense of being able to depend on a loved one creates a *secure base*—a platform from which to move out into the world, take risks, and explore and develop a sense of competence and autonomy. This *effective dependency* is a source of strength and resilience, while the denial of attachment needs and pseudo self-sufficiency are liabilities. Being able to reach out to and depend on reliable others and internalize a "felt sense" of secure connection with others is the ultimate resource that allows our species to survive and thrive in an uncertain world.

5. The key factors that define the quality and security of an attachment bond are the perceived *accessibility, responsiveness,* and *emotional engagement* of attachment figures. These factors can be translated into the acronym A.R.E. (In clinical work, I use A.R.E. as shorthand for the key attachment question that arises in couple's conflict, "Are you there for me?")

6. Separation distress arises when an attachment bond is threatened or a secure connection is lost. There are other kinds of emotional bonds based on shared activities or respect, and when they are broken a person may be distressed. But that distress does not have the same intensity or significance as when an attachment bond is called into question. Emotional and physical isolation from attachment figures is inherently traumatizing for human beings, bringing with it a heightened sense, not simply of vulnerability and danger, but also of helplessness (Mikulincer, Shaver, & Pereg, 2003).

7. Secure connection is a function of key interactions in bonded relationships and how individuals *encode patterns of interaction into mental models* or protocols for responding. One's sense of general attachment security is not a fixed character trait; it changes when new experiences occur that allow one to revise cognitive working models of attachment and their associated emotion regulation strategies (Davila, Karney, & Bradbury, 1999). It is possible then to be insecure in one relationship but secure in another. Working models are primarily concerned with the trustworthiness of others and the entitlement to care—that is, the acceptability of the self. They ask both, "Can I count on you?" and, "Am I worthy of your love?" They involve sets of expectations, automatic perceptual biases that trigger emotions, episodic memories, beliefs and attitudes, and implicit procedural knowledge about how to conduct close relationships (Collins & Read, 1994). These models, in their most unbending and automatic form, can distort perceptions in interactions and so bias responses. They are experienced as reality, as "just the way things are," rather than as constructed.

8. Those who are securely attached are comfortable with closeness and their need for others. Their primary attachment strategy is then to acknowledge their attachment needs and congruently reach out (e.g., matching verbal and nonverbal signals into a clear whole) in a bid for an attachment figure to make or maintain contact. When this figure responds, this response is then trusted and taken in, calming the nervous system of the one who reached out. By providing one with such an effective strategy, attachment security appears to buffer stress and potentiate positive coping throughout life.

9. If others have been perceived as inaccessible or unresponsive, or even threatening, when needed, then secondary models and strategies are adopted. These secondary insecure models can take the form of vigilant, hyperactivated, anxious ways of engaging with others and regulating attachment emotions or of avoidant, dismissing, and deactivated strategies. The first of these secondary models, anxious attachment, is characterized by sensitivity to any negative messages coming from significant others and by "fight" responses designed to protest distance and get an attachment figure to pay more attention and offer more reassuring support. On the other hand, deactivated avoidant responses, the next model, are "flight" responses designed to minimize frustration and distress through distancing oneself from loved ones who are seen as hostile, dangerous, or uncaring. Attachment needs are then minimized, and compulsive self-reliance becomes the order of the day. Vulnerability in the self or perceived vulnerability in others then triggers distancing behaviors. All people use fight-or-flight strategies at times in relationships; they are not dysfunctional per se. However, they can become generalized and habitual, rigidifying into a style that ends up constraining a person's awareness and choices and limiting his or her ability to engage constructively with others.

A third kind of secondary model arises when a person has been traumatized by an attachment figure. He or she is then in a paradoxical situation in which loved ones are both the source of and the solution to fear. Under these circumstances, this person often vacillates between longing and fear, demanding connection and then distancing, and even attacking when connection is offered. This type of response is called disorganized attachment in children, but is termed fearful avoidant attachment (Bartholomew & Horowitz, 1991) in adults and is associated with especially high distress in adult relationships.

The psychodynamic concepts of inner ambivalence, conflict, and defensive blocks are central to understanding the secondary models (and insecure strategies) described above. Avoidant children in infant research may look calm and contained, but are in fact highly aroused by separation from their mothers. Similarly, avoidant adult partners show little explicit emotional distress or need for others, but the evidence reveals that high levels of attachment distress exist for them at deeper or less conscious levels (Shaver & Mikulincer, 2002). Avoidant individuals are also less able to trust and benefit from the greatest resource we have for dealing with our vulnerability to stress and threat, the safe connection with special others (Selchuk, Zayas, Gunaydin, Hazan, & Kross, 2012).

10. Compared to child–parent attachment, the bonds between adults are more reciprocal and not so dependent on physical proximity; cognitive representations of an attachment figure can be effectively evoked to create symbolic proximity. Bowlby also identified two other behavioral systems in intimate relationships (particularly adult relationships) besides attachment: caretaking and sexuality. These are separate systems; however, they act in concert with attachment, and attachment is considered primary—that is, attachment processes set the stage for and organize key features of these other systems. Secure attachment and the emotional balance resulting from this security are associated with more attuned attention to another adult and more responsive caregiving. This security is maintained of course, on a continuum and is not a constant steady state but varies somewhat in specific relationships and situations.

Security is also associated with higher levels of arousal, intimacy, and pleasure and more sexual satisfaction in relationships (Birnbaum, 2007). Sex, a bonding activity in humans, has an emotional signature that varies with different attachment styles and the strategies for dealing with emotions and engaging others that accompany those styles. More avoidantly attached individuals tend to separate sex and love, focusing on sensation and performance in sexual encounters, while those who are more anxiously attached focus on affection and sex as a proof of love rather than on the erotic aspects of sexuality (Mikulincer & Shaver, 2016; Johnson, 2017a).

THE IMPACT OF SECURE CONNECTION ON MENTAL HEALTH

Secure attachment, as a style or habitual engagement strategy, has been linked in systematic research to almost every positive index of mental health and general well-being outlined in the social sciences (Mikulincer & Shaver, 2016). On an individual level, these indices include resilience in the face of stress, optimism, high self-esteem, confidence, and curiosity, tolerance for human differences, a sense of belonging, and the ability to self-disclose and be assertive, to tolerate ambiguity, to regulate difficult emotions, to engage in reflective metacognition, and to grasp different perspectives (Jurist & Meehan, 2009). The essential elements of this picture are an ability to regulate affect effectively in a way that maintains emotional equilibrium, an ability to process information into a coherent integrated whole, and an ability to maintain a sense of confidence in oneself that fosters decisive action. Even in the face of trauma, such as the events of 9/11, secure attachment appears not only to mitigate the effects of such experience, but also to foster posttraumatic growth (Fraley, Fazzari, Bonanno, & Dekel, 2006).

On an interpersonal level, these indices include a capacity for sensitive attunement to others, empathic responsiveness, compassion, openness to people who are perceived as different from oneself, and a tendency to altruistic action. When we can maintain our emotional balance, the research indicates that we are simply better at sensitively picking up on other people's cues and need for support and then responding in a caring way that they can take in and accept. When we are secure, we have more focused attention and more resources to offer to others. In contrast, more anxiously attached people tend to become preoccupied with managing their own distress, or they offer care that does not fit the needs of the other. Avoidant individuals dismiss their own needs and those of others, expressing less empathy and reciprocal support. They tend to turn away from vulnerability in themselves and others.

When we have a safe haven and secure base with loved ones, we are also better at dealing with differences and conflict. A secure connection shapes balanced, adjusted human beings who then have better relationships with loved ones and friends, which then foster ongoing mental health and adjustment and a greater ability to relate to others.

For the purposes of this book, it is especially important to note the impact of secure attachment on emotion regulation, social adjustment, and mental health. These were Bowlby's prime concerns. In terms of mental health, it is clear that attachment insecurity increases vulnerability to the two problems most commonly addressed in therapy, namely depression and anxiety. Exactly how this process occurs depends on individual clients but, in general, it begins for the attachment scientist with the process of emotion regulation. Secure people are more able to attend to and stay engaged with distressing emotions, without a fear of losing control or being overwhelmed. They do not need to alter, block, or deny these emotions and so can use them adaptively to orient to their world and move toward the fulfillment of their needs and goals. They can also recover faster from negative feelings like sadness and anger (Sbarra, 2006). I like to think of effective affect regulation *as a process of moving with and through an emotion, rather than reactively intensifying or suppressing it, and then being able to use this emotion to give direction to one's life.*

On the other hand, it is clear that insecurity is a significant risk factor for maladjustment. Anxious and fearful avoidant attachment are particularly associated with vulnerability to depression and various forms of stress and anxiety disorders, including posttraumatic stress disorder (PTSD), obsessive–compulsive disorder (OCD), and generalized anxiety disorder (GAD) (Ein-Dor & Doron, 2015). The severity of depression symptoms has been linked to insecure attachment in over 100 studies. If we look at different forms of depression, anxious attachment seems to be related to more interpersonal forms characterized by a sense of loss, loneliness, abandonment, and helplessness, whereas avoidant attachment is associated with the achievement-oriented kinds of depression, characterized by perfectionism, self-criticism, and compulsive self-reliance (Mikulincer & Shaver, 2016; see tables of studies pp. 407–415). Attachment insecurity is also related to many personality disorders—borderline personality disorder being particularly associated with extreme anxious attachment, and schizoid and avoidant personality disorders with dismissing avoidant attachment. Insecurity has also been linked to externalizing disorders, such as conduct disorders in adolescents, and antisocial tendencies and addiction in adults (Krueger & Markon, 2011; Landau-North, Johnson, & Dalgleish, 2011).

The literature linking attachment processes and PTSD are particularly fascinating. PTSD symptom severity in patients after cardiac surgery, (Parmigiani et al., 2013), among Israeli military veterans and prisoners of war (Dekel, Solomon, Ginzburg, & Neria, 2004; Mikulincer, Ein-Dor, Solomon, & Shaver, 2011), and individuals who were sexually or physically abused as children has been linked to high levels of insecure attachment (Ortigo, Westen, DeFife, & Bradley, 2013). A prospective study recently showed a clear causal link between attachment processes and the development of PTSD (Mikulincer, Shaver, & Horesh,

2006). The severity of PTSD intrusion and avoidance symptoms after the 2003 U.S.–Iraq war was found to be shaped by levels of attachment security measured before the outbreak of hostilities. Anxiously attached people showed more intrusive symptoms, and avoidant people more war-related avoidance symptoms. There is evidence that an attachment-oriented couple therapy approach can help trauma survivors, including those abused by attachment figures in childhood, to shape satisfying relationships (Dalton, Greenman, Classen, & Johnson, 2013) and that when this approach is used trauma symptoms seem to decline (Naaman, 2008; MacIntosh & Johnson, 2008). Dragons faced together are fundamentally different from dragons faced all alone!

Both John Bowlby (1969) and Carl Rogers (1961) believed in the client's innate desire to grow toward health. The image of health that emerges from attachment science fits particularly well with what Rogers, a key figure in the history of psychotherapy and in the development of the humanistic model of intervention, called existential living (1961), that is, an *openness* to the flow of experience and living every moment fully. The core characteristics of a fully functioning person are, according to Rogers, *organismic trusting,* which involves legitimizing and affirming the validity of one's own inner experience and using it as a guide for action; *experiential freedom,* which involves being able to actively choose different courses of action and take responsibility for these choices; and *creativity,* which involves being flexible and open enough to embrace the new and generate growth. Rogers concluded that a "fully functioning person" experiences greater range, variety, and richness in life, essentially because "they have this underlying confidence in themselves as trustworthy instruments for encountering life" (p. 195). This confidence is the gift that secure connection to others offers. The evidence for wide-ranging positive effects and the dangers inherent in chronic disconnection is considerable.

So, I am not surprised when I see a dramatic shift in Adam, my client in family therapy. Just three sessions ago, Adam seemed to be the epitome of a hostile, avoidant, and delinquent adolescent. But a moment after his father, Steve, openly reached for him and wept at his own sense of loss and sense of failure concerning his son, Adam told him:

> "Well, I was mad all the time. I felt useless, a pathetic loser, and it seemed like you saw me that way too. So there was no point in anything. Why bother? But, when we can be like this, closer even, then I start to think that you want me, like as a son. Somehow this helps me handle my feelings and not be so overwhelmed, and so angry all the time. It changes everything. It's like, I matter to you. I told mom the other day, now maybe I can turn things around. Maybe I can learn and be the person I want to be."

COMMON MISCONCEPTIONS ABOUT ATTACHMENT

Perhaps because attachment theory has developed and been consistently refined over a number of decades, and because the first research focused on mother–infant bonds, there are a number of common misunderstandings that often arise when mental health professionals refer to adult attachment. These misconceptions fall into four broad subject areas.

Dependency: Constructive or Destructive?

For many years developmental psychology described the transition to adulthood in terms of a rejection of the need for others and the ability to define the self and act independently. In clinical circles, dependency unfortunately became associated with a host of dysfunctional behaviors that attachment theorists characterized as somewhat extreme forms of anxious attachment, arising in a context wherein attachment fears are constantly being triggered. Labels such as enmeshment, codependency, and lack of individuation were, and still are, used to describe any number of behaviors in clinical practice. In fact, attachment theory posits that human beings define themselves *with* others, not *from* others, and that the denial of the need for supportive connection with such others is an impediment to growth and adaptation, rather than a strength.

A key contribution of attachment theory is the concept that a secure base with others enhances a strong sense of self, self-efficacy, and resilience to stress. Secure connection allows for the growth of effective, constructive dependency, where others can be a valued resource that nurture a positive, articulated, and coherent sense of self. Countless studies on parent–child and adult bonds support the links between connection with dependable others and the ability to define the self in this way (e.g., Mikulincer, 1995). Both anxiously and avoidantly attached people often adopt a controlling stance toward others; the former may have difficulty directly asserting themselves but use high levels of criticism or complaint, while the latter usually take a more directly dominant stance (see Mikulincer & Shaver, 2016, pp. 273–274, for a summary of the adult studies).

As Mikulincer and Shaver (2016, p. 143) state in their seminal book on attachment in adulthood,

> When one is suffering or worried, it is useful to seek comfort from others; when suffering is alleviated, it is possible to engage in other activities and entertain other priorities. When attachment relationships function well, a person learns that distance and autonomy are completely compatible with closeness and reliance on others.

The point here is that there is no tension between autonomy and related-ness.

Secure connection fosters the ability to confidently encounter the unknown. The secure base model is like a script that sets up specific "if this, then that" expectations that enhance exploration (Feeney, 2007). I often use a personal example to illustrate this point. How did my own secure attachment with my father help me decide, as a young woman of 22, to leave England and cross the Atlantic to Canada, where I knew no one and had only a tentative idea about how I would survive? First, my father's accessibility and responsiveness had shaped my perception of others as trustworthy and my belief that, because others could be counted on when needed, the world was essentially a safe place. The connection with him and his validation over the years had also enhanced my sense of competence and confidence. He consistently accepted my mistakes and struggles and responded to my uncertainties with reassur-ance and comfort, teaching me that I could survive uncertainty and fail-ure. More than this, he assured me that if I found life in North America too difficult, he would find the money so that I could come back home to him. He taught me that risk was manageable.

On a more general level, this focus on the secure base function of attachment gives attachment theory crucial relevance outside the tra-ditional areas most clearly associated with parent–child bonds. Some therapists have minimized attachment, suggesting its sole functions are simple protection and the management of fear at times of threat; they thus conclude that attachment theory is less relevant for adults. The secure base concept outlines how an ongoing sense of felt security with irreplaceable others provides a platform for optimal development, growth, and resilience *throughout life,* as well as the ability to maintain emotional balance and deal competently with stress in life's inevitable crises and transitions. Confident that support will be available, secure individuals are able to take calculated risks and accept the challenges that lead to self-actualization. They also literally have more resources at hand, such that they can dedicate their attention and energy that would otherwise be used in the service of protective and defensive maneuvers, to personal growth.

Models: Fixed or Flexible?

A second apparently common misconception about attachment theory is that it is deterministic, that it is almost exclusively concerned with how the past, specifically a person's history with his or her family of origin, dictates this person's personality and so predicts the person's future. Bowlby is often associated with analytic and object relations perspectives, approaches that stress how early relationships structure unconscious models that then play out in a client's future life. However, Bowlby used the adjective "working" when he spoke of such models and suggested that all of them can be adaptive in specific contexts, as long as they remain fluid and can be revised when appropriate. Over the years, it has become clearer that these models are more fluid than early attachment theorists suggested and can be expected to change, especially as the result of new experience. For example, in one study, 22% of partners changed their attachment orientations in the period from 3 months before marriage to 18 months after marriage (Crowell et al., 2002). In general, individuals with high levels of attachment anxiety are the most likely to change. It would seem that avoidant individuals, who tend to be less open to new experience and information, would be less likely to change—although a recent study of an attachment-oriented couple therapy (Burgess Moser et al., 2018) found that avoidant partners did indeed change their models of attachment by a small amount after every session. There is also evidence that working models of attachment can change in individual therapy (Diamond, Stovall-McCloush, Clarkin, & Levy, 2003). In summary, childhood experience indeed influences development, but its trajectory can be changed, unless models become rigid and exclusionary, so that new experience is avoided or dismissed, or negative patterns of interactions with loved ones consistently confirm these models' most negative elements.

Exactly how past interpersonal experiences might shape the present is also important. Attachment science suggests that early experience organizes a person's repertoire of responses to others, as well as their own affect regulation strategies, and their models of self and other. These can evolve and change, or they can act as self-fulfilling prophecies. Adam tells me, "I never expected to be loved, you see. I felt like a fraud. My lady had just married me by mistake. So I hid out all the time and never let her in. And of course, she left!" Another simple way to understand the perpetuation of disconnection from others is that while it is natural to long for loving connection (since this longing is wired into the mammalian brain), it is difficult to know what is possible and to persist in working to create positive connection if you have literally never seen such connection in action. Adam notes, "I didn't even know people could talk like we do here. I didn't know that people could bounce back from feeling so angry, that it helped to talk about your feelings. No one in my family would do such a thing. But I am learning it here."

Sexuality: Separate from or Antithetical to Secure Attachment?

Some contemporary writers suggest that attachment has nothing to say about sexual romantic relationships, which in contemporary society provide the chief context for significant adult bonding. The argument is that attachment may address the familiarity that typifies so-called companionate love, but does not address the erotic aspects of love. In fact, it has been argued that since novelty and risk are the sine qua non of truly gratifying sexual experience, secure attachment may actually interfere with the optimal fulfillment of sexual needs.

This concern about sexuality and attachment is addressed in more detail in Chapter 6 on couple therapy. In short, though, the evidence is substantial enough to be almost irrefutable: child and adult romantic bonding are "variants of a single core process" (Mikulincer & Shaver, 2016, p. 18). The parallels are obvious; both early and later bonding involve the same repertoire of behaviors, such as gazing, holding, touching, caressing, smiling, and crying. Both involve intense emotions, pain and fear at separation, joy at reunion, and anger and sorrow when bonds are threatened or lost. In both, there is longing for contact, and comfort when that contact is offered. The quality of both parent–child and adult partner bonds is defined by the sensitivity, accessibility, and responsiveness of the loved one when bids for connection are made; successful bids then result in feelings of confidence, safety, and expansiveness and empathic responses to others. Loss of connection results in anxiety, anger, and protest behaviors, followed eventually by depression and detachment. Anxious clinging or defensive distancing can be seen in both adults and children and can become habitual, reality-defining responses.

If the essential nature of the secure base function of attachment is understood, there is no inherent conflict between the eroticism of romantic love and secure attachment. In research studies, secure lovers report more satisfaction with their sex lives and, in general, secure connection seems to foster full, relaxed engagement in sexual encounters. It is disconnection, specifically more avoidant attachment, that appears to negatively affect sexuality. Avoidant partners tend to be narrowly focused on performance and sensation during sex and report lower levels of sexual frequency and satisfaction (Johnson & Zuccarini, 2010). If passion is defined as attachment longing linked with erotic exploration and play, secure connection emerges as a key positive element in optimal sexual experience. Security maximizes risk taking, play, and the ability to let go and become immersed in a pleasurable experience. There is evidence that secure connection is particularly relevant for women, who are more physically vulnerable in sexual situations and so naturally tend to be more sensitive to relationship context during sexual encounters.

While sexuality can be distinct from attachment and recreational in nature, it is also routinely integrated into bonding scenarios. After all, many of us call sexual intercourse "making love." This reflects the fact that for mated mammals, who invest in their connection and work as a coordinated team to rear young together, sexual interactions tend to be bonding experiences. Orgasm releases a bonding hormone, oxytocin, and it is during sexual encounters that the synchronous physical attunement and mirroring behaviors so apparent in mother–infant interactions are most apparent in adults.

Attachment: Fundamentally Analytic or Systemic?

Finally, another misconception, among couple and family therapists in particular, is that since attachment theory emerged from an object relations perspective, as formulated by luminaries such as Fairbairn (1952) and Winnicott (1965), it is fundamentally an analytic approach. As such, it is assumed to be not systemic or truly transactional. In fact, John Bowlby was ostracized for much of his life as a heretic who challenged traditional analytic theory. It is also clear that new links are being formed between modern analytic perspectives and attachment theory, in that psychoanalysis has moved away from classic drive theory with its orientation to sex and aggression. Psychoanalysis has taken a "relational turn" (Mitchell, 2000), becoming more interactive and focused on an authentic encounter between therapist and client where there is an "interpenetration of minds" (Stern, 2004). The term "intersubjectivity" is now used, in analytic and other approaches, to explicitly link this encounter, where there is matching of the client's and the therapist's affective states, to the attachment perspective (Hughes, 2007). Nevertheless, the signature element of psychoanalysis is its emphasis on internal subjective states, whereas Bowlby saw intimate relationships as the "hub around which a person's life revolves when he is an infant . . . and on into old age" (1980, p. 442). He was fascinated by the behavioral drama that goes on between people and, like Darwin, focused on what animals do to maximize their chances for survival, especially how they manage their vulnerability.

It makes sense then that Bowlby clearly set himself the task of integrating a systems approach that emphasizes interpersonal interactional patterns and circular feedback loops, what he termed the "outer ring" of behaviors, with inner cognitive and emotional processing, what he termed the "inner ring" of responses (Bowlby, 1973; Johnson, 2011). As I and others have suggested elsewhere (Johnson & Best, 2003; Kobak, 1999), one of the great strengths of his perspective is its breadth, the fact that it clarifies the key patterns of reciprocal feedback loops generated by the habitual responses of self and important others. Systemic therapists have been criticized for concentrating on constrained and constraining patterns of interaction or dances between intimates to the exclusion of the lived experience of the dancers. Attachment theory elegantly puts these two together. Patterns of interaction and their emotional consequences confirm and maintain a dancer's subjective construction of a relationship and sense of self in that relationship. These constructions then set up the interpersonal responses that organize the interpersonal dance. Thus, the demanding stance taken by my client, Andrew, to his wife, Sarah, is his usual way of dealing with his emotional panic when he begins to feel rejected by her. Unfortunately, his aggressive demands trigger Sarah's habitual withdrawal. The demand–withdraw pattern that then evolves confirms Andrew's worst attachment fears and his sense of inadequacy, perpetuating his obsessive pursuit of his partner.

Both attachment and classic systems theory (Bertalanffy, 1968) view dysfunction as constraint, that is, as a loss of openness and flexibility and a resulting inability to update and revise ways of responding in response to new cues. Rigid, constraining ways of seeing and responding are problematic. Attachment and systems theories are both concerned with process—the evolving "how" of things, rather than static, linear models of causality, and both are nonpathologizing. Clients are seen as stuck in narrow ways of perceiving and responding, rather than being defective in and of themselves. Attachment science adds to the systemic perspective, which tends to eschew inner experience, in that it posits emotional processing as the organizing element in stuck patterns of interactions with others.

THE DEVELOPMENT OF A RESEARCH BASE

Over the last half century hundreds of research studies on bonding across the lifespan with parents, children, adult partners, and even God, have created an enormous and coherent database that, for the first time, acknowledges and outlines the most basic element of our human nature: we are social and bonding animals. The first phase in the creation of this body of knowledge was when developmental psychologists started watching mothers and infants separate in a strange environment and then reunite, and finding reoccurring patterns in their responses. The Strange Situation is arguably the most significant psychological research protocol ever designed, even when we take into account basic conditioning studies on rats. What these psychologists found in studies of mother–infant bonding has already changed forever not only our parenting practices, but also our understanding of the nature of the human child. The second phase began in the late 1980s, when social psychologists began giving questionnaires to adults about their love relationships and finding the same patterns of responses to separation and reunion that showed up in the infant–mother studies. A developmental trajectory was identified (Hazan & Zeifman, 1994; Allen & Land, 1999) in which peers gradually replace parents as principle attachment figures. Researchers then set up observational studies. They began to code how adult lovers reached for and comforted each other when one of them was placed in a position of anxiety and uncertainty (Simpson, Rholes, & Nelligan, 1992), and found clear evidence for the three basic strategies, secure, anxious and avoidant, observed in the original bonding studies. They also found clear evidence for the adult equivalent of infant disorganized attachment, namely fearful avoidant attachment, where individuals flip between highly anxious and highly avoidant strategies (Bartholomew & Horowitz, 1991). It became clear that secure adults were able to disclose their anxiety, reach for a partner, and use comfort to calm themselves, and were also able to support and comfort their distressed partner, whereas adults who described themselves as avoidant, for example, pushed their partners away when their anxiety was triggered and also dismissed the other's need for comfort and care. Psychologists began to observe separation behaviors, such as partners' behavior at airports as they said good-bye to each other (Fraley & Shaver, 1998) and to study the general impact of attachment styles. For example, Mikulincer (1998) found that more security was linked to less aggressive hostility in arguments and less attributions of malicious intent to the other partner. He also found that more secure partners were more curious, more open to new information, and more comfortable with ambiguity (1997). Finally, studies outlining the impacts that are at the core of attachment theory were conducted for adults; attachment style was found to predict resilience in war situations, for example (Mikulincer, Florian, & Weller, 1993), and confidence and competence in career settings (Feeney, 2007).

This final wave of attachment research has vastly extended the understanding of adult attachment and its impact. It is hard to encapsulate the breadth of the research that has occurred in the last decade, but we can touch on some of the most interesting findings. Longitudinal prospective studies link attachment measured in childhood with behaviors and the quality of relationships in adulthood. As part of the many studies emerging from the University of Minnesota longitudinal project, Simpson and colleagues (Simpson, Collins, Tran, & Haydon, 2007) found that assessments of children's responses to their mother in the Strange Situation were powerful predictors of how socially competent these children were in elementary school, how close their friendships were in adolescence, and the quality of their love relationships with partners at age 25. However, let us also remember that even older studies show that the trajectory of childhood experience and its transgenerational impact can also be changed. Mothers who are anxiously attached, if they marry responsive men who offer them safe connection, are able to parent in a loving way, so that their children show secure responses to separation and reunion with them (Cohen, Silver, Cowan, Cowan, & Pearson, 1992).

The significance of attachment research now extends way beyond the boundaries of intimate relationships. In my book *Hold Me Tight*

(2008a), I point out that loving families are the basis of a humane society. Responsiveness to others is the essence of such a society. Secure attachment builds empathy and an altruistic orientation and a willingness to act on behalf of others. Numerous studies by Mikulincer and colleagues (summarized in Mikulincer & Shaver, 2016, Chapter 11) have demonstrated the link between altruism and empathy for others. These studies show, for example, that priming the attachment system with something as simple as pausing and recalling times when someone cared for you instantly reduces your hostility to people who are different from you, if only for a brief period. All the evidence suggests that active compassion and the willingness to help another, even if helping causes discomfort, are linked to secure attachment (Mikulincer, Shaver, Gillath, & Nitzberg, 2005). More avoidant people, on the other hand, report less empathic concern and are less willing to take responsibility for others' welfare or offer help to others (Drach-Zahavy, 2004), and more anxious people seem to feel empathy, but become caught up in their own distress rather than tuning in to the needs of others.

Secure attachment extends to such diverse areas as a person's relationship to his or her sense of God (Kirkpatrick, 2005; Granquist, Mikulincer, Gewirtz, & Shaver, 2012) and one's orientation to and experience in sexuality (Johnson & Zuccarini, 2010). The nature of prayer has been found to vary with attachment style (Byrd & Bea, 2001). Securely attached Christians tend to use a more meditative conversational style when addressing God, while the anxiously attached demand and petition for favors. Securely attached lovers report more varied motives for sex, but stress the desire for intimacy. They enjoy sex more, are more open to exploring sexual needs, and are able to communicate more easily and openly about sexuality.

ATTACHMENT CHANGE IN PSYCHOTHERAPY

It also seems appropriate to touch on the research on attachment changes in psychotherapy. What does it mean to try to measure and study change in attachment, which encompasses so many elements, such as emotions and ways of dealing with them, thought patterns and expectations, and specific responses? The most popular validated measure of adult attachment is the Experiences in Close Relationships Scale—Revised (ECR-R; Fraley, Waller, & Brennan, 2000), found in Appendix 1 at the end of this book. Reviewing the items may help the reader grasp the specific questions that both clinicians and researchers use to assess anxious and avoidant attachment. Secure attachment on this scale is represented by low scores on both anxiety and avoidance. Items offered for endorsement include statements such as "I worry that I won't measure up to other people," or "I find it difficult to allow myself to depend on my romantic partner." Readers may wish to use this scale to assess themselves to get a hands-on sense of how attachment is coded. Researchers also measure changes in specific behaviors toward others in interactions, such as conflict discussions, which can be coded on behavioral measures, such as the Secure Base Scoring System (Crowell et al., 2002). This measure codes factors like whether people can send clear signals about distress and what they need from another, and also whether they can take in comfort when it is offered and be soothed, as well as whether they can recognize another's distress and respond in a contingent fashion. We can also assess for shifts in one's state of mind regarding attachment and how attachment information is processed by interviewing a person about childhood attachments and recent losses, and coding his or her responses on the Adult Attachment Interview (AAI; Hesse, 2008). The interviewer might ask, "Can you give me five adjectives to describe your relationship with your mother?" In secure attachment, responses and narratives are flexible and coherently organized, and the person collaborates with the interviewer. In general, security on this measure in particular can be viewed as a measure of personality integration. Insecure narratives are characterized by vagueness, conflicting or contradictory responses, or digressions and silences. So Sam tells the interviewer, "My mother was amazing and affectionate. But of course she was never there anyway—too busy [he laughs], but that was fine. I don't really want to talk about this with you." Responses on this interview have been found to predict behaviors as diverse as coping with basic training in the Israeli army (Scharf, Mayseless, & Kivenson-Baron, 2004), negative mood management and conflict tactics in romantic relationships (Creasey & Ladd, 2005), and depressive symptoms and awareness and acceptance of emotions in impoverished adolescent mothers (DeOliveira, Moran, & Pederson, 2005).

As Dozier, Stovall-McClough, and Albus point out (2008), the vast majority of psychotherapy clients are insecure at the time they come for therapy, and there is some discussion as to whether particular models of therapy are a better fit for particular attachment styles (Daniel, 2006). While more secure attachment has been found to facilitate a positive therapeutic alliance, some suggest that a deactivating therapy, such as CBT, may be better for anxiously attached clients, whereas more intense, emotionally hyperactivating psychodynamic treatments might be better for dismissing clients who deny their emotions. Others suggest the opposite, that dismissing clients benefit from treatments that fit with rather than counter their style (Simpson & Overall, 2014).

We can also take account of the therapist's own attachment style. Secure therapists seem to be more able to be responsive and flexible with clients, both accommodating and challenging a client's "style"

(Slade, 2008). In individual psychodynamic therapy, changes toward more security have been found (Diamond et al., 2003; Fonagy et al., 1995). Attachment-based family therapy (ABFT; Diamond, 2005), which focuses on helping adolescents heal "relationship ruptures" has demonstrated significant results, reducing variables, such as depression, anxiety, and family conflict, associated with insecure relationships. In couple therapy, studies of emotionally focused therapy (EFT) show that couple therapy can significantly shift both anxious and avoidant partners in the direction of security and reduce the brain's response to the fear and pain inflicted by electric shock, as well as reducing symptoms, such as relationship distress and depression (Burgess Moser et al., 2015; Johnson et al., 2013).

However, we are getting ahead of ourselves since the topic of attachment and the creation of therapeutic change is, in fact, the subject of the nine chapters that follow. Although the impact of attachment theory on conceptualizations of personality, psychopathology, psychological health, and even psychotherapy over the past several decades has been nothing short of explosive (Magnavita & Anchin, 2014), there is still much room for growth. Toward the end of his life, John Bowlby noted (1988, pp. ix–x) that he was "disappointed that clinicians have been slow to test the theory's uses." I think he would still be disappointed!

We begin then, in the next chapter, to outline the implications of attachment science for the general practice of psychotherapy.

 ### TAKE IT HOME AND TO HEART

- Psychotherapy models and specific interventions and psychological disorders are proliferating daily. What is the best way for therapists to find a clear, effective path through this forest? How do we bring more coherence and order to the field of psychotherapy? One way is to prioritize empirical research and attempt, as expert technicians, to accurately match the model and intervention to the disorder. A second path is to simply stress the common factors involved in change and shape these in session. A third approach is to focus on commonalities, especially underlying processes, in the problems clients present and so dispense with long lists of labels for dysfunctions. A fourth approach is to find an empirically based holistic framework that captures who we are, how we develop as individuals and as social relational beings, and what our biological imperatives are, and then use this framework as a guide for intervention. This book suggests that the best way forward is indeed to dispense with long lists of labels for disorders and to adopt attachment theory and science as the basis for psychotherapy.

- Attachment is a well-substantiated developmental theory of personal-ity that gives priority to the role of affect regulation and connection with trusted others as the core defining features of mental health and well-being. The great strength of this perspective is that it links biology and interaction, message and mental model, and self and system, and outlines humanity's most basic needs and fears. It answers the age-old question, "What is love, and why does it matter so much?"

- Attachment security predicts almost every identified indicator of positive functioning, while insecurity is a risk factor for almost every identified indicator of dysfunction. Attachment security is the gift that keeps on giving across the lifespan. To change and repair ourselves, we had best know who we are. We are social bonding mammals, and coregulation of emotions and connection with others is our most basic survive-and-thrive strategy. It is our best guide to becoming safe, sane, and sound.

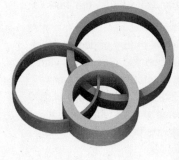

Chapter 2

Attachment Theory and Science as a Model for Therapeutic Change

Throughout adult life the availability of a responsive
attachment figure remains the source of a person's feeling
secure. All of us, from the cradle to the grave, are happiest
when life is organized as a series of excursions, long or short,
from the secure base provided by our attachment figures.
—JOHN BOWLBY (1988, p. 62)

In addition to the biological consequences of positive
relationships, our minds are also more apt to change when
linked to other minds. Having a witness activates mirror
neurons and theory of mind circuitry, making us more aware
of others and ourselves while reinforcing our identity.
—LOUIS COZOLINO AND VANESSA DAVIS (2017, p. 58)

Bowlby spent most of his life delineating the basic principles of human
bonding and the ways in which such bonds operate in our closest relationships to either foster optimal growth and balance or to prime dysfunction. This task was quite enough for one lifetime, and he found
little time to translate his work into a systematic theory of intervention.
However, he believed that, if therapy was successful, the change process
would culminate in experiences of *constructive dependency,* in which

the client's "working models of self and other," as he termed them, were clarified and made coherent and adaptive so that the client's potential for positive relationships with others was enhanced. Thus transformed, these models would form the basis of an integrated procedural map, an automatic if-this-then-that guide for emotionally and mentally constructing one's inner and outer world in a positive way that specifically leads to open, curious engagement with ongoing experience, flexible responding, and effective bonding with others. Bowlby stressed that the ability to relate to others and create close connections is the ultimate barometer of health and positive functioning. He stated, "The capacity to make intimate bonds with other individuals, sometimes in the care-seeking role and sometimes in the care-giving one, is regarded as a principal feature of effective personality functioning and mental health" (1988, p. 121). However, the original formulation of attachment theory did not spell out how a mental health professional can help clients move from distress and dysregulation into such "effective functioning" and the ability to be open and responsive to others.

In one of his final writings, Bowlby does state (1988, pp. 138–139) that therapy is about helping clients to reappraise and restructure their dynamic procedural maps or models of self and other. He suggests that this agenda presents the therapist with five tasks, namely: (1) to provide the client with a secure base, a "holding environment," in which to explore his or her pain; (2) to help clients consider how their manner of engaging in relationships actually shapes the situations that cause them pain; (3) to help clients examine the relationship with the therapist as a microcosm of this engagement style; (4) to explore the origins of this style in a client's past and the "frightening, alien and/or unacceptable" emotions that are primed in this process; and (5) to aid clients to reflect on how past experience constrains their perception of the world and so governs how they think, feel, and act in the present, and to then help them find better alternatives. In and of itself this portrait seems to describe a classic psychodynamically oriented therapy, albeit with a special emphasis on the survival function of relationships. But this brief summary of tasks misses what Bowlby added elsewhere in his conceptual comments and in his clinical case descriptions: a clear focus on the unique power of emotion and the corrective emotional experience that disrupts old patterns of behavior. The two most general clinical implications of attachment science are that harnessing the power of emotion within the client is the most potent way to promote change (indeed the word *models* in attachment theory is intended to be "hot," that is, loaded with emotion), and that change is inherently interpersonal in nature, sculpted by the emotional messages that occur in dialogue with another.

EFT: ATTACHMENT-DRIVEN PSYCHOTHERAPY

The process of healthy adaptation—the ultimate goal of therapy—based on attachment theory might be scripted as follows: A felt sense of connection with others (either through mental models, in which you engage with others on a mental level, or actual positive interactions) fosters emotional balance and regulation; this balance then potentiates the exploration and construction of coherent, adaptive inner worlds—of positive models of self and other; full, open, and flexible engagement with self, other, and the environment then becomes the norm; responsiveness fosters safe connection with others that renders the tasks of living manageable and constructs a sense of self that is competent to handle these tasks. Emotional regulation and engagement with others are at the core of this continually cycling process that occurs at a micro level in daily interactions and at a macro level across developmental phases.

The science of adult attachment has advanced to the point that it has begun to influence practice in therapeutic approaches that would seem, in their conceptualization, to have no obvious link to Bowlby's model, such as cognitive-behavioral methods (Cobb & Bradbury, 2003; McBride & Atkinson, 2009). Traditionally, attachment theory has been linked to insight-oriented dynamic treatments (Holmes, 1996; Wallin, 2007). But, in fact, humanistic *experiential* models of therapy offer the most consonant exemplar of modern attachment theory and science in action. These models grew out of and refined the psychodynamic model of change, especially with their clear focus on working directly with emotion. In particular, EFT, first developed for couples and families and therefore inherently interpersonal in nature, captures both Bowlby's original vision and key developments in modern attachment science, as outlined by social psychologists such as Shaver, Mikulincer, and colleagues (Mikulincer & Shaver, 2016). The most recent versions of EFT in its individual, couple, and family-practice formats, capture the essence of the attachment perspective and its concrete implications for intervention. Contemporary EFT does this in six important ways.

• First and foremost, the practice of EFT continually focuses on the active processing and regulation of emotion. Effective regulation here involves the step-by-step creation of emotional equilibrium and accompanying positive interpersonal emotional coregulation, both of which are at the heart of attachment theory. As Bowlby states (1979, p. 69), "Many of the most intense of all human emotions arise during the formation, the maintenance, the disruption and renewal of affectional bonds—which for that reason are called emotional bonds. . . . The threat of loss arouses anxiety and actual loss sorrow. . . . Both are likely to arouse anger . . . and the renewal of a bond . . . joy." Emotion is triggered most strongly by relationship issues, and coregulation with another is usually the most intuitive and efficient route to emotional equilibrium. Balance is attained by engaging with emotion fully and making it into a coherent whole, rather than leaving it denied, blocked, or fragmented, or, as Bowlby termed it, "alien." This is most naturally accomplished *with* another, even if this other is present only on a mental, imagined level. Systematically identifying the elements of emotion, namely, trigger, initial perception, bodily felt sense, meaning assignation, and action tendency or motivational urge (Arnold, 1960), allows specific emotions to be discovered, owned, and integrated. In addition, the client's relationship to his or her emotional experience changes as a result of identifying these elements and realizing that he or she actively creates this experience in the moment. In effective therapy, clients discover in an immediate, alive, and explicit way how their *manner* of engaging with their emotions shapes their suffering. New ways to engage with and regulate emotion can then become integrated into a more empowered and positive sense of self. This is an organic bottom-up process that arises from tuning in to one's "felt sense." Simply teaching top-down containment and coping skills to try to control emotion is considered insufficient.

• Second, the creation of in-session emotional safety is essential. Therapy has to be a safe haven for the client, and also offer him or her a secure base for the exploration of new and difficult emotions. Emotional safety is shaped by a particular kind of engagement with the therapist—a particular kind of alliance. This alliance must be one that makes clients feel accepted and understood at a visceral level. The therapist is a surrogate attachment figure who is able to be accessible, responsive, and engaged, much like a security-providing parent. The therapist has then to be genuinely emotionally present and willing to be seen, as proposed by Rogers (1961). Like a good parent, the therapist freely offers respect, compassion, and nonjudgmental regard, and normalizes any struggles the client may have. This kind of therapeutic engagement builds a sense of competence by frequent validation and titrated risk taking, offering soothing, reassurance, and comfort whenever a client is in distress. Therapists have to be able to tolerate strong emotions and stay curious and open in the face of their own uncertainty, and of client resistance and opposition. Bowlby himself spoke of tuning in to and empathizing with a widow's "unrealism" and sense of anger and unfairness at her loss. He did not suggest coaching her to be less angry or correcting her lack of realism.

In this kind of alliance, the therapist does not start out trying to change clients, but instead attunes to clients and meets them where they are. The therapist discovers *with* each client how his or her current dilemmas make exact and exquisite sense. As Harry Stack Sullivan points out (1953), much of what is ordinarily said to be repressed or suppressed is simply "unformulated." The constant emotional attunement of the therapist helps clients explore, formulate, and tolerate their inner world. The primary focus in therapy is not then on assigning labels for dysfunction, or even on the tasks of change, but on the always evolving personhood of the client. The therapist's central task is connecting with the client in a way that honors and expands this personhood. The clear outline of the EFT model also allows therapists to keep their own emotional balance so that they can remain engaged with the client while the client brings his or her full emotional experience, current dilemmas, aspirations, and challenges to the fore.

• Third, EFT and attachment both focus concurrently on the within and between. They integrate self and system, internal reality and interactional drama, context and client, grasping and working with how each constructs the other in the moment-to-moment process of living. Systemic transactional realities and inner emotional and mental realities constantly and reciprocally define each other. Internal aspects of a person, such as affect-regulation abilities, interact with the quality and nature of present close relationships in a dynamic manner. Dancer and dance, self and system coalesce into a holistic reciprocal reality. More specifically, in both EFT and attachment perspectives, the responsiveness and acceptance offered by key others (such as a therapist) is crucial in facilitating the recognition and ordering of personal experience into coherent meanings. These meaning frames then guide adaptive action.

In systemic models like attachment and EFT, causality involves a set of reciprocal feedback loops rather than a line running one way from a single cause to a single effect. These models bring constant attention to merging interactive between and within processes and how they define the client's reality. As Sullivan (1953) notes, "A personality can never be isolated from the complex of interpersonal relations in which the person lives and has his being" (p. 10), and a person achieves mental health to the extent that he or she becomes "aware of one's interpersonal relations" (p. 207). *In attachment theory and in EFT, the self is viewed as an ongoing construction, a process rather than an object, and one that is defined in interactions with others.* The experience and expression of emotion are key here. Emotion moves the individual, sculpting inner experience. Also, the expression of emotion is the primary organizer of the key interactions with significant others. The healthy self is flexible, balanced, accepting of self and others, and constantly in process. This view parallels Bowlby's definition of models of self as "working," when functional, working models are open to revision, as significant new experience occurs. In contrast, anxious attachment lends itself to a chaotic sense of self that is always trying to adapt to others, while avoidant attachment fosters a rigidly defined but fragile sense of self that is not open to new experience.

Bowlby stressed that we need to look beyond the individual embedded within his or her skin and see the individual as embedded in relationships. Modern psychotherapy has done relatively little of this; it has construed adjustment as physical and emotional self-regulation rather than as coregulation with others. It also construes adjustment as independence *from* others rather than constructive dependence *with* others. Bowlby (1973) spoke of people being embedded in two entwined feedback loops, or ongoing processes that structure inner experience and that shape interactions. Such patterns are self-sustaining: Affect regulation pathways and cognitive models bias perception and response; perception and response cue habitual ways to engage with others and constrain how they reply; their replies then feed back into affect regulation and mental representations.

• Fourth, attachment and humanistic therapies like EFT share a common understanding of health and dysfunction. Health consists of flexible and adaptive emotion regulation strategies that allow an individual to recover emotional balance when it is lost and deal constructively with vulnerability; positive, coherent working models of self and other that are open to revision when needed and set up realistic but constructive expectations; and a repertoire of behaviors to elicit connection with others and to respond to the needs of others. A healthy individual is able to accept and assert his or her needs with others and empathically respond to the needs of others. Dysfunction is viewed in terms of blocks to being open to new experience, to fully processing emotions, and to attuning to and engaging with others. The Rogerian view is that people will grow and heal themselves in an *organic* manner if given the right conditions. Similarly, attachment science argues that, given fertile ground and support, the individual will naturally embrace inherent longings for connection, reaching for others. If this reaching is responded to with recognition and empathy, then a cascade of positive effects can occur. The therapist is not then a composer rewriting a musical score for the client to lessen symptoms of discordance, but rather a conductor who knows that a full, vibrant song is already waiting to emerge. He or she simply guides and moves with the client to uncover it. Secure attachment does not simply provide comfort or foster equilibrium. The secure base it offers cultivates growth and aliveness.

Experiential therapies that arise from a Rogerian perspective (1961) and the attachment framework (such as EFT) are both compassionate and collaborative in nature, and they take a deliberate *nonpathologizing*, growth-oriented stance toward a client's difficulties. The therapist does not preempt the client's need to define his or her own reality and the unique formulation of that reality. Therapy is about discovery by client and therapist, rather than coaching by the therapist to reach already decided on, narrow criteria of improvement. Bowlby (1988) states, "The therapist's role is analogous to that of a mother who provides her child with a secure base from which to explore the world" (p. 140). The therapist is attuned and emotionally present—providing a source of affect regulation and constantly offering manageable challenges to promote growth in the here and now of the session.

• Fifth, EFT, humanistic therapies, and attachment science acknowledge the influence of the past, especially in terms of the development of sensitivity to threat and learned, habitual ways of dealing with vulnerability or of defending oneself. However, while acknowledging the impact of the past, in terms of intervention, EFT tends to stay with *present process*. The therapist tunes into experience or interactions as they occur in session and deepens awareness and interactions in the moment so as to allow new elements of reality to arise. For example, reflecting how a client changes the channel to abstract cognition every time anxiety is referred to by the therapist, and returning to this anxiety, so as to touch on the inherent threat that blocks the experiencing of this fear in the here and now. Modern attachment theory has also veered from an obsession with how the past perpetuates itself, mostly through the mechanism of working models of self and other, to an acknowledgment that these models are much more fluid than originally thought. Working models can and do change in many cases, for example, when people become happily married (Davila et al., 1999). Attachment science stresses that it is the constant *process of confirmation* in key present-day interactions that renders working models and affect regulation strategies stable and, in the case of negative insecure models, prevents the openness to the new experience that is necessary for positive revision. New (that is, *dis*confirming) emotionally laden interactions that occur in and out of therapy can then change these models and strategies.

A focus on the present requires attending to the "working" aspect of models of self and other, the process of *how* they are recreated from implicit memory and stay closed or open to revision moment by moment, rather than focusing too much on the cognitive content of such models. (An overemphasis on content sets up a change process oriented to the creation of insight, which is considered inadequate for significant change in experiential interventions.) For example, Ken accuses his wife of lying when she says she is sorry for hurting him and cares for him. Rather than pointing out that Ken has a working model, developed from past experience, of all others as unreliable and dangerous, the EFT therapist is more likely to say, "Right now, it is hard for you to take in your wife's comments—her caring. What happens to you when you hear her say

'_____'? What is it that is hard for you about letting that caring in for a moment? What will happen if, right now, for a moment you let that caring in?"

• Sixth, both the attachment and the EFT version of humanistic intervention are firmly grounded in empiricism, that is, in a continued commitment to the process of observation, the delineation of patterns of behavior leading to prediction, and the testing of the explanatory links that make up theory. In formulating attachment theory, Bowlby used ethology, the science of animal behavior that considers social organization from a biological perspective. He studied the work of Conrad Lorenz that explored how young geese imprint on the first figure they see and Harry Harlow's work with infant primates and their response to isolation. EFT interventions began with the intense observation of recurring negative emotions and interactions between adult partners and how these patterns changed as a result of specific therapist interventions. This grounding in the scientific method is not an academic issue, particularly when practice models proliferate so often on the basis of a simple idea or even on the basis of personal charisma and anecdote. At best, clinical intervention arises from the repeated examination of naturally occurring pivotal moments, which organize internal and interactional realities, and the decoding of the key elements of these moments. These pivotal moments can then be primed and choreographed in therapy sessions to obtain specific shifts in how clients construct their experience and interact with others.

EFT practitioners are true empiricists in that they attune to and constantly describe, as concretely as possible, what appears before them as it occurs, be this a person's struggle to define herself, the changing color of emotion, or a constantly recurring pattern of interactions between intimates—an interactional dance. The construction of meaning in session is explicit, is shaped in collaboration with the client, and is grounded in present reality. The attachment perspective offers a simple phenomenology and understanding of the hurts, fears, and longings that EFT therapists highlight and explore. The themes of abandonment, traumatic isolation, rejection, helplessness, anxiety, and inadequacy, and how they are dealt with by either shutting down and restricting experience or by becoming reactive and intensifying experience, are placed in an existential context and clarified by this perspective. The EFT therapist, guided by attachment precepts and science, has then a clear, empirically based map of common human misery and basic human motivation.

In summary, the natural integration of attachment science and a clinical perspective, such as EFT, offers clinicians the following: a map of the core aspects of a client's emotional life; a way of harnessing the considerable power of emotion in the service of change; a clear, specific outline of the therapeutic alliance as the context for growth; a focus on the self as a relational process; a clear view of what constitutes health as a therapeutic goal; and, a clear set of guidelines for how best to stay grounded and, in an organic manner that is consonant with the core elements of our human nature, create positive change.

THE SPECIFICS OF CHANGE: CHANGE EVENTS

Almost all therapy models frame the change process as occurring in basic stages, offering a first stage that involves some form of *assessment and stabilization*—a containment of negative intrapsychic or interpersonal symptoms—followed by a stage of *active restructuring* designed to lead to greater psychological adaptation, and finally a *consolidation* phase, wherein the clients become ready to leave therapy and maintain the changes they have made. In EFT, developed primarily as a couple intervention but always used with individuals and families as well, these stages are called de-escalation, restructuring attachment, and consolidation. Therapeutic models differ considerably, however, in the level of change aspired to, in how they understand the dynamics of change, and in what factors are considered necessary and sufficient to create significant shifts in therapy. CBT models, for example, highlight moments when a client accepts that specific thoughts are dysfunctional and challenges them with new thoughts and shifts in actual behaviors.

It is often hard to pin down exactly what creates change in psychotherapy. Some studies show that the theories of change inherent in specific accepted therapy models may not, in fact, be attentive to the key variables that occur in the actual change process. For example, one critical study found that focusing on changing "dysfunctional thoughts" did not at all predict success in CBT for depression; in fact, it was associated with negative outcomes (Castonguay et al., 1996). A positive alliance and emotional experiencing were associated with positive results. There is, however, a clear, empirically supported confluence between the change process inherent in attachment science and EFT, a humanistic experiential therapy.

From an attachment standpoint, a transforming change event in therapy involves the discovery, distillation, and disclosing of emotions, which then allows for better regulation of these emotions and enhanced emotional intelligence (Salovey, Hsee, & Mayer, 1993). In an attachment-oriented therapy, emotions that were alien are made familiar and meaningful and are integrated into the self. These events have the power to modify a client's models of self and other. New appraisals of behavior can then arise, and old, constricting expectations and beliefs can be challenged. New behaviors can be explored, and new risks can be taken in relation to basic needs for connection with others and a valued, empowered sense of self. Clients can begin to achieve a "working distance" (Gendlin, 1996) from emotion, and so use it as a compass to guide their adaptive responses. For example, Barbara has never allowed herself to feel angry at anyone or anything, and we explore how she always "dismantles and dismisses" her needs with others and any sense of entitlement to caring from them. As she engages with some of her pain, she discovers how her "acceptance" allows her to contain this pain, but keeps her "helpless and still—down and depressed." She begins to grieve for the losses of her life and her lack of expectations for herself. In highly emotional, imagined encounters with her father and husband, she risks feeling and stating her hurts and needs, finding a new sense of longing, and a new resentment, for her disparaging self and her dismissing loved ones. She begins to use her anger to assert and refine her needs and find her more assertive self.

Key change events in EFT for couples have been pinpointed, coded, and linked to positive outcomes and follow-up in nine studies (Greenman & Johnson, 2013), and illustrate the six principles of EFT already outlined. Future research will examine whether, as might be expected, these same change events also predict similar outcomes in family (emotionally focused family therapy [EFFT]) and individual (emotionally focused individual therapy [EFIT]) modalities.

These in-session change events occur in the context of a positive alliance, and they have been shown to consist of two key elements. These are, first, a deepening engagement with core emotional experience that restructures this experience and the person as an experiencing self who can define, tolerate, and trust her experience, and second, a new, more open, authentic engagement with others. Once clarified and refined to its core elements, emotional experience is expressed in a coherent way with a significant other (partner in EFT, family member in EFFT, or with the therapist or imagined other in EFIT). From many coded EFT sessions, it is clear that change events, as they evolve, also contain set steps or microelements. These are:

- The delineation of and active engagement with basic vulnerabilities and needs.

- The construction of messages that assert these needs coherently and directly.

- The development of the ability to take in comfort and affirmation from a supportive other.

- The development of the ability to give attuned support to another.

These change events happen in moments of constructive dependency that foster a coherent experience of and integration of self. In such moments clients are able to *accept* their vulnerability in a way that leaves them stronger and more flexible.

THE NATURE OF EMOTION

Before we can examine how emotion is accessed, reprocessed, regulated, deepened, and used to motivate clients in EFT, we must become clear about the nature of emotion itself. In this so-called "era of the brain," it is important to remember that "the brain is . . . a social and affective organ. Learning is social, emotional and conditioned by culture" (Immardino Yeng, 2016, p. 85). In itself, emotion is not an irrational response or simply a "feeling" that accompanies thought. Rather, it is a high-level system that integrates a person's awareness of innate needs and goals with feedback from the environment and the predicted consequences of actions (Frijda, 1986). Emotion is an information-processing system focused on survival. William James described emotions in 1894 as "adaptive behavioral and physiological response tendencies called forth directly by evolutionary significant situations," and modern science supports this view (Suchy, 2011). Both experiential and attachment viewpoints frame emotion as essentially adaptive and compelling, as organizing core experiences and cognitions about self and responses to others. Both also view problems in affect regulation as the core issue underlying the constricted responses that bring people into therapy.

Bowlby (1991) noted that the main function of emotion was to communicate one's needs, motives, and priorities to one's self and others. He would have resonated with the EFT concept that being tuned out of emotional experience is like navigating through life without a compass. The functions of emotion can be summarized thus.

1. *Emotion orients and engages.* Einstein noted, "All knowledge is experience: everything else is just information." What takes information to a level where we would describe it as an "experience"? The answer is emotional salience and active engagement with emotional cues. Emotion adds a visceral knowing and what Bowlby called a "felt sense" to any set of facts. By its nature, *emotion grabs our attention and guides perception.* It focuses us on what is relevant to our needs and wants, telling us what is salient, and engaging our attention in an absorbing way. You can be absorbed in listening to a lecture, but when the fire alarm rings your anxiety takes over and changes your world instantly. You are also tangibly aware of your need to escape the building.

2. *Emotion shapes meaning making.* Emotions have been termed the rudder that steers thinking (Immardino Yeng, 2016, p. 28). People who cannot access emotion owing to brain injuries cannot make rational decisions or choices (Damasio, 1994). They become caught up in pondering all possible alternatives. They have nothing to orient them to what they want and need—to give them a felt sense of what matters. Both experiential therapies and attachment theory also view emotion as priming internal models of self and other and the attendant sets of beliefs and expectations. Research suggests that affect may function as the "glue" that binds information within mental representations (Niedenthal, Halberstadt, & Setterlund, 1999). The emotional balance that comes with secure attachment and positive working models appears to result in the ability to construct and articulate coherent narratives about one's past relational world (Main, Kaplan, & Cassidy, 1985).

3. *Emotion motivates us.* It literally energizes us and primes a specific kind of action. The word *emotion* comes from the Latin, *emovere,* "to move out." Emotions are programs for action; anger, for example, usually primes movement toward something that is perceived as frustrating a goal or threatening well-being, and shame primes hiding and withdrawing.

4. *Emotion communicates with others and sets up their response.* This occurs rapidly and intuitively in ways that not only allow us to anticipate others' responses (and so coordinate tasks and solve problems collaboratively), but also potentiates emotional bonding and caregiving. The neuroscientist Marco Iacoboni in his brilliant volume, *Mirroring People* (2008), points out that our nervous systems are set up to be exquisitely sensitive to emotional nonverbal cues from others, especially cues such as facial expression and tone of voice. We are then programmed to mirror or imitate these cues, for example, with our facial muscles and, via the mirror neurons in our exquisitely social brains, to feel in our own bodies what we see in others. Affective expression, or at least how an interactional partner perceives this expression, then organizes the reflexive reactions and general response repertoire of that partner. Emotion is the music of the dance called a relationship. Working models of attachment are formed, elaborated, maintained, and, most important for the therapist, revised through emotional communication (Davila et al., 1999).

Not only are the functions of emotion becoming increasingly clearer, there also is now general agreement among theorists and researchers about the different kinds of emotion—the forms they take. There are six to eight core emotional responses (Ekman, 2003), although some theorists add specificity and expand the basic set to a few more, for example, expanding shame into guilt and disgust (Frijda, 1986; Izard, 1992; Tomkins, 1986). Ekman (2003) points out that these *core emotions* involve distinct facial expressions that can be recognized and ascribed common meanings across cultures and continents. Such emotions appear to be universal and to be associated with specific neuroendocrine patterns and brain sites (Panksepp, 1998). Emotions often have "control precedence" (Tronick, 1989), easily overriding other cues and behaviors, especially in important interactions with those we depend on the most. The core emotional responses can be most parsimoniously outlined as follows:

- *Approach emotions*
  - o Joy, evoking relaxed engagement and openness
  - o Surprise, evoking curiosity
  - o Anger, evoking assertion and moving toward goals

- *Avoidance emotions*
  - o Shame, evoking withdrawal and hiding
  - o Fear, evoking fleeing or freezing
  - o Sadness, evoking withdrawal or comfort

Obviously these emotions can be differentiated further. Shame, for example, has also been viewed by some theorists as including disgust and guilt at specific acts or thoughts. Sadness can include grief and be part of what we normally call hurt feelings. The emotion we refer to as "hurt" in and of itself is a conglomerate emotion rather than a core affect. It has been unpacked into its core elements, namely anger or resentment, sadness and loss, and a feeling of vulnerability or helplessness that involves fear (Feeney, 2005), specifically the fear of not being valued by key others and, therefore, deserted and rejected. While fear always involves a sense of threat and emerging helplessness, it can be expressed in the form of shutting down, or freezing, or a mobilized fleeing from danger.

Once we have set forth the elements that make up an emotion, the functions an emotion serves, and the different types of emotion, it becomes possible to reformulate emotional experience in a potent and positive way in a therapy session. The goal is not simply to regulate emotion into balance and even into a more integrated form, it is also to *harness* it in the service of the creation of new perspectives, cognitions, concrete actions, and attuned responses to others in the service of change.

CHANGING EMOTIONAL LEVELS

The concept of changing levels of emotion in therapy is as old as therapy itself. However, how to accomplish this and judging what the optimal or most functional level of emotional engagement is in a session, will vary wildly across therapy models. Although the attachment perspective has always valued emotion, research on emotion has become more differentiated, and its role in different forms of therapy more articulated than was the case when attachment theory was first formulated. Some attachment theorists have tended to emphasize calm, rational insight into emotion as a primary change mechanism in therapy (Holmes, 2001), while experiential EFT therapists attempt to create new, and sometimes intense, corrective emotional experiences rather than insight per se (Johnson, 2009). Some experiential therapists have identified some emotions as essentially maladaptive, especially when they are based on traumatic experience (Paivio & Pascual-Leone, 2010). In EFT, we focus rather on *how* emotion is constructed and regulated and how some forms of regulation are more flexible and adaptive than others. In order to shape optimal regulation that allows clients to harness their emotions for growth and aliveness, therapists have to ensure that clients are actively engaged with an emotional reality. This experience has to be primed, evoked, and actively engaged in session. A therapist most often cannot change this emotion from the outside by discussion, cognitive manipulation, or behavioral experiment. To change emotion you have to first allow yourself to feel it. Then you need to tolerate it, unpack it, take hold of its essence or distill it, and ultimately reshape it. The concept of *deepening* affect captures this process, helping the client go beneath the obvious and surface chaotic reactivity or numbed suppression. This involves switching from a reactive, automatic emotional response to a more profound, elemental, or core affect. The most common example here is that of the therapist who helps a client move from habitual rage or numbing to an awareness of the threat—the fear that triggers these more surface responses.

Just as Bowlby and Ainsworth (Ainsworth, Blehar, Waters, & Wall, 1978) focused on what happens in key moments when a vulnerable child is left by an attachment figure in a strange context, so the therapist tracks how emotion arises in a client, and how the client deals with that emotion in key existential situations when core vulnerability is present and compelling. The nature of this emotional vulnerability and how it shows up in clients' fears, longings, and pain is known territory for the attachment-oriented therapist so that he or she can guide clients into this space with confidence. (Chapter 3 outlines the specific interventions used in this process.) Explicitly existential models of therapy (Yalom, 1980) outline four universal life-and-death issues that elicit our deepest anxieties: Concerns about death, the finiteness of life, and the inevitability of loss; concerns about how to make life meaningful although transitory; concerns about choice and how to take responsibility for constructing a life; and, concerns about isolation and aloneness. Attachment incorporates this philosophical perspective on human vulnerability, but stresses the overarching primacy of emotional isolation as the core of helplessness. This isolation primes the sense of danger and links to the fear of death, primes a sense of meaninglessness (after all, if we do not matter to another . . .), and undermines the ability to be grounded and make clear choices. A felt sense of secure connection with others, on the other hand, is seen as our species main and most efficient way of effectively dealing with such existential vulnerabilities.

THE INTERPERSONAL: THE ENACTED ASPECT OF CHANGE EVENTS

If deepening engagement with core emotional vulnerabilities, especially with fears, unmet longings, sadness and loss, and shame or fears about the self, is the first key element of the change process in an attachment-oriented experiential therapy, the second element is that new facets of experience are explicitly rendered into action or enacted by the client. They are owned and expressed in an interpersonal context. Newly formulated emotional experience then becomes a transactional event. Emotion is discovered and distilled *with* the therapist and then played out in the session as an interpersonal response *to* a significant other. This other is usually an attachment figure (who is actually present or imagined), but occasionally it can also be the therapist in his or her role as a surrogate attachment figure. So, a client, Leslie, may access and explore the deep fear of being seen and denigrated by others that underlies her general antagonistic stance and scorn for closeness, but it is when she is asked to look into my face and share the fear that I, too, will betray and abandon her that this fear becomes tangible and truly owned.

This interpersonal aspect is a crucial part of the change events outlined and tested in EFT for couples and used in clinical practice with individuals (EFIT) and with families (EFFT); new emotion evokes new interactional responses to and from significant others. These interactional moves create, in session, a corrective existential drama of vulnerability and longing that can be dealt with constructively. In most cases, such a drama primes a more secure sense of connection in the client, or at least a coming to terms with loss that leaves a person open for new relationships. It is worth stressing that this enactment of an internal reality with a significant other is just as necessary in change events in EFT for individuals, as in EFT for couples or families. To those who think of individual therapy as essentially about improved intrapsychic, self-regulation strategies, working at this interpersonal level may seem unnecessary. But when working from an attachment perspective, it is necessary to keep in mind that attachment is all about the coregulation of emotion as the basic, or baseline reality, for human beings, with successful self-regulation emerging as part of this process.

The neuroscientist James Coan (2016) suggests that indeed coregulation, rather than solo self-regulation, is the baseline, normal, and most-efficient strategy for us as social animals. The brain appears to budget resources constantly and, at a neural level, simply expects supportive relationships to be available as a resource. It gives priority to social rather than self-regulation. Coan's brain scan studies (Coan, Schafer, & Davidson, 2006) of the positive effects of handholding by significant others on how individuals' brains perceive and respond to the threat and pain of electric shock parallel Bowlby's concept of the potent, positive impact of "contact comfort," and the idea that secure-base relationships literally create the perception of a safer world. Studies of visual perception also tell us that if we stand in front of a hill alone, our brain actually estimates the hill to be higher than if we have a friend standing beside us. The brain takes proximity to social resources into account even in basic perception processes (Schnall, Harber, Stefanucci, & Proffitt, 2008; Gross & Proffitt, 2013). The attachment concept that we are better together, sharing the load and the stress, seems to stand as a physiological fact rather than a sentimental statement. The evidence suggests that attachment figures, including relational partners, are incorporated into neural representations of self as vital resources that promote survival, the dilution of risk, load-sharing, and the regulation of negative emotion, and so carry an enormous existential significance. Interestingly, in terms of attachment figures being viewed as extensions of self, the brain apparently encodes threats to familiar others (in contrast to strangers) very similarly to how it encodes threats directed at the self (Beckes, Coan, & Hasselmo, 2013). This agrees with other findings that suggest that the loss of a partner is associated with immediate and persistent decreases in self-concept clarity (Slotter, Gardner, & Finkel, 2010).

It is also interesting to note that social affect regulation is a relatively bottom-up process, whereas self-regulation is usually a more costly, effortful, top-down process involving extensive cognitive and attentional processes to inhibit somatic responses that are already triggered (Coan & Sbarra, 2015).

All of this research has direct relevance for therapy. First, the EFT therapist pays most attention to the bottom-up process of decoding emotion as it occurs and helping clients order this emotion in the present moment. The therapist also stays attuned and emotionally present for the client as this process occurs, coregulating his or her emotional experience. With the therapist as a resource, the "hills" the client has to climb seem smaller.

Second, in interpersonal enactments, the therapist helps the client enlist attachment figures as aids in effective affect regulation. Exactly how this effective coregulation occurs is also becoming clearer. For example, sensitive maternal responses appear to deactivate a child's amygdala and activate the prefrontal cortex (Tottenham, 2004). As this becomes the norm, the stress system, or the HPA axis—the hypothalamus and the pituitary and adrenal glands, which trigger stress hormones such as cortisol—becomes tuned to a state of equilibrium and so is less easily triggered and easier to turn off (McEwen & Morrison, 2013).

It is also commonplace wisdom that we engage in internal dialogue with others constantly, but especially when under any kind of threat, where we use this dialogue to reappraise difficult experiences. An everyday example of such effective coregulation among people of faith occurs in the use of prayer designed to access God as a protective attachment figure (Luhrmann, Nusbaum, & Thisted, 2012).

In the much-studied classic change events in EFT for couples, newly formulated emotions are expressed to another in an engaged, open way that captures the essence of these emotions, without the need for avoidance, reactive blaming, or clinging. This often takes the form of acknowledging denied emotional wounds, asking for needs that are now owned to be met, or asserting the right to be heard and taken into account. This sharing redefines self and system—the position of the self in a key relational drama and the nature of the relationship itself. In this kind of enactment, key schemas or models of self and other are immediately accessible and are able to be reformulated. This change process is apparent in EFIT and EFFT. For example, Amy shows me that she now can turn to her "dominating, distant" mother, whom she can see in her mind's eye and who is present for her in this moment, and express her hurt and need with coherent clarity. As she does this, she tells me, "Right now, I experience myself as suddenly solid and as calm, and she does not look dangerous anymore. In fact, I see that she does not know what to do. She is scared of me. How about that! That's different. I am beginning to feel soft toward her, in fact. I wasn't such a bad kid. She just didn't know how to be a mom!"

Terry turns and tells his wife in Session 15 of EFT, "When I let myself feel this shaky feeling and put all my usual weapons down—my proofs of your failings, I feel really afraid. I realize that you may not want this softer, unsure part of me. I assumed that no one would want this Terry. But here I am now, in technicolor, and I want your reassurance so very badly. That you want to, that you will stay with me."

In an EFFT session, Tim tells his son, while his wife holds his hand, "I want to be a good dad. I just get lost in all the rules that I have in my head from my family. I am so sorry, son. I think I have let you down. That is hard to say. I don't want to lose you or hurt you. What I want is to find a way for us to be close. It feels strange, but it also feels good to say this." As he says this, his previously cool, defiant, and avoidant son finds himself weeping and reaches his arms out to his father. A cascade of inner and interpersonal change occurs.

In these change events fears are faced, needs owned and expressed, and old, automatic ways of regulating emotion, framing the self, and perceiving others are activated and revealed. They are in the process of revision.

The power of a so-called corrective emotional experience, often referred to in the psychotherapy literature, is made concrete and specific once it is placed in an attachment context. When such an experience works in session, a person is indeed fully emotionally engaged, but this emotion is now ordered and distilled, accepted as valid, and expressed to another with authenticity. The other is a witness to the emergence of rich, new experience and to the new manner in which a client is now able to piece together the mosaic of need and fear, self and other. Acceptance, be it by a surrogate attachment figure (the therapist) or by an actual attachment figure, is a potent validating force that affirms a client's vulnerabilities and needs, as well as his ability to actively reconstruct his experience with new awareness. This validation does not only consolidate new dimensions of experience and new relationship patterns, but also shapes a more competent experiencer who can define and trust his inner world.

In the next chapter I outline the core EFT processes and interventions that systematically set up transforming moments of change and the natural progression into the corrective experiences I have discussed. The words *natural progression* are used deliberately here in that, to the EFT therapist, it is apparent that this is an *organic* process, one that happens from the inside out. Just as a good physician knows how to help the body heal itself, a therapist who knows how to tune in to attachment and emotion, uses the power of naturally occurring processes to structure change.

 TAKE IT HOME AND TO HEART

- Intimate bonds with others are the basis of effective functioning and mental health. We can hold clients so they can better "see" their ways of engaging with others and the emotions that prime this engagement, and find constructive alternatives to their habitual responses. A key part of this process is to prime and regulate clients' emotions with them and help them find emotional balance.

- Experiential interventions, such as EFT, best reflect *the discoveries* of attachment science and turn attachment precepts into a map for intervention.

- Attachment leads the therapist to prioritize emotion regulation processes and the creation of emotional safety in session, which requires that the therapist be actively present and attuned, transparent and accepting. He or she has to work both within constructions of self and emotional realities, and on constructions of interpersonal patterns of interaction between significant others in the present moment. Constructive dependence leads to effective coregulation of emotion and the growth of a healthy coherent sense of self.

- Attachment offers a map of the phenomenology of key emotions, key self- and system-defining moments of interaction, and the necessary and sufficient elements of change.

- Stabilization, restructuring of attachment, and consolidation are the three stages of change. Deepening emotional engagement and choreographing new ways to engage with others are key to the change process. Emotions orient us, shape meanings, motivate, and communicate. There are six core emotions (joy, surprise, anger, shame, fear, and sadness), and the therapist uses them to reorient the client, shape new meanings, and motivate new responses and new ways of connecting to others. Corrective emotional experiences, particularly that of effective coregulation, redefine self and system in EFT.

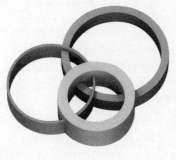

Chapter 3

Intervention

Working with and Using Emotion to Construct Corrective Experiences and Interactions

Our feelings are decision making algorithms that evolved to guide behavior toward what was historically most likely to promote survival and reproduction.
—MAIA SZALAVITZ (2017, p. 51)

Only when one feels an insight in ones bones does one own it. . . . The problem in therapy is always how to move from an ineffectual intellectual appreciation of a truth about oneself to some emotional experience of it. It is only when therapy enlists deep emotions that it becomes a powerful force for change.
—IRVIN YALOM (1989, pp. 22–23)

In his last book, Bowlby briefly describes a case of a young mother who was at risk of abusing her baby. Her therapist, knowing her history, offered suggestions as to how this mother must have, in fact, felt frightened, angry, and helpless as a child and longed for secure connection. The young mother was then able to express these emotions herself and thereby make progress in therapy and in her ability to parent (1988, p. 155).

A beginning therapist might see the example as just a regular therapy session, and that what actually happened was a simple attempt at insight induction. In fact, this presenting picture could have elicited many different kinds of intervention, especially with a loaded issue such

43

as a child at risk. We can only imagine the full picture of what happened and what changed for this young woman in this session. If this therapy hour generally resembled an experiential attachment-oriented approach to therapy, we can surmise quite easily what occurred.

- This young mother felt safe, held, and validated by this therapist; she did not feel judged and did not sense that she was being coached by an "authority" on how to change her behavior and so be a more competent mother to her child.

- The therapist guided the mother into her underlying fear and longing, core feelings that would most likely be triggered by her experience with her baby.

- Being able to explore her own experience as a child and touch her loss and her longing, this client was then more able to, in a visceral way, grasp the impact of her responses on her own baby.

- She might also have begun to feel more confident as an adult who could now acknowledge, accept, and make sense of her experience.

- She experienced a genuine supportive relationship with the surrogate attachment figure of the therapist, wherein she could find a relationship that met her own longing for *connection.*

- If she was able to continue to reflect on and integrate this experience, she realized that others may not always reject or desert her, and so her model of others expanded, and the possibility of turning to them as a resource became more tangible.

Carl Rogers, the father of experiential psychotherapy mentioned earlier, would probably have seen this session as a collaborative exploration of present longing and loss that expanded the mother's felt sense of her child and her emotional repertoire. It focused on evoking emotion and its power to guide actions toward others, rather than on changing cognitions per se or coaching behavior change. The emotions accessed were also specific: Anger, fear, and longing—the implicit flip side of fear and deprivation. And they were accessed in order to reorganize a key interpersonal drama. Bowlby would have framed this client's less-than-empathic response to her child as "perfectly reasonable" given her own experience, and Rogers would have begun in a similar fashion by extending acceptance and empathizing with this client's difficulty, offering her an attuned responsiveness that she had never experienced as a child.

Although they were both researchers as well as clinicians, neither Rogers nor Bowlby had access to the wealth of research that now exists on adult attachment, emotion and emotion regulation, and change processes in therapy. But they still managed to respond to their clients in ways that are consonant with current findings in these areas. Whether we are treating an individual, a couple, or a family, we can now outline a set of streamlined core interventions that reflect both the original formulations of Rogers' model and attachment theory, and also reflect modern clinical practice in experiential therapy and recent research on emotion and change in this model. In all three of the modalities just mentioned, change is an emotional and an interpersonal phenomenon. Since the later chapters specifically address these different modalities, in this chapter we will address intervention and how it aligns with pertinent recent research, in a broad generic fashion.

EMOTION AND CHANGE IN EXPERIENTIAL THERAPY

Experiential therapies have always paid particular attention to exactly how change occurs, with a spotlight on the active role of the client in the change process. If we concur with the premise of experiential therapies that clients are imbued with a self-actualizing tendency, then the overall role of the therapist is simply to kick-start this natural process of growth and guide clients past blocks as they arise. Working directly with emotion is a huge part of this kick start.

What we understand, we can actively sculpt, so this chapter will first elaborate on the nature of emotion and levels of emotion before continuing to discuss a specific metaframework for intervention and specific techniques used in EFT. It is important to note that the experiential perspective has always particularly privileged emotion as a major source of change and seen it as basically adaptive. Embedded in experiential models is a trust in the validity and worth of emotional experience that has often been missing in other models. Experiential approaches have avoided the earlier polarization in the therapy field, in which emotion was seen as either a potent geyser ready to explode—and should be vented in catharsis—or as a chaotic disorganizing force that had to be contained and controlled by reason or behavioral coaching.

Actually many clinical models that previously sidelined emotion are now viewing it more positively and attempting to address it in their treatment protocols. For example, the so-called third wave of behavioral interventions include the acceptance of emotion (Hayes, Levin, Plumb-Vilardaga, Villste, & Pistorello, 2013). A sharper focus on affect is now being incorporated into many different models of behavioral, psychodynamic, and interpersonal therapy. However, emotion still appears as much less central and as an essentially different animal in these models when compared to the experiential perspective. For example, emotion often seems to simply be named in the context of a predominant focus on thought or behavior. If addressed, it is as something to be regulated and contained with self-soothing techniques or used as one way to help generate insight.

In an experiential therapy, on the other hand, emotion becomes the primary focus of therapy. It is a target of change (being reprocessed and regulated more adaptively in therapy) and an agent of change (priming and reshaping cognition and action). Processing emotional experience is a key part of every session, and is used to guide people into new meaning frames, move them to new actions, or change how they reach for and respond to others. Experiential approaches—such as EFT, accelerated experiential dynamic psychotherapy (AEDP), focusing and process experiential psychotherapy, sometimes now referred to by the more generic "emotion-focused therapy" (and referred to in this book as PE/EF)—all systematically track, evoke, and actively shape emotion, even if there are differences in practice as to how emotion is tailored to create change (Fosha, 2000; Gendlin, 1996; Elliott, Greenberg, Watson, Timulak, & Friere, 2013).

More and more empirical studies on therapeutic change acknowledge the power of emotion to shift perspectives and open the door to new adaptive information about self and other. Emotion organizes our world and our relationships. In sadness, for example, we tend to not explore or respond to positive cues, and we often close down and close others out. We see differently and perceive different cues; we are physiologically organized differently compared to when we are mobilized in an emotion like anger. Under the influence of emotion, we process information and put it together into meaning frames in a way that fits with our physiological response, and we *move* differently in the world and relate to others differently. So, in a flood of anger, blood moves to my hands, and my heart beats faster; I notice and remember all the injuries received; see the line of your mouth as particularly contemptuous; and I lean toward you and raise my voice to "force" you to listen to me.

From the EFT perspective, the superior route to change in life and in therapy involves shaping new emotional experiences. Specifically, this "shaping" involves evoking and expanding emotional experience and awareness beyond surface reactive responses, and improving emotion regulation so that meaning making and behavioral responses can be more flexible and adapted to a specific context. *Working with emotion in EFT is an organic process in which technique can be held to a minimum, and the innate power of emotion itself can be used to take a client to another universe.* It is worth reiterating here that both Rogers and Bowlby explicitly believed that a good therapist essentially tunes in to and then fosters each client's innate capacity for growth. As Bowlby wrote, "The psychotherapist's job, like that of the orthopedic surgeons, is to provide the conditions in which self healing can best take place" (1988, p. 152). If we recognize that emotion is part of the biologically based, innate, and survival-oriented attachment system, then we can surmise that the change processes employed in EFT tap into what is known as biologically prepared learning. Evolution has equipped us to need just one experience of real disgust to forever veer away from the source of that disgust. Similarly, a felt sense of security and emotional balance, once experienced as a corrective self-healing shift (such as in experiential psychotherapy), stays with us.

Regulating Emotions

Before discussing the change process in an attachment-oriented therapy such as EFT, we should define emotion regulation. What exactly are we referring to when we speak of the regulation of emotion? Regulation is the ability to *access* and attend to a range of emotions, clearly *identify* those emotions, *modify* them by either reducing or amplifying them in oneself and another, and then *use* them to ascertain meaning, as well as to guide our thinking and actions in a way that suits our priorities in different situations. In session, the EFT therapist actively helps clients regulate their emotions, soothing or titrating emotional intensity and engagement, most often helping clients keep a *working distance* from emotion as it arises in the moment. Emotion is modulated—turned up or down—so that clients can stay within their window of tolerance, while moving into new territory with difficult feelings.

New concepts and ways of understanding emotion help us work with it more effectively, and many of these new ways offer an exquisite fit with EFT interventions. The work of Lisa Feldman Barrett on emotional specificity, or what she terms *granularity* (2004), illuminates the differences in how people experience, perceive, and understand their emotions. Feldman Barrett suggests that those who can put emotions into words, constructing their experience with a high degree of specificity and complexity in the face of intense distress, are less likely to use negative self-regulatory strategies such as aggression, self-injury, or excessive drinking. They also demonstrate less neural reactivity to rejection situations and generally suffer from less-severe anxiety and depression. One study found that recounting a difficult situation in a diary and precisely pinpointing the emotions that arose seemed to lessen stress and allowed people to cope better, compared to those who were less able to clearly specify and differentiate their emotional responses. The ability to articulate more finely tailored emotions seems to offer people more precise tools for making choices and effective problem solving (Kashdan, Feldman Barrett, & McKnight, 2015). Those who are diagnosed with major depression and social anxiety disorder show significantly lower levels of emotional differentiation than others, even when the intensity of their distress is accounted for. The positive effects on mental health of journaling about one's own emotional experiences also supports the idea that putting feelings into words serves a regulatory function in and of itself (Pennebaker, 1990b). Writing about them is just one way we can focus on making emotions concrete, and it specifically parallels the constant tracking, reflection, and *ordering* of the client's emotional experience that are key elements of EFT practice. Indeed, the EFT therapist also constantly renders elusive and vague emotional hints and whispers into concrete and specific experience. He or she is a granularity expert!

As mentioned, regulation can be more or less adaptive. It is now accepted that emotion regulation plays a critical role in the etiology and maintenance of psychopathology. Suppression, rumination, and avoidance are associated with a range of psychological disorders, especially problems of anxiety and depression, while more adaptive strategies, such as acceptance (leading to reduced experiential avoidance) and reappraisal are not (Mennin & Farach, 2007; Aldao, Nolen Hoeksema & Schweiser, 2010).

For example, depressed adolescents tend to disengage from their own feelings; they blame themselves for perceived rejection by others, tend to ruminate and catastrophize, and focus on themes of rejection, personal inadequacy, and failure (Stegge & Meerum Terwogt, 2007). Poor emotion regulation often renders interacting with others overwhelming, undermines any sense of efficacy in dealing with emotion, and generates an absorbing state where everything leads into depression and nothing leads out of it.

We can view emotion regulation strategies in terms of emotional intelligence. Salovey, Mayer, Golman, Turvey, and Palfai (1995) assume that emotions serve as an important source of information and that individuals vary in their ability to process this information. This processing involves the ability to attend to emotions and clearly make sense of and regulate them. For example, there are large individual differences in people's ability to infer emotional cues from another's face and voice (Baum & Nowicki, 1998; Nowicki & Duke, 1994) and, as noted above, people vary in the precision or *granularity* (specificity and complexity) with which they automatically perceive their own experience of emotion.

THE ROLE OF ATTACHMENT IN AFFECT REGULATION

In general, attachment security, a felt sense of connection to others, facilitates positive affect regulation strategies and processes (see discussion in Chapter 2). Such security fosters emotional balance. People high on the continuum of security are better at maintaining equilibrium at every point in an emotional experience. They are less easily triggered, tending to construe things in more benign terms and tolerate ambiguity better. They can attribute undesirable events to controllable, context-dependent, and temporary causes. They have learned that distress is generally manageable. In terms of physiological responses, they tend to less easily experience or stay caught in anxious hyperarousal, nor do they habitually numb themselves or shut down emotionally. They are better at exploring the meaning of an experience, and they trust and can use the information emotions give them to navigate and impact their world. They can also reflect on their emotional experience and order it—an ability most likely developed as a result of their experience in infancy of having a loving attachment figure. This caregiver was able to reflect on the infant's mental experience and represent it to them "translated into the language of actions that an infant can understand. The baby is thus provided with the illusion that the process of reflection of psychological processes was performed within its own mental boundaries. This is the necessary background to the evolution of a firmly established reflective self" (Fonagy, Steele, Steele, Moran, & Higgit, 1991). Their emotional balance renders secure individuals less likely to deny, distort, or exaggerate their emotional experiences (Shaver & Mikulincer, 2007). They can then be open to their emotions and those of others, express and communicate them, and use them as a guide to effective action.

In contrast, avoidant or anxious attachment fosters the "defensive exclusion" or suppression of emotion (Bowlby, 1980), or the intensification or chronic activation of emotion. Suppression, as already noted, tends to trigger a rebound effect. It is a fragile strategy that usually shatters under intense stress. Chronic activation can be seen in anxiously attached people, who become caught in emotion as in a web, ruminating on real or potential threats and generalizing negative experiences, so that one cue can trigger a flood of others, resulting in confusion and incoherence. It is easy to see why insecure partners are more prone to anger, hostility, and violence; this behavior is particularly true of those who are anxiously attached, but is also found in avoidant individuals, in spite of their attempts to deny vulnerability. It is particularly interesting that in the face of true existential threat, involving images and thoughts of death, anxious people become caught in rumination and heightened fear, while avoidant people suppress fear but show heightened implicit/unconscious reactivity to death cues. Both types of insecure individuals then tend to become more judgmental and punishing of others—in contrast to more secure people, who tend to deal with death anxiety by directing their energy into thoughts of symbolic immortality, such as creating a legacy, and increasing their desire for intimate connection with others.

Having expanded our understanding of emotion, let us now turn to an overview of change processes in EFT as an attachment-oriented intervention.

THE EXPERIENTIAL CHANGE PROCESS IN EFT

Studies of the process of change associated with successful treatment repeatedly point to two principal factors: The deepening of engagement with emotion and the creation of affiliative interactions with attachment figures (Greenman & Johnson, 2013). These findings support the formal theory of change in the EFT model.

Experiential attachment-oriented therapists take Bowlby's belief in the power of emotion seriously. The goal of every session is to change the way the client engages with his or her emotion experience. Therapists help clients tap into the wisdom of their emotions and use them to give direction to their lives, enabling them to order or regulate their emotions more effectively, to pinpoint their needs, and to grasp the specific ways in which the active construction of their emotional experience shapes their sense of self and key patterns of interaction with others. This part of the chapter will explain how to work with emotion to reach these goals.

Therapists need to be able to differentiate levels of emotional engagement so they can systematically evoke and recognize them when they occur in their clients. The measures used in research can help us pinpoint clinical phenomena. In EFT studies, the Experiencing Scale (EXP; Klein, Mathieu, Gendlin, & Kiesler, 1969) has been used to capture this concept of levels of emotional engagement and identify what deepening engagement actually looks like. The EXP measures client movement across seven stages of engagement. In the early stages, clients have low levels of engagement with their emotions; they make mostly impersonal, superficial, or abstract discursive remarks about their experience. Later, clients begin to recognize, explore, and make bodily feelings more explicit. Then, in the more advanced stages, new, corrective compelling experiences set up new meaning frames, and clients actively use emotion as a guide that takes them into new territory. As emotional experience deepens and is expressed through these stages, interpersonal connection in interactions between client and therapist, in imagined attachment figures evoked in the therapy process, and (in couple and family therapy) between attachment figures in the room, also becomes more open and authentic.

James, who complains of depression, tells me in a first session that all people are narcissists, and that this is so because of the political and economic climate. He has obviously used this speech before, and his tale is remote and distancing. This rather impersonal conversation would be coded as Stage 1 or 2. Later, as James's treatment progresses, he moves into Stage 3, exploring his relationship with his mother who is dying. He talks about specific events in adulthood when he felt angry and scolded, just as he did as a child, and then lists all the actions he took to contain the impact of these incidents, such as giving up on others and distrusting their positive intentions. As therapy progresses, James enters Stages 4 and 5, as he gives a more personal recounting of such events, setting out his assumptions in detailed personal statements. He now recognizes and pays attention to soft, vulnerable emotions in the session, pointing out that he feels "small" around his mother and wants to keep his armor on and "hide," even now when she is so frail. Ultimately, as he enters Stages 6 and 7, James actively explores and *discovers* his immediate feelings and his grief that he never felt loved as a child, the hopelessness and helplessness he felt then, and is able to outline the impact this emotional experience has had on his life. Emotional experience is now vivid and concretely felt, and James presents it in a way that evokes compassionate empathy in me. James can now tolerate and keep his balance in his vulnerability. He is fully *present*. New levels of awareness become a springboard into new motivational states, realizations, and existential positions. James tells me, "I can't grieve my mom. I never had a mom really [he weeps]. She never showed up for me. She couldn't do it, I guess. I grew up alone and thinking there was something wrong with me. That I can grieve—for little James who felt so cold and small in the world. And I am still hiding out. It's hard to hope again. Right now, I look at you and see that you are sad for me. That feels good, but I need to weep for a while. Maybe I want to go and find what I never had." James ends up being much more open to experience and equipped with emotional balance and trust in his newly emerging experience as a guide to future action. In attachment terms, his framing of this experience is *coherent*. The formulations here are expansive—the client is on a journey rather than being stagnant or stuck. This new level of emotional engagement changes the color of James's relationships, opening the door to more authentic connection with others, more compassion for himself and others, and the ability to risk, reach, and respond in close relationships.

It is possible to set out the elements of James's emotions in the affect assembly and deepening intervention (discussed later), weaving emotional experience together in an ordered, coherent manner. Doing that leads clients like James to becoming more deeply and fully engaged in their internal experience, rather than avoiding or suppressing it. In the process, the client's emotional range expands and new elements emerge, as when anger gives way to an awareness of loss and grief. (Later we will discuss how we help clients take this new level of emotional experience into their interpersonal world, in a process we call enactments.) More adaptive, flexible affect regulation also becomes part of clients' changing their models of self and other, their personalities if you will, and becoming more secure. As the attachment researchers Mikulincer and Shaver suggest (2016, p. 189):

> Having managed emotion-eliciting events or reappraised them in benign terms, secure people do not often have to alter or suppress other parts of the emotion process. They make . . . a "short circuit of threat," side-stepping the interfering and dysfunctional aspects of emotion, while benefiting from their functional adaptive qualities. They can remain open to their emotions, express and communicate feelings freely and accurately to others, and experience them fully without distortion. Moreover, they can expect emotional expression to result in beneficial responses from others.

In EFT, new emotional music translates into new dance steps and new levels of engagement with others. Later in this chapter, I describe the way the therapist continually sets up a cascade of shifts in a client's felt sense of emotion, which cues shifts in meaning and behaviors and then cues positive shifts in interactional patterns. This metasequence of interventions is termed the EFT Tango. The tango is used as a metaphor because it is a constantly fluid improvised dance to emotional music. This dance can be disjointed and result in distance, misattunement and discord, but can also result in physiological and psychological harmony and synchrony. Due to its improvised nature, the quality of a tango rests almost entirely on the dancers' attunement and connection. In tango, when a dancer is fully engaged with another, it is hard to tell the dancer from the dance. As he creates a new dance with another, James builds a new sense of self.

RESEARCH ON EMOTIONAL ENGAGEMENT IN THERAPY

What does outcome and process-of-change research tell us directly about the part emotional engagement plays in successful experiential psychotherapy?

In terms of couple therapy, nine studies of EFT have found that emotional depth and more open, engaged, and responsive interactions, coded as more affiliative on the Structural Analysis of Social Behavior (SASB; Benjamin, 1974) predict success (Greenman & Johnson, 2013). Change events in the restructuring stage of EFT, as defined by scores on the EXP and the SASB, have consistently been associated with positive change at the end of therapy and at follow-up. These later-stage change events in the couple version of EFT are described as *softenings,* since in these events more blaming partners can soften with their partner, disclosing fears and asking for attachment needs to be met. Such events are not initiated in session unless the more-withdrawn partner has gone through a similar process—that is, has re-engaged emotionally and is now more present and responsive. Research on this change process in EFFT has not been conducted, but many years of clinical observation tell us that the same processes occur between parents and children as occur between adult partners.

There are, of course, other kinds of change events, but they always seem to include deep emotional engagement. For example, bringing new, "hot" present experience into memories of past events as they are triggered in the session, transforms these memories, not by countering them, but by the assimilation of new material into past narratives (Schiller et al., 2010). As Alexander and French (1946) suggest, reexperiencing old difficulties while shaping new endings to them, on both intrapsychic and interpersonal levels, may be the secret of all significant changes in therapy.

Research also testifies to the power of working with emotion in individual therapy. Studies of PE/EF, which spring from the same root in experiential theory and so is similar to, although also different from, the more systemic and attachment oriented EFT, generally show similar results to CBT for problems of anxiety and depression. They also find that client depth of experiencing in therapy as measured by the ECR-R is consistently related to positive outcome. The higher the experiencing level, the better the outcome (Elliott, Greenberg, & Lietaer, 2004). A recent meta-analysis of 10 studies finds that while experiencing levels are higher in PE/EF than in interpersonal or cognitive-behavioral therapy (CBT) models, higher levels are associated with positive outcome in all three of these models (Pascual-Leone & Yeryomenko, 2016). An increase in client levels of experiencing from early to late therapy also seems to be a stronger predictor of outcome than the working alliance, and high emotional arousal plus reflection on that arousal distinguished between good and poor outcomes. This makes sense; deeper experiencing on the experiencing scale does not just measure arousal, but also measures a person's ability to make sense of this arousal. Early capacity for emotional processing (presumably reflecting existing innate abilities) was not found to influence outcome, but moving into increased emotional depth in therapy was predictive. In PE/EF imaginal confrontation with others (a basic technique employed in both EFIT and in PE/EF) using empty-chair work also predicted better client engagement in therapy and seemed to contribute to the reduction of interpersonal problems.

Furthermore, there is specific evidence that the depth of a therapist's experiential focus helps clients achieve deeper experiencing. Therapist empathy, attunement, and exploration impacted both the depth of client's experiencing and the complexity at which it was processed (Gordon

& Toukmanian, 2002; Elliott et al., 2013). The numerous studies summarized here all confirm the power of actively moving into and processing moment-to-moment emotional experience.

It is also worth noting that in all experiential therapies, the process of change is collaborative. In research using the NIMH study of depression data (Coombs, Coleman, & Jones, 2002), across both cognitive-behavioral and interpersonal therapy models, collaborative emotional exploration was associated with successful outcome, whereas a more coaching-oriented, directive process that deemphasizes emotion and focuses on cognitive themes and advice was not. Similar results were found in an earlier study by Jones and Pulos (1993).

Research on the process of successful therapy is a helpful guide to the processes that correlate with change and, therefore, to the direction to take in the moving drama of a session. This brief review has focused particularly on the role of emotion in change since this is so central to EFT. It is particularly helpful to be able to note key change events, or emotionally charged moments when a cascade of changes can occur. As a therapist, I can then work toward these events, deliberately choreograph them, and help clients to integrate the changes they instigate into their lives.

Note that there is a movement in psychotherapy to simply dismiss models, specific change processes, and techniques as irrelevant, and concentrate instead on so-called general or common factors, such as therapeutic alliance. For those who are specifically interested in this issue, or wish to read a summary of the elements deemed necessary for any effective therapy, see Appendix 2, which discusses these points as they relate to the content of this book. The position taken in this appendix, in short, is that so-called general factors are not so general and that, while we must know about them and take them into account, they do not provide enough direction for effective intervention.

THE HEART OF EFT INTERVENTION: THE TANGO

It is time to outline the basic set of interventions that the therapist employs again and again in all stages and forms of EFT. The conceptualization of an attachment-oriented psychotherapy leads naturally to prioritizing certain processes in session with clients, and calls for a particular sequenced set of therapist interventions to create these processes. Any set of interventions in an experiential therapy is, of course, improvised on and used with different pacing and intensity at different stages and in particular sessions. This set of interventions and associated client change processes is called the *EFT Tango* (see Figure 3.1, page 55), and is most easily described as a set of five "moves," namely:

1. *Mirroring present process.* The therapist attunes to, empathetically reflects, and clarifies cycles of affect regulation (e.g., numbing flips into rage which dissolves into shame and hiding) and cycles of interactions with others (as I hide, you harangue me and I shut you out more, triggering an increase in your aggression, and so on). The focus here is on how clients are, in the present, actively and most often without awareness, constructing inner emotional and interpersonal interactional realities into self-perpetuating cycles.

2. *Affect assembly and deepening.* The therapist joins the client in discovering and piecing together the elements of emotion and placing them in an interpersonal context that renders them coherent and "whole," often resulting in an expansion of awareness into deeper elements or levels of emotion.

3. *Choreographing engaged encounters.* Expanded and deepened inner realities are disclosed in structured interactions guided by the therapist, so that new inner processes become new ways of interacting with and relating to real or imagined others.

4. *Processing the encounter.* The new interactional responses are explored and integrated and also related to presenting problems. In

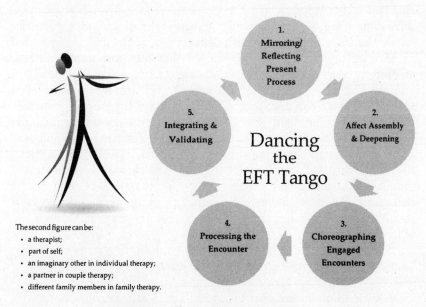

FIGURE 3.1. The five basic moves of EFT.

couple and family therapy any stuck or negative responses to another's new behaviors are contained or processed further with the therapist. In individual therapy a negative, nonaccepting response may come from another part of the self.

5. *Integrating and validating.* New discoveries and new, positive interactional responses are highlighted and reflected, and validation is offered, to build competence and confidence. This process highlights both inner experience and how it shapes interactional patterns in a self-reinforcing manner, and how the nature of this interpersonal connection reciprocally shapes inner experience and the sense of self.

Let us now look at these moves in a little more detail.

EFT Tango Move 1: Mirroring Present Process

Occurring in the context of a growing therapeutic alliance, the first step taken by the therapist is to offer the client an attuned, simple description of the process that is occurring in the present, in the presence of the therapist. Doing this requires tracking and collaboratively naming the experiential and interactional processes that occur—both those within the client and in interactions between the client and the therapist or a real or an imagined other in the room. It is essential that this be done in a descriptive, normalizing, and *evocative* manner (without evaluative comments) that fosters engaged exploration at the cutting edge of a person's experience or awareness of interactional patterns, rather than in an intellectually discursive or rationalizing mode. The client's emotional expressions or messages and associated thoughts, sensations, actions, and interactional moves and positions are tracked and reflected, beginning with those at the surface (mentioned explicitly by the client) and then carefully delving into those that are implied. Interactions, whether they are held in the client's imagination or played out with the therapist or with an attachment figure in the session, are described in simple language and framed as having their own dramatic momentum and self-sustaining nature. Each client is the author and the victim of the drama that is laid out and distilled to its simplest, most-essential elements. The therapist captures and reflects the drama as it unfolds, invites clients to stand back and look at it from a distance, and frames it as having a life of its own.

In an individual therapy session in the stabilization stage of therapy, Tango Move 1, mirroring present process, might look like this.

"I hear that you are very upset and angry at your boss, Sam. You feel unfairly treated and see this as leaving you in this dark fog of depression. If I have it right, you get caught in this space and become more and more angry, more and more down, till the spiral takes over your life. You didn't want to come to talk to me about this really—it's hard. It feels safer to shut everyone out—yes? [The focus is mostly on tracking within processes here but still moves into the area of connection and disconnection from others.]"

In a family session in the stabilization stage, Tango Move 1 might appear something like this:

"Sam [Dad], can we stop here a moment? So right now what is happening is you are telling your son he must do as he is told. Trying to reason with him, and my sense is this is hard for you. You do not think he is hearing you and so you are looking out the window as well. And Mary [Mom], you try to add to your husband's comments, pointing out to your son how difficult he is and how he is destroying the family. Tim [adolescent who is having huge temper tantrums and refusing to cooperate], you are gripping your hands together here and refusing Dad's request. Telling him *"No."* Is this right? [Tim nods his head.] Dad reasons with you but stays kind of distant, mom pleads and repeats the rules, and you sit in anger and refuse to do what they want. Dad does what dads do—asks you to cooperate, Mom gets upset and pushes you, and you get angrier and angrier. And this dance has taken over the whole family."

EFT Tango Move 2: Affect Assembly and Deepening

How do we help clients discover their emotional experience in a way that is tangible and relevant to them? We focus on the core elements of emotion and then put them together. That is, we *assemble* them *with* the client into a whole that creates a sense of completeness, a "Yes, that is it—that is how I feel, and it makes sense" experience. This then opens a door for further discovery and a deepening awareness of more hidden or unacknowledged emotions. Assembling a client's affect is a relatively simple concept, but proves to be extremely useful in clinical practice. To address emotion effectively and systematically, to be able to turn it up and turn it down, or to order it when it is chaotic can seem like over-whelming tasks. This is perhaps why directly working with emotion has tended to be dismissed or sidelined in many therapy models. It is useful to remember that, as discussed in Chapter 2, there are really only six basic emotions: Anger, shame, sadness, fear, joy, and surprise. The softer emotions, sadness, fear, and shame, are most often less accessible than the others. Clients often present with reactive anger or a numbed-out lack of feeling (which shows up in repeated intellectualization and shallow, detached descriptions of problems).

As briefly noted in Chapter 2, we can think of emotions as comprising components or core elements. The most-parsimonious delineation of the core elements of emotion is provided by Magda Arnold (1960). Arnold's synopsis of elements is a powerful tool that allows the therapist, piece by piece, to discover, delineate, and unfold an emotional response, distilling its essential nature. The therapist's job is then to help clients shape this experience into a unified coherent whole and link it to habitual ways of engaging with self and others in their lives. The process itself not only raises awareness, but also improves emotional balance. The phrase "What we can name, we can tame" comes to mind. The elements of emotion that Arnold lays out are:

- Trigger or cue

- Initial perception

- Body response

- Meaning creation

- Action tendency

This final element moves emotion not only into the realm of personal motivation, but also into the interpersonal realm. Emotion organizes actions toward others, and emotional signals set up and constrain the actions of others to the self. These signals also set up habitual interaction patterns, or "dances," that then feed back into and frame the experience of each of the dancers. Each emotion is linked to a discernable action tendency. So anger is an approach emotion that sets up the assertion of needs and the removal of blocks to satisfaction; sadness elicits support from others and withdrawal in the service of letting go; shame elicits hiding; surprise elicits exploration and engagement; joy provokes openness and engagement; and fear elicits fleeing, freezing in paralysis, or a fight response. *Emotion can then be elicited to literally move people into specific kinds of action.*

The process of eliciting and unfolding each of these five core elements, and then assembling them into a simple, tangible whole, brings implicit emotion out in the open, where it can be recognized and identified, explored further, added to, and deepened. Each element has first to be evocatively probed for and made concrete, and then linked to the other elements. The process of unfolding can begin with any element, but often begins with the therapist noticing and slowing down an obviously significant but unheeded emotional response (e.g., a brief shift in emotional expression) and attempting to pinpoint the stimulus (core element 1) that cued this response with reflections and evocative questions.

With a couple, the eliciting process might look like this:

THERAPIST: Can you help me, Dan? You just turned away and shook your head there, as Marnie talked about her hurt. What happened there? What is it that has you shaking your head like this?

DAN: I think it's that voice she uses.

He identifies the *trigger* for the beginning of his habitual withdrawal from his partner. Previously, the therapist has found that if she simply asks Dan about his feelings, Dan dismisses the question or says he does not know. However, when this therapist asks more specifically what triggered a particular behavior, Dan is able to answer. The therapist then invites Dan to engage in an *experiential search* for the other elements of his current experience. She focuses on *body response*.

THERAPIST: Can you help me? What does your body feel like when you turn away; what does it feel like right now?

DAN: (*Looks blank.*) I just shut down. I don't feel nothing at all. Nothing.

The therapist then probes for the initial general "take," or *perception*, which is often vague.

THERAPIST: So, you want to shut down, something here doesn't feel good?

DAN: Oh, it feels bad, bad, like get me out of here, so I turn away.

Dan now gives his initial perception and his *action tendency*, which is to flee.

The therapist summarizes the above elements, and then continues by focusing on *meaning*.

THERAPIST: So you hear her tone, and it feels like something bad is going to happen. What do you hear in her voice?

DAN: She says she is "hurt" all the time, but all I hear is "You have screwed up again. You are just a screw up, period."

Now the therapist has all the elements and can piece together this emotional response with Dan by reflecting it as a whole, putting it into the context of his ongoing attachment relationship with his wife and his sense of himself in that relationship. The therapist constructs Dan's emotional response with Dan, enhancing specificity and "granularity" as she does so. Dan becomes absorbed in this process and, as he finds order in his experience, his window of tolerance widens. He can then start to own and integrate this experience. The therapist then provides affirmation of Dan's ability to do this and for the "reasonableness" of his experience. *Being able to grasp, make sense of, and trust one's own experience is the ground on which positive adaptation stands.* Once Dan can do this, he is asked to share it with his wife in the next step of the Tango (see Tango Move 3).

This discovery and assembly process regulates emotion at the same time as it elicits and distills it. As they occur, key emotional responses are made coherent and integrated into self and system. Once therapists have a core set of emotions to work with and a clear list of the elements that make up any emotion, they can put all the pieces of a complex emotional response together and place it in context of the interpersonal attachment dramas where this experience occurs. In this way, reprocessing and expanding emotional awareness becomes a relatively simple and predictable task. This new formulation of emotion can then be used as a source of relevant new information about the nature of self and others and the constraining force of one's fears, as well as providing clarification about one's needs. It is also a source of motivation and a way to signal to others. It's as if we hear new music, and naturally find ourselves moving differently.

However, assembly is not the whole story; it is the prelude to the next part of Tango Move 2—deepening engagement and exploration of emotional experience. Once emotional elements are named and made sense of, the therapist concentrates on increasing engagement with deeper core emotions. The therapist directs Dan's attention to his body response in the moments when he hears criticism and threats that his wife may leave him and responds by going "still" and "numb." Dan is surprised to find that his heart is pounding and he feels breathless, "almost as if I was scared," he says. Then he adds, "Maybe I am, but that would be ridiculous." These deeper emotions, most often fear and its attendant helplessness, shame, or sadness, may be relatively easy to access and engage with, or they may emerge only with significant effort. The pace and level at which this "deepening" is done depends on the openness and ability of the client to recognize and tolerate emotions that are unfamiliar, fragmented, or frightening. They also depend on the stage of therapy and solidarity of the therapeutic alliance. The therapist often simply touches on or leads into a "new" and deeper emotion, and then guides the client into the process of distilling the essence of this emotion (or acknowledging blocks to this process). Once this is done, then the therapist will encourage the client to stay with and explore the emotion on a deeper level. The goal is to discover and clarify the emotional reality—the engine of fears and longings behind the narrative that the client constructs regarding his problems and dilemmas.

In couple therapy in the stabilization stage, this deepening might look like this:

> THERAPIST: So, Paul, you are getting "riled up" as you put it right now, yes? As you try to explain to Mary that she is always too busy for you, you get more and more upset. You prove your case, but then you look down and sigh. Can you help me understand that sigh? Is it an echo of what you said last week, that sinking feeling that you don't matter to her? That has to be so painful—and it's like there is nothing you can do?
>
> PAUL: (*Nods and turns away to weep.*) I am alone here—again. It hurts. Always alone. Do I even have a wife—a person who gives a damn?

Or in individual therapy in the restructuring stage, it would appear like this:

> THERAPIST: Carol, can you stay with that image of your mom wagging her finger at you? What is happening here? Is this one of those times when you, as you put it, "die inside"? It's like she is never going to accept and cherish you. What happens at this moment?
>
> CAROL: It's scary. What's the point? (*Hunches down in her chair.*)
>
> THERAPIST: Yes, and that sparks despair in you. There is nothing you can do. No matter what you do, how hard you try, she can't seem to give you the love you need. You say to yourself, you will never feel this kind of love.
>
> CAROL: (*Weeping.*) That kind of love is not for me, but I can't breathe without it.

EFT Tango Move 3: Choreographing Engaged Encounters

In this step the client's internal drama moves into the interpersonal realm, and she or he is guided to share with a significant other the assembled and distilled (and sometimes deepened) emotional realities engaged with in Tango Move 2. In the course of the client's sharing that emotional experience with a significant witness, a new or *expanded emotional reality is made explicit, concrete, and coherent,* and the client comes to own it.

This other is actually present in couple and family interventions, but may be the therapist or an imagined attachment figure in individual therapy. This other may be emotionally accessible, responsive, and engaged, may be unable to be so engaged, or may even be hostile. In either case, the client's connection to this other is explored, moderated, and directed by the therapist. Whether the encounter is positive or negative, new emotional music invites the client to try a new kind of dance with this other person, often at a different level of connection. Sharing newly accessed vulnerability with such a significant other expands a person's behavioral repertoire and also has the potential to elicit new positive responses from the other. Sharing such vulnerability with an imagined parent who then responds with rejection, enables a client to start asserting her need, accepting her loss, and taking a new position with this internalized parent. Asserting an emotion with another also deepens engagement with this emotion and allows it to be integrated. In this enacted drama, models of self and other are also open for revision.

Tango Move 3 can be viewed as a form of exposure therapy. In a safe environment, with the protection and direction of a professional, clients embark on challenging interpersonal encounters in which they may have been wounded or threatened in the past, and negotiate this territory differently and with different consequences. As in formal exposure therapies, the therapist titrates the risks a client takes and often "slices the risk thinner" by suggesting, for example, "Perhaps this is too hard. Can you simply just tell him then, 'It is just too hard to tell you about . . . I cannot do it right now'?" These encounters can also be viewed as a key ingredient of a corrective emotional experience, wherein key life dramas are returned to and transformed.

In individual therapy in the restructuring stage, Tango Move 3 may look like this:

CAROL: (*Depressed; has her eyes closed.*)

THERAPIST: So, Carol, can you see your mom? Can you tell her about this desperation? (*She does this with deep feeling.*) Can you tell her just how hard this is for you and how it leaves you with, as you said, with no oxygen, always fighting for breath or looking for ways to not feel—to numb? (*Carol explores her "numbness" and "aloneness."*) What do you—that numb part of you—want to tell her?

CAROL: (*To the therapist.*) I want to tell her I had to shut down cause this hurt so much and cause I thought it meant that there was something wrong with me. But shut down is no way to live your life!

THERAPIST: So close your eyes and when you can see her, tell her, tell her that.

In a family session in the early stabilization or de-escalation stage, the intervention would look like this:

> "Jacob, you are saying that you are always angry and mad. This is what your family sees; but that underneath the mad you are really sad and alone and scared that your dad doesn't want you, that you are not the son he wants. How could he help you with that? Can you tell him about that—being sad and scared?"

EFT Tango Move 4: Processing the Encounter

In Tango Move 4, the therapist reflects and summarizes the process of interaction—the transactional drama that arises from the client's newly accessed emotions being directly shared in an engaged way. With the client, the therapist explores what enacting this emotion was like, and how the responses of the other (whether therapist, partner, family member, imagined attachment figure, or even disowned part of self) were heard and integrated. Blocks to hearing the other's experience or response can then also be explored. So, in couple therapy, if one partner dismisses the message offered by the now more open and vulnerable other partner, the therapist will intervene and "catch the bullet" (see Chapter 6), working with this person's difficulty in taking in, accepting, or responding to an unfamiliar message from this person. New emotional experience becomes a new interactional drama, and now this drama has to be reflected on, explored, mined for meaning, and integrated into models of self, other, and relationship. The provision of safety, structure, and reflection offered by the therapist allows for the building of momentum; clients can take greater and greater risks in these dramas and process the new information and experiences that arise effectively.

In a family session in the stabilization stage, Tango Move 4 may look like this:

> THERAPIST: So what was it like to reach out your arms to your dad and say, "I want a dad—I want you to come close"? That was pretty brave. (*Jacob says it feels good to say this.*) What was it like for you to hear this, Sam?
>
> SAM: It moves me. It moves me, Jacob. But I get this wobbly feeling inside. I don't know how to do this—how to be a dad, so I kind of freeze. I'm failing you. It's sad and scary too. I want to be your dad.

The therapist asks Sam to say this again, and continues to follow this thread into further elucidating the sense of incompetence that blocks Sam's responsiveness to his son.

In couple sessions in the restructuring stage, Tango Move 4 would look like this:

THERAPIST: Paul, what is it like to tell Mary, "I do get mad. You are right. I am so alone here and there is nothing I can do"?

PAUL: It feels good, solid. Ground under my feet. It's right. I don't want to be alone, and I am trying to get her to see that.

The therapist asks Mary what it feels like to hear this:

MARY: I am a bit confused. I never see Paul as vulnerable. I can hear it. I can hear it. I guess I kind of spark his rage—just by my silence! Who knew that?

In individual therapy in the restructuring stage, a Tango Move 4 intervention might look like this:

THERAPIST: (*To Carol, who has been imagining an encounter with her mom.*) How does it feel to say to mom, "I am not going to creep around and beg for your love anymore. I needed it, and you couldn't give it. It wasn't about me." (*Carol beams and flexes her muscles.*)

CAROL: (*Laughing.*) It's new; it's dynamite, that is what it is.

EFT Tango Move 5: Integrating and Validating

In the final move in the process of new and deeper engagement with one's own experience and with significant others, the therapist reflects the whole process of the previous four moves from a metaperspective and highlights the key significant moments and responses, using them to validate each client's strength and courage. The message clients receive from this intervention is that they can change their ways of experiencing and dealing with emotions, understanding themselves and others, and begin moving in the key relationship dances that define their lives. In Tango Move 5, the therapist brings coherence and closure to the whole tango process, so that it becomes a building block for continued progress in therapy. The therapist also builds on the positive emotions often expressed in this move, heightening and finding images for them. Positive emotions have been shown to broaden attention and conceptual breadth, increase creativity, relax vigilance, and so motivate approach and explore behavior (Frederickson & Branigan, 2005). Ideally, the Tango sequence ends with a moment of positive *balance and accomplishment*. Indeed, neuroscientist Jaak Panksepp (2009) actually refers to experiential therapies as affective balance therapies. Each time this tango sequence unfolds, it then creates momentum for change and boosts clients' sense of mastery and confidence—they can understand their inner life and their relationships, and they can shape and change both.

In individual therapy in the stabilization stage, this move may look like this:

> "That is amazing, Carol, you have just taken all your 'weakness,' as you call it—all your pain—and faced it, stating it clearly to your mom, and now you are beaming at me! Seems like you can deal with this now. You have found the oxygen you need."

In family therapy in the consolidation stage, Tango Move 5 could go like this:

> "Wow, guys. This is amazing. Jacob, you just stepped past your anger and asked your dad for what you needed, and Dad, you hung in and told Jacob you were not sure what to do, but then you reached back to him. Fantastic—in your bones you do know how to be a dad! And Mom, you stayed quiet here and supported your husband with kind words and helped all this to happen. You all took a new step out of your old dance today."

This EFT Tango process orients the therapist. When a therapist finds herself lost or confused, she can simply return to this core process as a metaframework—a basic set of foundational interventions—and begin to orient herself again. Bear in mind that all five moves of the Tango are not always fully played out in a session. Each of them, especially in the most intense sessions in the restructuring stage of therapy, could take up a large part of a session itself. In the softening change events explored in research studies of EFT for couples and in EFFT, Tango Moves 2, 3, and 4 are intensified and often repeated a number of times to shape specific new levels of reaching and responsiveness. This repetition of deepening emotion, enacting it with another, and processing the encounter are often done to choreograph new, secure bonding scenarios. (Softening change events deserve special attention, and are discussed further in later chapters.)

Once the basic sequence of these moves in the EFT change process is mastered, then therapists can improvise with creativity. Knowing how to access and work with emotion in the affect assembly and deepening process, how to shift interactional patterns in highly charged encounters, and how to shape new, constructive attachment experiences all empower the therapist so that he or she can be authentic and present in session; indeed he or she can play! In all of these processes, therapist and client listen to and modulate the emotional music, shape new interpersonal moves, and choreograph specific dances of safe connection to evoke adaptive shifts in self and system.

The Therapist's Stance in the EFT Tango

For the therapist, the five moves of the Tango framework for intervention unfold at many different levels. The challenge of offering effective therapy is to be completely present and engaged on an authentic personal level, while also keeping different levels of professional awareness, such as the structure and direction of one's interventions. The relational context—implicit messages about the relationship between therapist and each client—is the platform on which all of the EFT change processes are based. First, the therapist is attuning to and resonating with the emotional music of the session and using feedback from her own emotions to move into an empathic state with clients and their dilemmas. She is present and genuinely engaged with each client.

Second, the therapist is constantly monitoring and actively maintaining the safety of the alliance between her and each client. For example, she might state a reflection of problematic behavior in an especially soft and accepting manner to a very sensitive client, adding a validating remark immediately after. She deliberately offers relational messages that define the session as a safe haven where risk is titrated and relentless empathy is offered. (This stance parallels the role of the loving parent who provides safety and soothing in the face of the tidal wave of life.) The therapist attempts to be *accessible, responsive,* and *engaged* (A.R.E.; remember these are the three main factors of a secure bond mentioned in Chapter 1) with each client, and when this felt sense of safe connection is lost, the therapist pauses and prioritizes the repair of the rift.

Third, each therapist is a curious explorer of the client's world, a process consultant who stands with clients, moment by moment, as they touch and organize their experience, finding the fragmented, denied, and avoided elements in that experience. The safety of the alliance allows the client to attempt a new level of engagement with his emerging experience *as it occurs and is being encoded in the brain.* Neuroscience suggests that this deeper engagement allows for the optimal shaping and reshaping of neural circuits as they are being challenged (J. A. Coan, personal communication, June 18, 2008).

Fourth, the therapist is routinely reflecting on the whole process of the session and linking it back to the stages and processes of therapy and to the client's treatment goals. He or she acts as a secure base in the therapy session by setting up challenges at the *leading edge* of each client's comfort zone. For example, a client will then be asked to go more deeply into a difficult or traumatic event, or to try engaging with an attachment figure in a way that triggers basic existential vulnerabilities.

Fifth, both therapist and client often collaboratively explore the dilemmas of being human, not as expert and pupil, but as two human beings who struggle to learn how to live, as living sweeps them onward. So the therapist can step aside from the expert role and paint a picture of how the client's dilemmas are universal and how clear answers are often hard to find. The therapist can even use limited self-disclosure as part of this intervention.

In short, the EFT change process requires a specific kind of therapeutic alliance in which the therapist is emotionally and personally present, and this presence provides the context for transformational change.

GENERAL EXPERIENTIAL TECHNIQUES

Having established a broad perspective on who we are as human beings, the common dilemmas we all face, and the core processes in change, we are ready to delve into the specific interventions used in EFT. While the subsequent list offered is useful, it is important to remember that when these techniques are combined they interact and mesh to construct different interventions, just as discrete ingredients combine to make different kinds of bread. Reflection, for example, can be empathic and soothing, a summarizing tool to use in the service of creating coherence, or even a confrontation if it is describing behaviors that a client does not want to own. Specific techniques mentioned below are used in any or all of the Tango moves, but some techniques may better fit and, therefore, be used more frequently with, different moves. For example, the EFT therapist takes every opportunity to use reflection and validation from the first encounter with clients until the last handshake. Evocative questions are also used generally as part of the model but are particularly useful in the affect assembly and deepening move of the Tango.

Individually Oriented Interventions

• *Reflection* of emotional processing as it occurs. The goal is to focus on inner experience and make it explicit, concrete, tangible, and alive. Bowlby spoke always of significant inner experience as a "felt sense," that is, an embodied experience, rather than focusing just on cognition or information processing.

Example

"As you tell me that you are now fine with how this loss of your best friend occurred, I notice how very still you are, and how you seem to be holding the arms of the chair very tight."

• *Validation* of habitual emotional regulation strategies and perspectives, stuck places, and attachment longings and fears. The goal is to affirm and *normalize* clients in their struggles, protective stances, and attempts to grow, fostering a sense of constant safety in the therapy session and reducing the debilitating sense of aloneness or shame many clients associate with their problems.

Example

"This must be so hard for you, Tim. As you say, you are in foreign territory here. You have never had the experience of staying with and making sense of your feelings, and what worked for you in the past was just to distract yourself and turn off. So, of course, that is the first place you go."

• *Evocative questions and responses* to elicit underlying emotions and thoughts—ways of constructing experience. Key moments are replayed and key experiences that shape self and system are delineated from the most basic elements of experience—sensations, perceptions, and emotions—that is, from a bottom-up, rather than from an abstract, top-down cognitive perspective.

Example

"What just happened to you, when I commented . . . ?"; "When does this sinking feeling, this helpless feeling come up for you in your life?"; "How do you do that—just 'turn stuff off,' as you say?"; "Where do you feel that in your body right now?"; "How can your partner help you with that feeling in this moment?"

• *Deepening engagement in inner experience* by heightening the salience of a moment or a response and delineating the response further. Repetition and evocative imagery are particularly useful here. It is useful to think of skillful repetition as wearing away at the muscle required to suppress emotion and also as gradually rendering what is new and strange more and more familiar. This deepening technique is a key part of the Tango Move 2, but it is also a general experiential technique. For example, a therapist might use a particularly powerful evocative image in setting the tone for and bringing drama to an enactment (Tango Move 3).

Example

"I hear you. This feeling of wanting to hide, to just keep everyone out, is so compelling. It's urgent. So part of you says, 'This is life and death.' Life and death. If someone sees you, something dreadful is going to happen—yes? You can't risk that. It will be terrible—a catastrophe. You are not sure you would survive—being really seen. It's dangerous?—yes, dangerous. The only way is to be invisible. Unseen, that is, safe. It's protection—but protection that becomes a prison."

• *Interpretation* at the leading edge of a client's experience. Here the therapist ventures an extension of the client's expressions. Care is taken that such conjectures are framed tentatively. If the desire is to increase intensity and deepen engagement, then these interpretations can be offered in a proxy voice—that is, they are framed as if the client himself is stating them.

Example

"So, can you help me, Jim? When your son reaches for you, you kind of freeze up—yes? That is what happened just now. You go still and silent. You don't know how to respond perhaps? This is not a dance you know—you didn't grow up with people making these kinds of appeals and others responding. Perhaps you say to yourself, 'If I move, I am going to get this wrong. I am going to blow it with my son and my wife and everyone will get upset with me. I will hear that I have failed again. Best to be quiet and hope this blows over.' Is that it?"

Interactionally Oriented Interventions

• *Tracking and reflecting interactions* and interpersonal dramas as they occur in session between intimates, in a client's narrative, or in imaginal encounters. The goal is to identify and outline significant responses and the patterned steps that typify distressing or stuck places in these interactions and to bring into high relief the nature of self-generating cycles of interaction.

Example

"So, this happens a lot. You are insisting and pushing for her to hear your point of view. You want a response. But she 'refuses' to be persuaded and 'dismisses' you. And the more she shuts you out, the more you push and demand, until you are completely exhausted."

• *Reframing* in order to shift the meaning frame of an interactional response or cycle. The desired shift might be from helplessness to agency, from negative and dangerous to positive, from critical and hostile to desperate. Reframing is used at moments of emotional intensity when negative interactional cycles are being addressed. The goal is to shift a client's perspective from a problem-reinforcing mindset to one that expands awareness and acknowledges underlying attachment vulnerabilities.

Example

"Your father would get 'big and loud' and tell you that you were just a bad kid in these situations, and there was nothing you could do. And this figure of your father stands behind your husband, Bill, and you hear the same condemnation. [Client nods in agreement.] But Bill is calling to you because he needs you to turn toward him right now. He is loud because he is desperate for your help; because you are so important to him, not because you have made a mistake. He is asking for your help. Can you see that?"

• *Direct choreographing of interactions and responses* can be used in three ways. First (in Example 1) in order to pinpoint reoccurring problematic interactional responses that are resistant to change. This technique helps bring them into the light, so they become clearer and more easily modified. Second, the therapist might also use direct choreographing to exemplify and dramatize new responses; after all, what is admitted to another becomes more real. Third, this technique is used frequently (but especially in Tango Move 3) to turn new emotional experience into new signals to others that then potentially evoke new responses, and so set up new kinds of corrective interactions.

Example 1

"So as you say, you have only anger for him right now. So you cannot do anything but tell him his mistakes, even when he explains how much this hurts him. Can you simply tell him, 'Right now, I cannot hear your hurt. I am so angry, I want to push you off balance; maybe I want you to hurt, to know I can hurt you. So I keep lashing out at you'?"

Example 2

"So you are talking about feeling small in the moment before you move into making all these threats. Can you simply tell your mother right now, 'I do threaten you, but in the moment before I puff up and threaten, I feel so so small'?"

Example 3

"So can you hold onto that amazing crystal clear statement and turn your chair, look into his face, and tell him, 'I show you my armor and tell you my reservations, but inside I am so scared to risk and ask for your love. A voice in my head says you will not want that small, scared me'?"

The exact nature and quality of all these interventions depends on the specific context in which they are used. Whatever form these interventions take, it matters how they are conducted.

Tone: The "How" of the Technique

In any intervention that privileges secure connection between therapist and client, the nonverbal communication from the therapist—how things are said—is of crucial importance. At moments of emotional vulnerability when clients are risking new levels of engagement with inner experience or with others, the therapist interacts with clients keeping the acronym RISSSC in mind. The elements in this acronym stand for:

1. Repeat
2. Imagery
3. Simple words
4. Slow pace
5. Soft voice
6. Client's words

Clinical wisdom from many years of working with highly distressed individuals, couples, and family members has shown again and again that these stylistic features make a difference in therapy. Clients, for example, will most often not take the risk of deepening their engagement with their vulnerabilities or hanging out at the leading edge of what is known to discover new territory, if the therapist proceeds too fast, uses many abstract intellectual words, or speaks in a raised or impersonal, externally oriented tone of voice. It has become somewhat of a cliché in EFT training for novice therapists to murmur the mantra "Soft, slow, simple." If we need a model for this style, we only have to turn to an image of a security-priming mother interacting with an anxious child. A parent can be making positive comments, but unless she calms the child's nervous system, that is, unless the pace is slow and the prosody is soothing, the positivity is most often lost, and the child's response is difficult to predict.

As suggested above, repetition is offered not in the spirit of skill building, but in the spirit of aiding real listening. For example, James Gross (1998a, 1998b) points out just how much effort the suppression of emotion involves, so therapists are wise to make reflections and interpretations as evocative as possible and repeat them a number of times. After some five or six evocative repetitions (e.g., calmly restating a client's reluctant admission of possible inferiority), which, contrary to the client's expectations, do not trigger any catastrophes, the client's fearful resistance begins to wane. Suppression then simply dissolves. Repetition is also absolutely necessary to enable the client to orient to and take in strange, foreign information. Using the client's words also evokes acceptance and familiarity. Images also move us emotionally and pull us in, capturing complex realities in simple, powerful ways.

This chapter has outlined a metaframework sequence of interventions (the moves of the Tango) and associated processes of change, as well as more general microtechniques in an emotionally focused attachment model. The next six chapters set out how change occurs in individual, couple, and family therapy in more detail. Throughout those discussions we will refer back to the EFT Tango and the general techniques spelled out in this chapter.

 TAKE IT HOME AND TO HEART

- Attachment privileges the place of emotion in human functioning and change. Attachment and attachment interventions are all about the regulation of emotion and the creation of *emotional balance*. We help clients change how they regulate their emotions and we also use emotion to "move" people—to evoke and shape new behaviors. This movement is an innate, organic, and biologically prepared process.

- Discovering and ordering one's emotions, adding granularity, and making sense of key recurring emotions is an essential part of the change process. Constructive affect regulation shapes constructive dependency on others and the growth of the self.

- Working effectively with emotion requires that we expand our capacity to differentiate levels of emotional processing and to know how to shape core corrective emotional experiences, which always involve both inner shifts and shifts in the relationship with significant others. Change is within and between.

- The change process in an experiential attachment-focused therapy can be distilled into a metaframework for intervention and change processes known as the EFT Tango. The therapist's accurate, relentlessly empathic responsiveness is the basis for the five moves of the Tango, which involve the reflection or mirroring of present processes that make up inner and interpersonal realities; the assembly and deepening of emotion; the choreographing of new, more engaged encounters with significant others; the processing of these new encounters with significant others (imaginal or real); and the validation of this new experience, which fosters integration into a relational system and sense of self.

- The therapist uses general Rogerian and systemic techniques, such as evocative questions and choreographing new interactions, in the EFT Tango process and throughout the therapy sessions. The constant creation of safety is essential. Risks must be titrated by the therapist's tone, soothing presence, and attuned contact, as clients reconstruct new inner and outer realities.

- The EFT therapist finds his or her own secure base in the attachment perspective, a clear sense of the nature and power of emotion as a crucial part of the change process, a metaframework for intervention, and a set of techniques that integrate the systemic and interpersonal with experiential realities. The therapist knows where he or she is going and is able to use exactly what the client's nervous system recognizes as crucial and compelling, namely, emotion and new, more constructive ways to engage with those who matter most in the service of change.

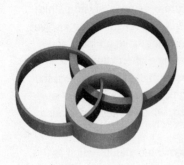

Chapter 4

Emotionally Focused Individual Therapy in the Attachment Frame

Expanding the Sense of Self

We need the eyes of others to form and hold ourselves together.
>   —DANIEL N. STERN (2004, p. 107)

I saw the angel in the marble and carved until I set him free.
>   —MICHELANGELO

A felt sense of secure connection with others and a coherent and integrated sense of self that empowers a person in the face of life's challenges are two sides of the same coin. The ongoing construction of selfhood is a process that occurs within the web of close interpersonal relationships that shape a life. From the attachment point of view, ongoing personality development involves a number of key processes, namely, the structuring of habitual emotion regulation strategies or styles that become especially pertinent under conditions of threat or uncertainty; the formation of a number of "hot" existential meaning frames (e.g., emotionally loaded expectations and causal attributions) that mesh with and arise from working models of self and other; and the creation of a behavioral repertoire and specific protocols for engaging with others. These developmental processes are highly interactive, and they are always colored by our felt sense of connection with others.

The image of health offered by attachment science offers the therapist a clear goal in terms of individual psychotherapy. Specifically, the ideal outcome of attachment-based therapy is an individual who is balanced emotionally, mentally open, flexible in terms of action, deeply engaged and alive and, above all, able to learn and grow. Bowlby depicted healthy working models of self and other, for example, as subject to constant revision and change in the light of experience. The research linking positive intrapersonal and interpersonal attachment variables to security is extensive (see Chapter 2). Here we review that research briefly, as it applies to treating individual clients.

THE INDIVIDUAL IN THE CONTEXT OF INTIMATE BONDS

Overwhelmingly, the evidence supports the belief that the lack of secure connection with others limits and constrains us. Cognitive closure, the kind that limits creative problem solving, can be observed in more insecure individuals even when the context facilitates positive feelings and relaxed exploration (Mikulincer & Sheffi, 2000). Those who are avoidantly attached seem to dismiss signs of safety to maintain cognitive control, and the anxiously attached respond with impaired creativity to positive cues, such as retrieving a happy memory, seemingly mistrustful of safety signals. In terms of models of self, avoidant individuals seem to prioritize self-enhancement over task engagement and so have a hard time acknowledging mistakes and revising decisions or plans. Anxious people's struggles with self-defeating beliefs and worries about rejection also tend to impair full engagement in goal-oriented behavior (Mikulincer & Shaver, 2016). This kind of data counters the long-held idea that to grasp, define, and help to shape a mind or a personality, it is sufficient to focus on the individual as a single entity isolated from the interactional reality of his or her social bonds.

The goal of EFIT is essentially the same as for EFT for couples and EFFT for families, namely, to give clients an integrative corrective emotional experience in which they explore new ways to engage with their own experience, with others, and with the existential dilemmas of life. All this is accomplished in a context wherein present responses are viewed in the compassionate light of the limited-survival and affect-regulation choices offered in the past. The EFIT therapist takes the stance that in life, we do what we know to get us through the night, and then, ironically, often remain stuck in these constrained strategies and perspectives in the light of day.

Attachment in Individual Therapy

How do attachment theory and science fit with the field of individual intervention? The attachment perspective is beginning to be used more and more as a theoretical and pragmatic basis for individual therapy interventions in clinical practice in EFIT and in accelerated experiential dynamic psychotherapy (AEDP; Fosha, 2000), and at least as part of a general theoretical backdrop in approaches such as interpersonal therapy (IPT; Weissman, Markovitz, & Klerman, 2007) and process experiential/emotion-focused therapy (PE/EF; Elliott, Watson, Goldman, & Greenberg, 2004). All of these approaches can be classified as either psychodynamic or humanistic experiential in nature. However, they vary with respect to many factors, such as the role of the therapist; the techniques used; whether a systems theory approach focusing on circular causality is integrated into the model (as it certainly is in EFT); the intensity and use of the connection between client and therapist; the parsimony and clarity of formulations and interventions and the centrality of attachment science in treatment; and last, the level of empirical validation. For example, in the practice of the AEDP model, outlined by Fosha (2000), it seems as if there is a greater emphasis on working with positive emotion than in EFIT and a more analytically deprived approach to the formulation of dysfunction. All approaches consider how traumatic experience from one's past, particularly when inflicted by attachment figures who are expected to offer safety and support, affect the manner in which present experience is encoded and integrated in ways that lead either to growth or to dysfunction. They also acknowledge the key role of emotion in human functioning. (If the reader wishes to look at the differences and similarities between the EFIT model proposed here and the more psychodynamic IPT and experiential PE/EF models, chosen for comparison for the sake of clarity and because both of these interventions have been tested in outcome studies, these comparisons are discussed in Appendix 3.)

There are, of course, other notable contributors linking attachment and the practice of psychotherapy. Peter Costello (2013) poignantly describes how basic choices about who we are and can be evolve in an attachment context. He suggests that we decide with caregivers what we can see and name, what will happen when we are lonely and afraid, whether it is best to voice or stifle our vulnerability, and how best to get a response from others. These scenarios are then written in our neurons and neural networks and become automatic; they are simply who we are!

THE ATTACHMENT ORIENTATION TO DEPRESSION AND ANXIETY

Attachment insecurities are associated with a general vulnerability to mental health issues in general and to the development of depression and anxiety disorders in particular. It is an almost impossible task to pinpoint the specific mechanisms that lead to specific disorders. The principle of multifinality (that is, many roads lead to the same destination) tells us that one individual with a particular attachment history and placement on the continuum of either anxious or avoidant orientations will develop one set of symptoms, while another similar individual will develop another set. Distal risk factors such as separation from parents, more proximal risk factors such as patterns of affect regulation, and moderators such as the nature of present relationships and ongoing stress, all work together to determine the trajectory of dysfunction (Nolen-Hoeksema & Watkins, 2011). Attachment theorists do suggest (Ein-Dor & Doron, 2015) that avoidant attachment is more likely to be linked to so-called externalizing disorders, such as substance abuse and antisocial disorders, and that clear associations also exist between the distress and fear associated with attachment insecurity and internalizing disorders, including depression, anxiety disorders, and PTSD.

Bowlby himself suggested that, in general, "clinical conditions are best understood as disordered versions of what is otherwise a healthy response" (1980, p. 245). Withdrawal and immobilization can be functional responses to impossible or dangerous situations where vulnerability is overwhelming (Porges, 2011), such as finding oneself dependent on a dangerous and unpredictable attachment figure. Easily triggered anger and hypervigilance are likewise functional when the alternative appears to be that one is inevitably dismissed or deserted. The disorder appears when such responses become generalized and global and cannot be revised.

In terms of depression, Bowlby speaks of the "disorganization" that follows loss, and notes how, when combined with helplessness, it seems to trigger depressive responses. The best protective factor in his view is a sense of "competence and personal worth" (1980, p. 246). He further elaborates that depressed individuals commonly describe themselves with four adjectives, namely, lonely, unlovable, unwanted, and helpless. These clients often see themselves as failures, and usually narrate a history of close relationships in which they could never meet the expectations of others and so never experienced being valued just for themselves. They do not then feel truly entitled to compassion and care. As my client Jen says, "I could never please my dad no matter what. Whatever I did, it was never good enough. And I guess I just kind of took that in and got used to that frame. Now I treat myself that way too. I criticize myself for everything." Loss, failure, and self-criticism demoralize and depress. No matter what the precipitating factors may be, the attachment perspective parallels the model of depression proposed by Hammen (1995), where intrapsychic response and interpersonal dysfunction trigger, maintain, and exacerbate each other. Susceptibility to depression, triggered by personal history, stress, or negative models of self and other then shapes maladaptive interpersonal behaviors that undermine relationships and add momentum to the depressive response.

These themes are common to anxiety, too, but in anxiety disorders there is not the same loss of positive emotions that is found in depression, and immobilization is often replaced by agitation and greater sensitivity to threat (Mineka & Vrshek-Schallhorn, 2014), although extreme anxiety can also result in paralysis and an inability to move and act. The rejection sensitivity and relational stress that come with anxious attachment also predict depression (Chango, McElhaney, Allen, Schad, & Marston, 2012). Anxiety functions to warn us about potential danger and triggers the protective mechanisms; as such, it can be extremely useful and enhance performance. But if the warning siren is too loud and always on, it becomes self-perpetuating and self-defeating and a problem in itself.

The four key elements of dysfunctional anxiety are (Barlow et al., 2014; Barlow, 2002):

1. Frequent and intense negative emotion and less clarity about and acceptance of this emotion.

2. Vigilant information processing biases and intolerance for uncertainty or ambivalence (also found in depression).

3. Avoidant strategies for dealing with emotion and the use of suppression when negative emotion does occur; such emotion is more likely to be seen as uncontrollable and intolerable. Unfortunately, suppression creates a rebound effect and increases or maintains negative emotions and physiological arousal (Hofmann, Heering, Sawyer, & Ashaani, 2009). Avoidance has been called the kryptonite of all mental health disorders since it prevents corrective experience from occurring and paradoxically sensitizes us to whatever it is that we are avoiding. In generalized anxiety disorder (GAD), worry or compulsions can be seen as ways of avoiding the distress of anxiety and depressive symptoms, and also as being maintained by the chronic avoidance of engagement (Manos, Kanter, & Busch, 2010).

4. The generalization of negative reactions to the experience of fear itself—the fear of fear (especially seen in panic disorders). The interpretation of negative experience impacts its intensity, duration, and consequences. A sensitivity to anxiety resulting in a heightened sense of threat or danger and intensifying attributions predicts the onset of depression and anxiety disorders (Schmidt, Keogh, Timpano, & Richey, 2008).

In general, it matters how experience is processed. It is *how* one relates to feelings of anxiety or low mood that is crucial rather than simply the frequency of negative emotions. The way of interpreting and responding to negative emotions often paradoxically serves to increase and maintain negative emotions in anxiety and depressive disorders. *Negative ways of viewing and dealing with distress form a self-perpetuating feedback loop that leads into the construction of further distress.*

Clearly different anxiety problems and mood disorders share many common features. These shared features, particularly emotion regulation issues and interacting process variables common to both disorders, are set out in Barlow's model of a unified protocol (UP) for emotional disorders. This model delineates the common structure of anxiety and depression (Barlow et al., 2011), and outlines how these two problems can be combined into one joint category, namely *negative emotional disorder*. The UP model fits well with the focus of attachment theory and attachment-oriented interventions such as EFT. Both approaches see a sense of uncontrollability and perceived danger as the core common factors in anxiety and depression. This uncontrollability is also exacerbated by ineffective affect-regulation strategies like suppression that intensify the problem. Both the UP model and EFT include a general focus on gradated exposure, in which fear-inducing or painful experience can gradually be felt and processed in new ways, and attention is given to shaping new pathways for emotion regulation and increasing the client's use of social support.

More specifically, the therapist using either the UP or EFT will:

- Ask about emotion and examine typical coping techniques, as well as the action tendencies linked to the emotion.

- Attend to helping clients alter their perceptions of threat and their ability to cope by, for example, addressing and reducing catastrophizing.

- Encourage more acceptance of emotions in general.

The UP model reflects the reality that the comorbidity rate of depression and anxiety disorders is high (Brown, Campbell, Lehman, Grisham, & Mancill, 2001), and that the features of one kind of disorder seem to act as a risk factor for other disorders. Treatments for one disorder also seem to produce significant improvement in other disorders, even when they are not addressed in therapy. A wide range of emotional disorders also respond equivalently to antidepressant medications, indicating a shared pathophysiology. Barlow also suggests, in a way that parallels research on attachment, that a heightened sense of unpredictability and uncontrollability can be associated with brain functioning created by early adverse experiences, or it can be learned, manifesting in different pathways leading to different specific kinds of anxiety issues or mood problems (Barlow et al., 2014). These problems are viewed then as relatively trivial variations of a broader syndrome—negative emotion disorder. The delineation of this general concept of negative emotional disorder fits with the more parsimonious and nonpathologizing stance of attachment science and of EFT as an experiential therapy. It identifies and operationalizes a problem in a client, without forcing his or her presenting difficulties into a formal diagnostic system, such as the DSM or the ICD.

Where the theoretical framework of the UP approach does not fit so well with attachment science is in Barlow's proposal that the common determining factor in setting up these disorders is temperament and trait neuroticism. I suggest that attachment theory and science offer a much more convincing explanatory framework. The way treatment is delivered in the UP also differs from EFT, in that the UP model presents a much more coaching and cognitively oriented and behaviorally based frame using extensive homework and exercises than is offered in EFT. (The UP model is termed both "traditional CBT" and "emotion focused" in the treatment manual. From the point of view of EFT, while there is more attention paid to emotion in UP than is usual in behavioral models, using these generic labels for intervention here is simply confusing rather than clarifying.)

CASE FORMULATION WITH EMOTIONAL DISORDERS

In this book the focus of intervention is depression and anxiety—also referred to as "emotional disorders." How does the attachment-oriented clinician view such disorders? We answer that by discussing the EFT approach to case formulation.

There are two principles that generally clarify the process of case formulation in EFT across modalities. First, the point of an experiential therapy is not to *fix*, as in find immediate solutions for the symptoms clients present at the beginning of therapy. As stated in the basic text on couples EFT (Johnson, 2004), the therapist is not a coach who corrects misguided assumptions or teaches skills or a wise creator of insight. In light of this, it is worth noting that the EFT therapist is a process consultant who accesses and walks into painful experience *with* clients (as in the old adage, the only way out is through), and collaboratively joins with them in processing this experience more fully. As Rogers suggests (1961), the process of therapy is one in which the therapist and client can "enjoy discovering the order in experience" (p. 24). The normalizing of our limited ability to process our experience in the most constructive way, due to our blind spots resulting from our history and our inevitable struggles in the face of life's demands, is perhaps the key feature of the humanistic experiential, or person-centered approach.

This approach, in many ways, is at odds with the whole attempt to define and categorize mental health issues and problems in formal diagnostic systems, such as the various reiterations of the DSM. The descriptive labels used in such systems can be helpful in orienting the therapist. Also, brief formal questionnaires tied to the diagnostic entities in the DSM and other systems, such as the Beck Depression and Anxiety Scales (Beck, Steer, & Brown, 1996; Beck & Steer, 1993), can be used as an aid and a way of opening a discovery process with clients. In couple therapy, the Dyadic Adjustment Scale (DAS; Spanier, 1976) can be given at the beginning of therapy, but a newer measure, the Couples Satisfaction Index (CSI; Funk & Rogge, 2007) also seems useful. However, in general, assessment is an ongoing part of treatment, and what is poignant or truly problematic for clients will emerge as part of the process of therapy.

Second, assessment focuses on process, not just content. The first session in EFT consists of creating a safe environment and a collaborative alliance, an invitation to engage with the therapist in an open manner. The therapist elicits from clients their stories and their agendas for therapy. As suggested by attachment science (Main et al., 1985), the way in which clients tell their stories and engage with others, be it the therapist or others in the session, is at least as informative as the content of the interview itself. The therapist pays attention to the nonverbals, the emotion expressed and how it is regulated, the general coherence of clients' stories in terms of meaning, and the terms in which the self and others are generally described. It is clear that more securely attached clients are able to be more specific and coherent, as well as more reflective about assigning meaning to their experience. Anxiously attached clients become easily overwhelmed by emotion and present more extreme and fragmented narratives, while avoidant clients tend to skim the surface of experience, change the topic, or deflect questions and present as detached, as they recount potentially painful events without reflection or engagement. *How* an experience is encoded and presented is then often more telling than the *what*—the actual information given by the client. As discussed in the last chapter, the depth of experiencing and the *granularity* of emotion expressed attunes the therapist to the client's habitual processing style.

This initial engagement process is a genuine act of discovery (part of the three D's of EFT—discover, distill, and disclose, discussed in Chapters 2 and 3) on the part of the therapist and client. The curiosity and open discovery process will be curtailed if the therapist is caught in rigid cognitive frames around diagnosis or is committed to finding the element of experience that his or her dominant theoretical framework decrees is paramount. Hence the cliché that if we have nothing in our kit but a hammer then everything becomes a nail. For this reason, experiential therapies aspire to be "client centered" and to enter into a genuine encounter with the person of the client, rather than becoming mesmerized by the problem as presented. This discovery process is particularly crucial when working with clients from different cultures or different economic, racial, and sexual backgrounds. So, a Japanese couple teach me what the concept of honor means in Japan and how this impacts the messages that may be sent to a partner. A rape survivor teaches me what happens for a woman like her after this kind of trauma and how she makes meaning out of this event. The universals, emotion and attachment, make for common ground even in the face of significant cultural differences in how these variables may be expressed. The EFT therapist basically undertakes the task of being a permanent student in what it means to be a human being. Clients are the experts on their own experience, and central to the art of the EFT therapist is to become better able to sensitively attune to, hold, and capture that experience.

As I mentioned earlier, EFIT is best suited to address issues of depression and anxiety, including the aftereffects of traumatic experience and existential issues that arise from such experience, especially those concerning interpersonal connection and negative relationships. In terms of treatment inclusion and exclusion criteria, the therapist's ability to provide a safe environment is a determining factor. EFT as an approach is usually a short-term therapy, which requires a certain ability to maintain focus and engage with the therapist; psychosis or antisocial personality disorders make such engagement unlikely. In situations where risk factors are significant, such as chronic addictive behaviors, severe chronic depression, or a high suicidal risk, it may be more suitable to involve other professionals offering specialized interventions and/or medication, working in tandem with an EFIT therapist. If a client has been given specialized treatment for a problem, such as addiction, and wishes to enter EFIT, the therapist will liaise with the other therapists involved (with the client's permission of course). The therapist has to feel confident that the client can tolerate engagement in the EFIT process safely, and that he can adjust the pace and intensity of intervention to the client's window of tolerance.

In addressing all presenting issues, the therapist is concerned with the developmental narrative of a client and how it has shaped working models of self and other. Case formulation and engagement in EFIT includes an emphasis on the following issues:

- Affect regulation challenges and cycles of high reactivity or numbing and dissociation.

- Somatic issues, such as momentary dissociation or body pain and discomfort.

- Blocks to effective, coherent meaning making that supports agency and positive models of self and other.

- Blocks to adaptive action wherein, for example, ambivalence or conflict result in paralysis and stagnation and emotion is suppressed, fragmented, or denied.

- Negative models of self, wherein the self is seen as unworthy and unentitled to care, as a failure, ineffective or helpless, and sometimes as so unacceptable to others as to be outside of the fold of human connection.

- Negative models of other, wherein there is a conviction that others are dangerous or at least unreliable, unpredictable, and sources of inevitable abandonment and rejection.

When negative models of self and other are dominant, trust is an enormous risk, undertaken only when the wired-in longing for emotional connection and the pain of isolation become front and center. These "hot" adverse models are not absolutes, of course, and appear on a continuum but, if they are significantly negative, leave the individual in a world where constant vigilance is essential and emotional regulation swings between hyper- and hypoarousal. In the face of such oscillation, growth and flexibility are then impeded and the process of potential revision of working models is undermined. Choice and agency become impossible, and reactivity to immediate cues takes over the client's life; the ability to reflect on and make choices to reshape one's experience or relationships is lost. Part of the corrective emotional experience that is essential to change in EFIT sessions is that emotion and meaning become clear and ordered, leading naturally into a heightened awareness of both the implicit choices that make up a client's life and new choice points that lead in new directions.

No matter what the presentation, the apparent dysfunctionality, and the nature or number of diagnoses, the therapist always actively searches for the *strengths* of each client and articulates those strengths. In some cases, just to have survived, struggled on, and sought out help is a huge testament to courage. The therapist's nonpathologizing stance is often the first step in clients' abilities to accept themselves and truly explore how they shape their world. As the therapist enters into the client's frame of reference, helping him or her clarify and focus on what is important (Rice, 1974), key concerns about self, relationships with others, and existential dilemmas naturally emerge.

The formulation of the key problem to be addressed in therapy is a collaborative effort, not one imposed on the client, and is a part of solidifying a therapeutic alliance. One client may come just to see if it is even possible to talk to a mental health professional about her life; another may bring a more extensive agenda for negotiating a life transition without succumbing to debilitating anxiety. Occasionally clients present with incongruent goals that have to be questioned and revised with the therapist. Some clients start individual therapy aiming to affirm that their perception of a negative relationship or impossible partner is accurate. The more explicit, concrete, and realistic the articulation of the goals of therapy, the better. When the client's goals are clear, the therapist can respond genuinely regarding his or her ability to lead the client toward his or her stated goals. If this is not possible because the goals are incongruent with the goals of EFT, then the therapist points this out. For example, an EFT couple therapist might suggest to a military veteran and his wife that he accept a referral to a psychiatrist for possible medication and/or work in EFIT sessions. This individual work would focus on the veteran gaining control of his flashbacks of traumatic war experiences, as preparation for beginning EFT couple sessions with another therapist.

All through the case formulation process the EFT therapist focuses on *present process*. The therapist is not looking for character traits or to apply set labels to clients, but rather attempting to engage with each client in an open, curious way in the present moment. The goal is to explore how this person is constrained by patterns in her own ways of processing her experience and ways of relating to others. The attachment-oriented experiential therapist, following the lead of Rogers and Bowlby, believes clients have an innate desire to grow and find ways to get their needs met. If seen through a compassionate, survival-focused attachment lens, the client's behavior is always perceived as "reasonable." Working from that mindset, the therapist naturally focuses on following each client's pain, making it tangible and making explicit the blocks to positive functioning that clients unwittingly create or allow to overwhelm them.

STAGES OF INTERVENTION

As noted previously, the EFT model proceeds through three stages: *Stabilization* (which is called *de-escalation* in EFT for couples, for the obvious reason that to create stability it is necessary to de-escalate negative interactional patterns); *restructuring;* and *consolidation*. Stabilization shapes a strong therapeutic alliance and a new level of emotional balance, constructing a secure base for further exploration and engagement with unfamiliar and/or painful experience. During restructuring, engagement in therapy deepens, and corrective experiences revise models of self and other, bring new coherence to emotional processing, and shape new interactions characterized by constructive dependency. Consolidation then takes a metaperspective on the process of therapy, integrates the changes in self and system that are now apparent into the client's life and existential choices, and builds resilience to prevent relapse.

We will now look at the elements of these stages and typical EFIT interventions in a little more detail. The basic EFIT interventions are the same as outlined in Chapter 3. At times, variations in intervention do occur in a particular modality, and these variations will be discussed in the following chapters. We will then briefly discuss the repetitive core process of the EFT Tango that occurs across stages (see page 55 in Chapter 3) in the EFIT process.

Stage 1: Stabilization

The essential elements of Stage 1 in EFIT, stabilization, are:

• Joining with the client in formulating treatment issues and goals and formulating how they arise from the client's life narrative, history of relationships, and style of engagement with the therapist, and in discovering with the client his or her strengths and vulnerabilities. The assumption is that these issues will always reflect issues in emotional regulation, interpersonal connection, and negative models of self and other.

Typical Intervention

"So, you are able to look at your life right now and see these key problems, even though it is hard to name and face them, and what you are hoping for is that we can find ways to turn down this sense of anxiety you have around meeting others and find ways for you to feel more confident and at ease with people. Do I have it right?"

• Building a stable safe haven and secure base (in the alliance), while acknowledging any ambivalence the client may have about it.

Typical Intervention

"How can I help you to feel safe in the session with me? I hear that your last therapist seemed to 'lecture' you and that did not work for you. I do not want you to feel that here. Would you tell me, please, anytime when it feels like I am lecturing you? The goal here is for you to find your own truth and direction."

• Discovering with clients how they prime and maintain their depression and anxiety, first, by tracking and outlining recurring patterns in how they shape their inner emotional world. The therapist clarifies processes of emotion regulation (most simply, noting how clients turn emotion up high, turn it down, or try to turn it off), and the meaning making that arises in this process. Second, the therapist outlines with clients the habitual patterns of engagement in interpersonal relationships that are shaped by the action tendencies inherent in their emotions (most simply, noting how clients turn toward, away, or against others). The therapist listens to content issues and the narrative of the client's life but sorts continually for these process variables—patterns in the inner ring of emotional processing and the outer ring of interpersonal responses.

Typical Intervention

"So, what happens to you when a potential friend calls and suggests you meet? What do you feel/do in that moment or even as we talk about it here? Sounds like your 'unsureness' comes and you freeze—go numb as you said, and then you turn the friend down? It seems too risky—is that right? It's so natural that when we long for something and it suddenly appears, we hesitate and doubt and find that we cannot bring ourselves to reach for it. But then you are alone—yes? And you feel safer for a moment. So this kind of confirms that it's better not to take risks—others are just too dangerous." [The self-sustaining feedback loop of emotional music and the dance with others are made clear.]

• Make emotion more granular, and vague or disowned responses explicit, specific, and concrete. This may entail a simple process of focused reflection and evocative questioning with some clients or a much more elaborate structured assembly of emotion with others. We can think about this process in terms of the E for emotion: We evoke, engage, explore and expand, elucidate, and actively encounter emotion.

Typical Intervention

"Can you help me here? You say that you really don't pay attention to your feelings in these situations. You just want to fix the problem. But as you talk about this, you jiggle your leg very fast and look at the floor. Your body does this when we begin to talk about your wife getting mad at you. I think you said, 'She gets this look on her face.' In that moment, what do you see in her face—in the moment before you try to 'prove' that what she is feeling is wrong?" [The therapist is outlining a trigger and body response that occur before a problematic response to another.]

• As emotional experience begins to evolve, it brings with it new action tendencies and new meanings, which the therapist validates, heightens, and turns into enacted responses in imaginary encounters with key figures in the client's life. These figures are not hard to find. As Irvin Yalom points out (1989), the therapist has to "get acquainted with the characters that people your client's mind."

• Clients usually find tremendous relief in being able to make sense of their emotional lives and feeling truly heard by a validating other, and also experience a sense of efficacy in being able to integrate emotional response, meaning making, and interpersonal response into a whole. The therapist helps clients integrate all of these processes into a secure base—a sense of direction for their growth. Interactional response and pattern, narrative, and the process of emotional regulation are all put together in a way that offers the client a sense of balance and control that begins to translate into new awareness and actions outside the session.

Typical Intervention

"So, let me see if I have this right? You are finding that when the 'dark cloud' comes for you, you can see it more clearly and predict how it will start to open the door to the voice that tells you that you are 'worthless' and 'always on the outside' with others. But sometimes now you don't move into hiding from others and giving up, you start to comfort this disheartened part of you and tell yourself, 'everyone feels this way sometimes' and reach out to your friend. Is that it? That shows so much strength. Can you close your eyes and tell your friend about this right now?"

At the end of the stabilization stage clients will typically be:

• More balanced emotionally, that is, less reactive or less numbed out and more aware and accepting of their emotions, especially fears, vulnerabilities, and longings, and more active in terms of reflecting on them.

• More discovery oriented and open about their inner experience and interpersonal encounters, and more able to allow the therapist to take them to the leading edge of experiences and encounters.

• More able to focus on and outline patterns in key encounters with significant others (including the therapist) and enter into an engaged emotional narrative or imagined encounter with such others.

- More able to integrate the emotions and responses of self and others into a coherent meaningful narrative that is linked to the symptoms that brought the client into therapy, and the ways in which the client defines self and others.

All of these changes, which occur in the context of a growing therapeutic alliance, result in a client experiencing a new sense of hope, efficacy, and direction. Gary tells me after six sessions:

"I feel calmer somehow. Not so freaked out all the time. It feels good coming in here now, not like I am taking some test or something. My friend told me last night that I was less touchy, so that is good. I am for sure less depressed—realizing that lots of people would have gotten down and edgy in my situation, losing my job and girlfriend all in one go. Maybe I am not so strange. In the last session when I found myself really picturing her telling me she was leaving me and hearing that . . . well . . . a kind of disgust in her voice, I could feel how that pulled me into some kind of panic. It was good to tell her, 'You don't really know me.' That stayed with me all week. I think this is all about always taking other people's word about who I am. I get the pattern here. Maybe I don't have to do that so much, but I sure get stuck there."

Stage 2: Restructuring

The essential elements of the restructuring stage of EFIT are:

- The emotional exploration of core themes and triggers which are now deepened, and encounters with inner emotions and representations of others become more intense and take on a more existential tone. The therapist stays longer with the process of really engaging emotions that have been previously outlined and assembled, and may use more conjecture and intensify this conjecture by speaking as the client in the client's voice (using proxy voice), as well as asking him or her to take greater risks in imaginary encounters with elements of self and with others. The client is usually now in unfamiliar territory and may access very difficult emotional experiences both from him or her past and present life. The therapist typically uses repetition and images, especially evoking the key emotional phrases that the client has already shared, which we term *emotional handles,* to hold the client in the experience. An attuned EFIT therapist is careful to structure these experiences so that they are challenging but not overwhelming or outside of the client's window of tolerance. Emotion is deepened in some moments and contained in others, depending on the client's ability to stay engaged and regulated in the face of a felt sense of vulnerability. Typically it is here that deep feelings of attachment longing, abandonment, and rejection emerge, along with fears of catastrophic isolation and emptiness.

All of these emotions are normalized within the attachment frame; the reassurance offered by the therapist who simply states some version of "This is just how our brains/nervous systems are made—this is just who we are—all of us" is always potent. *Our frailties become proof of belonging.* In these sessions, core definitions of self and other become available and more open to modification, and core experiences of sadness and loss and shame and fear are more fully engaged with.

Typical Intervention

"Can you stay with this feeling, this sense of falling through space. Can you really feel that—the sensation of falling, of no control, of helplessness? This is when that terrible phrase echoes in your head—you don't matter—your pain doesn't matter. That is so so hard—to feel that. Never feeling seen and accepted—precious to those you loved. So terrifying. [The client is nodding and acquiescing all through this and has touched on all this before, even if superficially.] This is when, what did you say?—'I die inside' [The therapist uses a proxy voice—speaks as the client.] When the only thing to do is, as you say, to 'zone out into nothingness and give up.' What is happening as we stay here for a moment? [The client weeps and says, 'Alone, alone alone.'] Yes. And this is the pain that had you putting up this façade all these years—performing but with this loneliness inside. What is happening now as we bring all this together and speak it out loud?" [The client states, smiling through her tears, "It's strange. It hurts but it also feels so good—to pin it down somehow."]

• As the process of attunement to new elements of self and other becomes more explicit, the therapist structures expanded emotion into deeper and deeper encounters with parts of self, the therapist, and representations of key figures in the client's life. These encounters now take the client into new territory where different emotions emerge and new patterns of thought and responses take shape. Finding new dimensions in oneself and encountering others in a new way begin to influence each other in an evolving process that is synthesized by client and therapist into a more coherent and constructive whole. Fresh imagined encounters with others shape a different emerging sense of self and vice versa. Attachment needs and fears are now encountered and owned in the present in a visceral way. The interpersonal dramas enacted here may involve encounters with very rejecting or dismissing figures in the client's life and so may need to be repeated a number of times on different levels of engagement before they can be truly tolerated and responded to in a new way. Critical incidents and traumas may be replayed but experienced from a position of efficacy rather than helplessness.

Typical Intervention

[In soft, slow voice.] "Whose voice is this that you hear right now? If you close your eyes, is this part of Kelsey [the client], or your dad or . . . ? [Kelsey says, 'No. It's my mom again.'] Right—this is the Judge again—yes? Sometimes the 'harsh' part of you joins in and sometimes it sounds like your dad who wanted you to be the big lawyer, to prove yourself. But when you really listen, it sounds most like your mom. Maybe the voice you heard when you told them you had failed the exam? [She weeps.] Can you stay with me here? [The therapist lightly touches the client on the outside of the knee.] Can you just breathe with me and feel your feet on the floor, your back against the chair. Right. ['Holding' client and containing emotion— long silence.] This is worth weeping for, isn't it? If you close your eyes, can you see your mom . . . what would you like to tell her? [The client says, 'I don't know,' and weeps more intensely.] Can you tell her, 'I hurt. Just like the time I failed the exam and you laughed at me and labeled me as pretentious—as getting above myself for trying—as not one of the family'? [The client does this, changing the words to her own; she weeps.] This is so hard. So hard to touch. But you are nailing it—courageously saying what is true for you! What does your mom do? [The client says, 'She smiles but it's mean. She is cold and still—like she cannot hear me. Like I am not there.'] She doesn't see you—you're hurt. Like it doesn't matter? [The client weeps and nods.] You have been alone with this hurt all your life— hiding it and trying to 'perform'? But your pain does does does matter, doesn't it! [The client nods emphatically.] Can you tell her? Right here. [The client pulls her shoulders back, and begins to tell her mother this in a clear, coherent manner.] Wow—that is pretty clear! You sound so strong! Like you have your feet on the ground. Can you tell her again?"

• The more intense emotional experiences and potent enacted encounters with attachment figures—and the often despised parts of self—begin to take on a quality of flow (Csikszentmihalyi, 1990). Flow is defined as an experience in which one is completely focused, tuned into what one is doing, and utterly *absorbed*. This is defined as essentially a positive, enlivening experience, in spite of immense effort or challenge, such as when one is caught in playing a piece of music or dancing, in which the process seems to take over and shape the dancer.

Here the client is fully engaged and creates, with the therapist, a powerful corrective emotional experience. *In this experience, vulnerability is embraced and owned in a way that leaves the client feeling more whole and more balanced, and ironically, more powerful.* The therapist's job is to direct this process, refocusing the client in the face of detours, such as tangential memories or intellectual discussions, helping the client distill and synthesize the new experience effectively, as well as encapsulate the new sense of self and other that this experience offers. Clients find themselves more empowered in defining their own experience and in imaginal interactions with attachment figures.

Typical Intervention

"What happens when you touch that sore place now? You said it's more 'manageable—not so overwhelming'—yes? So, can you close your eyes and tell that small hopeless part of David how that feels? . . . That was great, David, so real and strong. You are telling him he doesn't have to be so scared now . . . that his fears are natural, but now you have found your strength and know how to comfort him . . . you know what he needs . . . Can you tell him—show him it's okay? . . . As you do that, you sit up taller and your voice seems deeper. This is the 'grown-up' part of David calming the more vulnerable part. How does it feel to do this—to be able to do this?"

So what does the completion of Stage 2 look like? For Gary, who we listened to earlier at the end of Stage 1 dealing with his anxiety and depression, completion might be described as follows:

"Things feel different. After our session, I went home and just before falling asleep I kind of found myself talking to my older brother again—the one who everyone adored, including me. Got really sad, just like in the session with you. I so wanted . . . I ached to be his special buddy. Heard him telling me, 'You just can't make it, Gary, silly little bro. You don't have what it takes man. Just crawl back into the shadows—get back behind me.' But instead of getting all agitated, I just felt all this huge sadness for that dream—that longing, here in my chest. To be like him. With him . . . so so wanted his approval! And sad that I am not him, never will be so glamorous, shiny, popular. But then I heard your voice and that part of me that says, 'Well, maybe Gary doesn't have to be some shiny glamour boy. Maybe I don't have to be afraid of not living up to the big-brother standard all the time. I can tell him, I am different—not behind— just different.' That was kind of a weepy moment. [Laughs.] My mom always said I was the softer one, and I took that as a bad thing.

But it isn't, really. Think I have learned to like my softness in these sessions, and I am going to go out and see my mom next week and tell her that I see now how she tried to support me."

Gary is not just less anxious and less depressed, he is balanced, assertive, and tuned in to his vulnerabilities and his needs. He is empowered.

Stage 3: Consolidation

The essential elements of Stage 3 in EFIT, consolidation, are:

• The therapist helps the client translate the discoveries made in therapy into new positions regarding pragmatic problems and relationships in her or his everyday life. New solutions naturally arise from revised working models and a new ability to use emotion as a *compass,* elucidating needs and preferences. Significant decisions can now be approached with more confidence and new solutions can be formulated. The therapist's main role is to validate the client's new confidence and sense of agency.

Typical Intervention

"Before you would have simply tried to agree with your boss and hide your feelings, but now something new is happening. You can handle your fear differently . . . you told him no! You refused! And then you set out what you wanted to happen . . . This is a new kind of approach. If you can do this, then the work problems start to change—yes?"

• With the client, the therapist collaboratively creates an overview of the client's therapeutic journey and present reality with regard to the clinical issues presented in first sessions. This overview is formulated into a simple evocative narrative that is directly relevant to the client. It particularly articulates and stresses the client's strengths and new ways of engaging with difficulties and again normalizes the struggles the client has been through in terms of existential realities and universal dilemmas (Yalom, 1980). Changes in emotion regulation, cognitive meaning frames, behavioral responses like avoidance, and levels and forms of interpersonal engagement are all presented and made vivid. The therapist also helps the client create a vision for the future wherein such issues can be managed in an effective way so as to minimize the possibility of relapse and help ensure that new growth-producing paths are taken. The therapist celebrates the client's ability to unlatch from old self-reinforcing patterns of experiencing and relating, and also fosters the client's ability to mentally represent the therapist as a supportive surrogate attachment figure that can be let go of, but also held in mind.

Typical Intervention

"You have come so far, James. From, as you put it, 'terminal wimpdom' into confronting all those fears and finding that you can stand tall. In the last few weeks you have . . . [Lists four specific shifts and new ways of engaging others.] You took on all those old stories about who James is and turned them around. This is so hard to do. So many of us struggle with this our whole lives. And you were able to reach out and ask your lady for support and tell her you want to be with her in the future. The old James just couldn't face that! How do you want James to be in the future—what do you see him doing, especially at times when potential 'wimpdom' comes into play?"

What does the end of Stage 3 look like for Gary? He tells me:

"I have withdrawn my application for that job. It doesn't really suit me. It was more about trying to be like my brother. I am looking for jobs that are in tune with my feelings about who Gary is—who I want him to be. That feels really good. I went out on a date, too, and found that I was less anxious—felt less pressure to be shiny! Think the title of this story has been Anxious Gary and his search for the dad he lost when he was really tiny—and how he put his brother up on a throne. I shared that with my mom and she gave me a big hug."

THE TANGO MOVES IN EFIT

Stages and interventions are mostly standard across modalities and, if we consider the core recurring change process that happens in every session of EFT (regardless of modality), we note that this process is also generic. Recall that the moves of the Tango are mirroring present process; affect assembly and deepening; choreographing engaged encounters; processing the encounter; and integrating and validating. In this section, I describe what the four moves of the Tango might look like in EFIT.

EFT Tango Move 1: Mirroring Present Process

Dave tells me that he cannot make decisions, like buying a car, or even letting his wife buy new cushions, because of his GAD, for which he has been hospitalized three times. He tells me he wants a solution, and soon, before his wife leaves him! I sit with him and track the inner and inter-personal process that occurs when he even thinks of making a decision. He tells me about his past life growing up with an unpredictable, dangerously violent father and depressed mother and always being told that the abuse directed toward him was his fault for being more like a girl— "Daniella" than Dave. As he talks about this we also begin to track how when his wife, Frankie, bought cushions home, he looked at the receipt and immediately flew into a rage. His wife told him he was impossible to be married to and left the house. I use reflections and questions such as, "And how are you feeling as you say this?" or, "Can you slow down and help me understand what thoughts came up for you as you looked at the receipt?" or, "This is what happens—sounds like it happens a lot, you are waiting for something to go wrong and, when it does, all this rage comes up—yes?" Dave shares that once he calms down he "decides" that indeed he is a "complete screw up and his dad was right—he is a wimp and a failure," so then he withdraws for days and hides out in the basement. In spite of Dave's attempted exits into long content stories of past decisions suddenly reversed, we identify an inner drama consisting of Dave taking a stance of vigilance in a "dangerous" world and feeling an urgent need to be in control, followed by a trigger where he finds he is not in control, and a move into rage, followed by numbing and avoidance. The more he worries about everything being under control, the more he looks for danger and finds it. The more he explodes and draws rigid lines to try to assert his control, the less room or confidence he has to make decisions or trust others to help him, and the more he worries! Attempts at self-protection become a prison.

We track that same drama as it unfolds when after countless weeks of checking out a car in minute detail, he begins to sign the buyer agreement and then suddenly becomes alarmed, finds something wrong with the car, and angrily storms out of the store. We outline, step by step, the same kind of recurring pattern with his wife. He monitors their contact and, if she is a few minutes late joining him to watch a TV show, he jumps up and berates her. She withdraws, and he demands explanations and pursues and blames her. She explodes, tells him that he is impossible and that she should not have married him and goes to sleep in the attic for a few days and ignores him. He then feels worthless and "sucks up" to her, but the whole thing then happens again. The more demanding he is about their time together, the more she withdraws, and the more she withdraws, the more he rages and demands and decides that he is an inadequate partner. We conclude that this "dance of danger and doom" has taken over their relationship, and as a result, he is always worried that she will, in fact, leave him, and so he "has to" constantly check out their connection. My alliance with Dave seems to be easy, and I share with him that this all sounds exhausting and sad. He works so hard just to try to feel some control and safety in his mind, in his world, and in his relationship, which is so natural given that he grew up in constant danger. He agrees. Each time we return to these descriptions in therapy they become clearer, and Dave's acceptance that he is stuck in this kind of self-perpetuating dance of doom increases.

EFT Tango Move 2: Affect Assembly and Deepening

As Dave returns to his inability to make yet another decision, his endless weighing of the odds, and his inability to risk and choose, I simply stay with his emotions. He says that he only really feels anger. I slow him down and ask him to stay in the moment before he moves into "rage." As he lifts his hand to sign for the purchase of a car, what happens? I move into asking questions about the five elements of emotion. I ask the following questions and receive the following replies:

SUE: What do you feel in your body at this moment?

DAVE: I feel my heart pounding, and I hold my breath.

SUE: What meanings/thoughts arise with the emotions, what do you say to yourself?

DAVE: I hear this voice say, "You are going to screw up here. How do you know this is right? This is a mistake. You can't be sure. You will screw up, and it will be awful," and I can't decide. I can't take the leap.

SUE: What action do you want to take, what does your body want to do?

DAVE: I want to go over all the alternatives again and again and again. But that doesn't work. I want to run, get away. But then I am a wimp, pathetic. I have this general anxiety disease thing.

SUE: What is the most catastrophic thing that could happen here? [This addresses the implicit perception and adds to the meaning frame.]

DAVE: I will lose money—fail—fail again. It will all be hopeless.

I summarize this exchange and suggest that he somehow turns this all into anger, perhaps to find some sense of control or appear strong, or he becomes caught in how impossible this all seems, so he is frustrated and tense. Dave replies, "All of that, but mostly I just know how to do that—the anger bit. Feels stronger for a minute, I guess." I go back to his words, "I will screw up—mistake—want to run." He goes very quiet as I repeat these elements and again put them together. Then he says, "I guess I'm scared, aren't I—scared I will never get it right?" I ask him how he feels as he admits this, and he says, "Paralyzed—so I just freeze and get the hell out of the situation." We look at how this music plays with his wife and when he has to make a decision. Together we distill the experience in terms of Dave always being on the verge of panic; he flips between angry attempts at control and the flight or freeze up response. He can never simply trust himself, and he is also ashamed, judging his terror of making a mistake as "weakness." He tells me, "This is strange. Putting this all together like this. It's like a foreign land suddenly becomes real, kind of recognizable . . . familiar."

EFT Tango Move 3: Choreographing Engaged Encounters

I ask Dave how he feels telling me all this. He looks away. He asks if I think he is some kind of freak. I validate that he grew up without anyone safe to tell him he could trust himself, make mistakes, and still be loved, and that I see how brave he is to face these things and tell me about them. He weeps. I normalize his attachment wounds and the impact of the biting rejection that shaped him in his early life. I ask him who else might judge him as not able to make decisions, as a failure or a wimp? First, he speaks of his dad and how demeaning he was, but it is when he mentions his wife that his facial expression and voice change. We stay here, and we look at what happens to him when Frankie does not come and watch TV just when she said she would and then, after he berates her, shuts him out. We explore how helpless and "out of control, scared" he feels. She is the only one he has ever "kind of" trusted. We now begin to go through the steps of creating engaged encounters. These include intensifying the client's core emotions into a concrete "felt" reality that becomes an absorbing state; distilling the essence of this experience into a brief, cogent message to be given to a significant other; directing the client to begin this encounter and, if necessary, refocusing and offering direction to the client. This task is done in a way that regulates the client's emotions, as this person engages with them more deeply.

In the session with Dave, I now *heighten* his engagement in this emotion by repeating the images he uses, distilling core meanings, and "holding" him and evoking safety with a low and slow voice, and with my attuned tracking of his experience. I then ask him to share his fear and helplessness with the Frankie he sees as he closes his eyes. With my help to frame the formulation of the message in concrete, simple, and on-point terms, he speaks to his wife, "I am never sure of myself. Never sure if you love me—if I am ever good enough with all my rages and hang-ups. So I push you to respond—I want you to make me feel more sure. But when you turn away, then I have no control—I am scared—terrified." Dave weeps. He is completely immersed in the reality of this encounter.

I validate and normalize his fear in attachment terms. I ask him to tell me what Frankie replies to his disclosure, and he smiles and reports that he sees her as comforting him and "loving me after all—even if I am wimpy." He beams at me through his tears. (Later in another session we shape an encounter with his abusive, demeaning father and the mother who did not protect him, and finally, with his careful but about-to-panic self, who is always telling him that he is about to prove himself a fool and a failure and so will be abandoned.)

EFT Tango Move 4: Processing the Encounter

I reflect the encounter with Frankie and we explore Dave's response to her imagined offer of comfort. He states that he feels good about opening up and risking with her and "knows" that she is "gentle" with him when he can be "soft," instead of angry or pushy. This comfort calms and reassures him. I ask him how he feels about directly talking to me about his soft side and if he still worries that I see him as a "freak." He laughs and says, "Just a little maybe, but it feels good to be here with you. Safe. I feel seen and it's okay." I reiterate his wife's willingness to respond to Dave's vulnerability, and also validate that this is not where his brain naturally goes because so much of his early experience was devoid of this comfort when danger loomed. I want to make sure that he can indeed take in this comfort, so, at my invitation, he closes his eyes and listens again to her comfort, tells me what he sees in her face and how his body feels. I want this experience to be more accessible for him when panic looms.

EFT Tango Move 5: Integrating and Validating

I sometimes refer to this move as "Tying a bow on it," and that is what we do here. We summarize the process that has just occurred, focusing on the emotions that emerged and how Dave dealt with them differently, taking new risks and exploring this new territory, and pinpointed the meanings that he was able to formulate. I validate how hard it is to have confidence in yourself and risk making mistakes if you have learned in your early years that there is good reason to be wary and watch for the coming doom. I also validate his strength in being able to look at the fear of being unworthy and the hurt underneath his rage. Dave tells me, "Right. If I can touch that before I leap for my weapons, well, maybe I can ask for my wife's help with that softness rather than push so hard—push her away." I reply, "You are a clever man, Dave. New emotional music pulls new steps from us—moves us into a new dance."

The best outcome in EFT is not just that symptoms of emotional disorders subside or even that this impacts other less-than-functional behaviors, but that the corrective experience of therapy shapes a more secure, coherent, and resilient sense of self and a more secure sense of others as responsive attachment figures. The goal is to open the door to all the myriad strengths associated with this security and the flexible resilience that is its main feature. Attachment science offers us a map for ongoing growth from the cradle to the grave. It offers us a guide to the emotional *safety* that generates a *sound* connection with self and other. This safe and sound connection to one's own emotional life and to others, held in the mind or in actual encounters, is a place where the self continues to grow and expand throughout life—so that the client is able to live fully and well.

A HOMEPLAY EXERCISE

For You Personally

This exercise is in four parts. First, can you identify the closest person to you and/or the person with whom you experienced the most positive connection in your life—a special person? It might be someone in your past or a present relationship. It may even be an image of a spiritual figure that epitomizes your religious beliefs. Now also choose a familiar acquaintance in your everyday life.

Second, can you search for a vivid and upsetting personal memory and pinpoint a trigger for this memory? For example, I remember the moment in a strange town as a child when I realized that I was lost, and I also remember standing in an empty hospital room watching my child being wheeled away for an emergency operation. The trigger for the first one is a sudden squeezing in the chest and the thought that no one knows where I am and I cannot find my way home. The trigger for the second one is the image of the hospital building where this occurred.

Third, can you sit quietly, close your eyes, and trigger the upsetting memory? Now imagine the acquaintance that you just identified comforting you. Rate how comforting this is on a scale of 1–10. Now trigger the memory again and imagine the special person coming to comfort you. Rate how comforting this is on a scale of 1–10.

Fourth, stay with the memory of this special person comforting you, and let the drama unfold. What exactly does this person say or do? How does your body react and your thought processes shift? Does your sense of what to do—how to act—change in any way?

What is the key message that you hear from this special person? Can you imagine using this message to find comfort in a distressing situation that might arise in your life now?

In many ways this exercise parallels parts of the EFIT process and it also parallels a study on attachment by Selchuk and colleagues (2012).

For You Professionally

A depressed client, Martin, tells you the following:

> "I know you will say that this has happened before, and I guess it has, but I got just wiped out by a woman again—at a party on Saturday night. So I just crawled off with my tail between my legs as usual, and then spent the next day listing all the reasons why I seem to have such a total failure rate with women. It's hopeless. I am just not what women want. It's just never going to work for me. Some of the women there were friendly enough, I guess, but . . . well I tried coming on to one of them, made a sexy remark or two. Disaster. She just changed the subject on me. I felt so stupid that I felt sick. So I just up and left the party. What is the point! It is just the way it is with me. I can't stand this anymore. Maybe I should just blow my head off or something." [Laughs, but then closes his eyes.]

How might you, in very simple terms, reflect this (Tango Move 1) in a way that helps Martin begin to see this drama (i.e., how the way he deals with his anxiety at the party and after he leaves confirms and maintains all his worst fears) and also validates his painful feelings and conclusions?

The "diagnosis" Martin arrives with from his doctor is depression, but we can also see the key elements of debilitating anxiety here, intense emotion and vigilance to threat, coping mechanisms and attributions that exacerbate the problem, and avoidant strategies related to inner feelings and interpersonal situations.

How would you then help him systematically assemble his emotions here (Tango Move 2), using the elements of trigger, initial perception, body response, meaning creation, and action tendency?

Try writing out what you would say. (This is play so there are no wrong answers!)

 TAKE IT HOME AND TO HEART

- Attachment offers the clinician clear ways of understanding emotional disorders (as outlined in Barlow's UP model) that fit with current research on depression and anxiety.

- The attachment-oriented, experiential therapist discovers with the client's reality with this person, both how the client constructs his emotional reality and his interactions with attachment figures. The focus is on the present process that unfolds in the session. Empathic responsiveness based on sensitive attunement is the key to this process.

- The therapist is a surrogate attachment figure who shapes a safe haven and secure base in the session, distills the client's strengths, and finds the logic in the client's stuck patterns of inner processing and interactions, and then gradually leads the client into new ways of constructing emotions, framing models of self and other, and shaping interactions with significant others.

- EFIT proceeds through the stages of stabilization, restructuring of attachment, and consolidation.

- The process of the generic EFT Tango is easily applied in individual therapy; much of the process, such as assembling and deepening emotion, is the same as in other modalities. However, unless an attachment figure from the client's life is invited into a session, Tango Move 3, setting up enactments to alter interpersonal patterns, occurs with representations of attachment figures that come alive in the session or in encounters with the therapist.

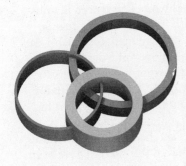

Chapter 5

Emotionally Focused Individual Therapy in Action

A case was referred to me for individual therapy by another therapist. The client, a woman, had just started couple therapy with her, and appeared to be really stuck, almost hysterical, and completely unable to share or engage with the therapist or her partner in session. Couple therapy seemed to be just too difficult at this time, but the therapist was concerned for this woman's well-being. The client agreed to see me and have all sessions taped and transcribed, and the excerpts used here.

FERN: THE BACK STORY

Fern marches into my office with a bright but fixed smile and tells me, in a rush, that she wants to see me because she had just started couple therapy with her husband, Dan, after 13 years of marriage and then 6 years of separation. She then shares that she knows couple therapy will not work because, "It's just too hard for me to talk about stuff. There are things I just cannot get over that I don't talk to anyone about." Fern tells me she is 46 with a job as a supervisor in a bank and is living with her adult son and her dog, usually seeing her husband on the weekends. On the commonly used Beck Depression Scale she scores 22, and on the Beck Anxiety Scale, 35; both of those scores are in the moderate range (a score of 20–28 marks moderate depression, and 22–35 marks moderate anxiety on these scales). However, Fern certainly seems exceedingly anxious, even for a first session.

Once the introductions are over and we start to talk, Fern suddenly shifts from superficial niceties to crying copiously, but tells me at the same time that she isn't sure she wants to revisit or share the "painful stuff" that she keeps inside. She says she has always experienced her husband as distant, and that when she lived with him, she would regularly plead with him to "show me you want me and love me," to which Dan would usually reply, "I don't want to talk right now." She describes how she felt excluded from the family of three adolescent boys from his first marriage who lived with them most of the time. They spoke Spanish to their father, and he replied in Spanish, continually leaving Fern feeling like "I wasn't part of anything." After 7 years of increasing distress in this relationship, she quietly tells me that she had been "fooled and conned" by a man who sold her a car. She believed this man to have been separated from his wife, and had a 6-month affair with him, resulting in her leaving Dan. When the man's wife found out about the affair, he immediately and completely cut Fern off and refused to even talk to her. She weeps as she tells me this, and says that she "cannot get over this" and "cannot talk to anyone about it, because I am so ashamed. I was such a fool." She proceeds to tell me that her family and Dan's publicly and virulently judged and condemned her for this affair, to the point where she lost contact with both. "I look like I am in control," she says. "I am a good employee at work. I put on a big front, but inside . . . I can't sleep. I can't look when I drive by car dealerships. I can't breathe when I think about this, and I am obsessed with it. Think about it all the time. I broke all my rules, went against all my values. But I should be over this by now—be able to just get over it! I can't do this anymore."

I inquire about her attachment history with her family, asking her to whom she used to turn for comfort and with whom she felt safest and could count on when growing up. I suggest that she tell me about an incident when she felt close and safe in her family. She does not answer my questions, but instead stares at me blankly. She then proceeds, in a breathless rush, to tell me that in her family, which was very musical, she was the most talented, but "nothing was ever good enough for my dad, who liked my sister's music performances better. He always pushed me into really hard competitions. I had to be better, but I never got the approval even when I won!" In spite of her protestations that she does not want to talk, Fern goes directly to her emotional dilemmas. She is easy for me to connect and resonate with. I can feel her anxiety about talking to me, but also the pressure she is under to confide in someone about her pain, and her nonverbal expressions are easy to read. She also responds instantly to any compassionate or reassuring remarks that I make. I find myself thinking, even early on in the first session, that she is hungry, starving even, for the affirmation and belonging that was apparently missing in her family of origin. In terms of emotion, when I ask her directly, she is able to give me a list, albeit at first, in a mechanical remote manner. She lists a mix of anger at herself, shame at her "crime" and her inability to get over it, and sadness that the affair and breakup happened. I am struck by her sense of loss, helplessness, and inadequacy, as well as her self-criticism, all of which would logically set up and maintain her anxiety and depression. But most of all, it is her agitation that stands out. I sense that she has run out of the energy needed to push her feelings aside. I follow Fern's lead and relate to her at the level she presents in session.

Let us now look at my work with Fern over seven sessions, focusing on the bare-bones process (with more superficial content omitted), as Fern and I dance through a typical course of EFIT together. In the initial stage of stabilization (the stages of therapy as they appear in EFIT are laid out in Chapter 4), I create a safe haven by reflecting the key elements of her reality and validating and normalizing her pain in an attachment frame. I try to be accessible, responsive, and engaged.

SESSION 1

The key concern in the first session is, of course, to make an alliance and to empathically reflect Fern's pain and how she relates to it. Indeed the emphasis in this session is the first two moves of the EFT Tango, mirroring present process and affect assembly and deepening.

> SUE: So, can you help me, let me know if I have this right. You tell yourself you should just be able to "turn this off." You hurt and are constantly frustrated with yourself—kind of critical of yourself for hurting? (*Fern nods.*) You have been carrying all this guilt and pain and dismay for years, all by yourself, telling yourself to hide it and not "burden" others with it. Never turning to others for comfort and feeling caught in all these feelings and alone with them. Is this right? [Reflect present process—emotional and interpersonal and place in an attachment frame.]

> FERN: Yes. You got it. I shared some stuff with a friend but . . . I don't want people to know the reality of it.

> SUE: The reality. [Attachment gives me a clear map to the rather chaotic reality she is describing, her needs and fears, and this facilitates my ability to attune to her.] Hm—I think you are telling me that the reality is that, when you lived with your husband, you were starving—starving for attention and validation, to know you were seen, loved—special to someone. You didn't feel this with your dad, your husband, or your family,

and suddenly someone turned up and gave you that feeling and it was irresistible. Like coming out into the light from darkness. You just couldn't turn away. You reached for it. But it was a lie, and you lost even the thin thread of connection you did have. And you also blame yourself—you have punished yourself for years and years for your hunger—the fact that you reached?

FERN: (*Tears up.*) Yes. Yes. That man gave me compliments, compliments! He told me I was beautiful! It was all a con. [She then goes into lots of details about the deception, about how she should have seen through it, and about how her husband found out and her family judged her. I listen, summarize, and return to the need that propelled her to reach out for this man.]

SUE: You longed for this—to feel special and held and seen for so long—so long and then it was a con—a lie. That hurts so much!

FERN: (*Speaking fast and with agitation.*) He just walked away from me and refused to talk—never explained anything! Why did I allow this to happen to me? I am so embarrassed by this.

SUE: Hm—(*Softly and slowly since Fern is very upset.*) You are so strong to come and share with me so openly—to take this risk—of being embarrassed here, maybe judged by me. (*Fern nods.*) You are caught here in this spiral of continuing hurt. You reached for the connection you desperately needed and found yourself—find yourself even more alone, and then you blame yourself for letting this happen and then for not just being able to bounce back. You judge yourself, as well as feel judged by others! So hard, and this makes you even more upset, more alone, struggling to put on a front all the time. Hurts to be so alone with all this pain and doubt about yourself. (*Fern weeps.*) [We are moving fluidly mostly between Tango Move 1, mirroring present process, and Move 2, affect assembly and deepening, and touching on underlying emotions as much as is usual in the stabilization stage.]

FERN: (*Softly.*) I don't tell people—I can't tell Dan. I just stay away from my family.

SUE: So what is it like to tell me this stuff—are you worried I am judging you right now? What do you see in my face? [Tango Move 3: choreographing engaged encounters.]

FERN: (*Tentatively.*) I feel understood! Seems like you are safe. But it's hard to take that in. I don't usually . . .

SUE: Yes—you are used to—you expect—judgments, condemnations even, and you judge yourself. So it must be strange to come in here and risk—to tell me all this and begin to feel understood—hard to really take in. [Tango Move 4: processing the encounter.]

FERN: (*Weeps again.*) I just told you more than I ever told anyone! How could I have been so stupid!! Sometimes I just sit in the car and scream. It keeps coming up—I see a car that reminds me . . . I try to bring myself down but . . . nothing works really.

SUE: [I summarize the discussion again—Tango Move 5: integrating and validating.] This is constantly triggered, isn't it! This isn't just something that happened years ago. It is still happening now, and then it triggers you blaming yourself, which is another pile of hurt. I have just met you and heard your story, but my sense is that all of us, all of us, when we are starving for love and affection and need to know we matter to someone— that we are accepted and acceptable—we will turn toward it when it is offered—like a plant turns toward the sunshine—it's irresistible for us. It is just the way we are made. It seemed that you were suddenly offered what you longed for all your life and so you reached for it. You wanted to believe that man so much that you broke your own rules. And then you judged yourself—that is what you had been taught to do in your family. So you have carried this pain and shame for 6 years all by yourself—wow! That is so hard—too hard. We can't work through this kind of hurt all on our own; it's too much. You hurt, you were already raw, and then you were abandoned and rejected, deceived. And then you decide that perhaps this is what you deserve and you hide. So it just goes on and on. You hurt and can't forgive yourself for not being a perfect wife— person—for not just being able to live by the rules, no matter what. So you beat yourself up and hurt even more. Do I have it right here?

FERN: Yes—I failed here. I committed adultery and betrayed my husband. That is what my sister said. (*Long pause.*) But I don't want to feel this way anymore—can we make it go away? It's ridiculous!

SUE: Well—we can look at it together and we can change it together, so you don't feel like you have to be some kind of superwoman- saint–judge–perfect person all the time. So you can maybe understand and forgive yourself a little. It feels sad to me, your story, not ridiculous at all . . . but very sad. We are not wired to deal with this kind of experience by ourselves—not feeling entitled to be heard and held. Does this feel okay for me to say this? Perhaps the sentence for Fern is over now?

FERN: I feel like you get me. Perhaps we can do this. (*Smiles. She is also appreciably calmer than when she walked into the session.*)

If we look, not just at the metasequence of the EFT Tango, but also at the experiential, more microinterventions here, then we can see focused, attuned reflection of emotional processing and interpersonal patterns; validation and evocative questions; deepening engagement with images and repetition; conjecture that is simple and stays at the leading edge of the client's felt experience; the creation of new kinds of enactments/interactions (with the therapist); and interpersonal reframes.

SESSIONS 2 AND 3

In the next two sessions, Fern and I list her "crimes," namely, "adultery, hurting my family, hurting my husband, and of course, betraying myself." We particularly focus on reflecting present process (Tango Move 1), explicating her own inner dialogue and emotional dance with her sadness and shame, and how it translates into her inner and actual dialogues with others. We outline how very high her expectations of herself are and how she would never dream of being as hard on someone else as she is on herself. We talk about the Ruthless Judge she hears in her head, modeled on her father; as Bowlby said, we do as we have been done to. She now judges that she "failed" at music, with her family, and most of all in her marriage. We externalize her negative thoughts as The Judge who tells her, "Your pain didn't matter in the past, and it doesn't matter now—you deserve to hurt."

We sometimes stay with assembling and deepening emotions (Tango Move 2) around her "crime" and all the specific accusations that the Judge directs at her: that she was blind as to the game she was caught in with her lover, that she hurt her husband, that she hurt her husband's family. Using a typical EFIT evocative question, I ask, "What happens to you as you tell me about this—what are you feeling, right now?" In answering she begins with a surface, reactive response of anger at herself, but she moves to an awareness of an "ache" in her chest—after I ask her, "What is happening in your body right now?" This grows into a sense that she could sob, and when I ask, "What do your thoughts say to you right now?" she talks of hearing an inner voice tell her, "You are responsible; it's all your fault." She says this voice provokes a desire to run away and hide from everyone. Let us see how this assembly process moved into deepening.

SUE: [I summarize our discussion and then ask for more specificity.]

Can we go back a moment? Can we stay with the ache in your chest and the "sob" that you sensed was there. There is pain here—yes? Part of you constantly chastises yourself for turning to another man and hurting people, and part of you gets ready to weep in pain? Am I getting it? (*Fern nods.*)

FERN: (*Suddenly calm and speaking intellectually now.*) I am not a bad person. How could I have done this? It's a mystery to me! How could I have done this? [Exits from deepening, but this seems pertinent, so I follow her. I can come back later.]

SUE: I believe you. It is clear that you are basically a very serious, responsible, caring person. You are someone who has tortured herself for years for this one time of hurting people. [As a positive attachment figure, I frame Fern's sense of self in compassionate, accepting terms.] But you really don't understand how this happened. So some part of you maybe decides you must be just defective—flawed somehow?

FERN: YES—exactly. The judge says I must just be a bad person or just stupid maybe. And my family confirmed that—my dad and my older sister especially; my mom and brother were just silent. [A sense of being desperately alone and also bad/unworthy, and so deserving this isolation is perhaps the most toxic stuck place we can shape for ourselves.]

SUE: And that really hurts—to feel so judged—so rejected at a time when you were so vulnerable. Also some part of you agrees—says they are right, and that hurts even worse.

FERN: Yes. My two close friends were supportive but . . . I have high expectations of myself I guess. But I get mad at my sister when she comes on so judgy with me.

SUE: [Where to go? What resonates with me is "mystery" and "ache." So I follow this resonance using my own emotions as a guide.] Hm—part of all this agonizing and obsessing about what happened and what it means, if it means something dreadful about you, is that your actions are still a "mystery" to you?

FERN: [A long digression unfolds about how she is in control in her life, and how she should learn the lesson from this. I listen but hold onto my focus, waiting for a chance to return to the emotional channel.] But I judge myself for what happened—even if I don't understand it. I failed somehow. I try to figure it out all the time but . . . it's an obsession. There is no way out of this feeling—of failing.

SUE: Well, my sense is that it's hard to figure out in your head, but deep down—in your gut—you know what happened—that you turned away from your husband to reach for someone else, in spite of your sense that this was something foreign to who you were. There was something here that made all the high expectations you had of yourself kind of unimportant. You said that your relationship with your husband was "rocky" and that the man was so "flattering."

FERN: (*Instant tears and agitation.*) I was invisible in my relationship with Dan. Invisible with his kids—in my home. I didn't exist . . . but I should have tried harder to fix that. But . . .

SUE: Hm. (*Touching Fern on the arm to soothe her and keep her focused.*) Invisible. You have told me that he was abandoned by his first wife for another man and that he was very withdrawn always in your relationship, and you would spend all your time knocking on his door. I hear that you were alone, shut out. That drives people crazy—it's unbearable. They are in a relationship, all their longings primed by the presence of the person they love, but there is no response! This person does not show up! And suddenly someone was there—wanting you! You are looking skeptical—let me guess. The Judge says, "Inadmissible defense."

FERN: (*Laughs.*) Exactly. (*Goes still and quiet.*) But, it feels like my responsibility. Dan even says it was his fault too but . . . [She dismisses her own pain, so now I want to highlight it.]

SUE: [I decide to press the replay button and refocus.] Can we go back to your feelings? What happens to you when you say, "I was invisible—alone?" (*Fern weeps.*) I think you said there was no talking—Dan and his kids even spoke in a different language at meals, one you couldn't understand. And Dan dismissed or seemed to ignore your pleas around this. You said it was all a big "zero"—yes? It was like he wasn't there—you were emotionally separate. You had no partner.

FERN: (*Weeps.*) That's not how you treat someone you love. (*Weeps more—I ask her again what she feels.*) I feel so sad, sad, sad. I was so lonely, with four other people in the house! I tried so hard to be a good wife, a good mother. (*I reflect and repeat her words in a quiet, slow voice.*) It's like I was dismissed—I didn't matter at all. Like I didn't deserve to be loved at all. (*Curls into a ball in the chair and sobs.*) I can't get my breath.

SUE: (*Soft, slow voice—reaching and touching Fern softly on the outside of her knee.*) Yes. So painful. Not deserving, starving, desperate to be seen and held. Just like with your dad, trying hard, but no response, no affirmation. That is too hard, yes?

Like no one cares about Fern? What would you do, Fern, when this happened? What did your body tell you to do?

FERN: I would start to feel sick and feel this ache, an ache in my heart, and then I would get up and leave. I would leave the room and no one would come after me. No one cared. I was clearly so so *not* needed there. I tried so hard.

SUE: Yes. It hurt too much. So you would flee—leave. To find some safety, to get away from the pain—a pain you still feel. (*Fern nods.*) An ache in your heart. To be invisible—alone. So you had to leave. Fern, can you look at me please? (*Fern looks.*) You had to leave—Yes? Years of this ache in your heart, trying, but never getting recognized. This is a pain that drives all of us crazy, makes us all feel like we are, helpless, dying. You had to leave—you were starving. But you hung in and hung in . . . tried harder . . . until someone offered you caring, and you turned toward it like a plant turns toward the light. Yes?

FERN: (*Shifts into different voice—more cognitive and declarative.*) But that is no excuse though, is it?

SUE: (*Smiling—touching Fern's arm.*) I think his honor, the Judge, just showed up! Excuse. You need an excuse to flee from this agony? Every neuron in your brain is wired to tell you that this pain is unbearable. When we call and no one answers, we get desperate, panicked. Every neuron starts to sing, "Somebody see me—act like I matter. Like I exist." [I validate, using the clear understanding of her pain and fear provided by attachment theory.]

FERN: Yes—I was desperate—like I was going to be alone forever. (*Quietly.*) I don't think I deserved that. [This is the core existential threat—the catastrophe—that isolation will be never ending—we will always be alone.]

SUE: Right. If you close your eyes, can you see the Fern who tried and tried to get Dan to open up to her—the Fern who sat at the dinner table excluded and alone. So alone. Can you see her, can you see her pain? (*Fern nods.*) Can you close your eyes and tell her, "You are so hurt—you don't deserve to be so hurt." Tango Move 3, choreographing engaged encounters, this time with Fern's vulnerable abandoned self.]

FERN: (*Moves into this imaginal encounter seamlessly. Her eyes are closed.*) It's so lonely for you. Desperate. You tried so hard for so long. You joked, you hugged, you explained, you got mad, you . . . you didn't deserve that. You couldn't just stay there . . . you were . . . nonexistent.

SUE: (*Softly.*) Yes. Nothing you did took the ache away. (*Fern shakes her head.*) The fear that you would never matter—always be alone—as if you did not exist. [I summarize her existential panic.] Until one day, a stranger—a man—comes along and he smiles at Fern.

FERN: He knew just what to say. He was warm. He would give me compliments—compliments—for just showing up!!! It was so nice, really nice!

SUE: Like the sun came out—you had longed for those compliments, that recognition, for so so long. (*Fern nods.*) Like suddenly you are special to someone. You matter. He is pleased to see you. He sees you! How does it feel, Fern, right now?

FERN: My heart is bursting—relief.

SUE: How could you turn that down, Fern? No one could. Starving, and suddenly—a feast. Hope. What you have always longed for right there. You reach out your hand . . . So human . . . so natural. . . . He says, "Come," and you turn toward him. (*Fern is weeping and smiling at the same time.*) What is happening as I say this? Can the Judge take this pain, this need, into account? Extenuating circumstances—it's called "being human." Does he see the whole picture now? How could you not respond? [I am modeling compassion, and also shaping Fern's deeper engagement with her pain and its meaning to evoke self-compassion.]

FERN: (*Laughs.*) Right. Right. It's like if someone is on fire don't blame them for leaping out of a burning building. I see it. [She offers a wonderful summarizing image here. She then recaps our discussion with my help. Repetition is necessary for full engagement and the embedding of new frames alongside the old, well-trodden pathways of thought and response.]

SUE: So, can you close your eyes again and see Fern, alone and in pain? What would you like to tell her—about the "mystery"— about what you are learning about her reaching for the man?

FERN: (*Weeping.*) You hurt so much. You were dying. Desperate. How could you not respond? He played you. He saw how much you needed love. You just had to reach for it, to go with the hope. [We now summarize what we discussed and agree that the Judge in her mind seems to be somewhat silenced for the moment. Fern agrees to go home and try to write a narrative describing the entire process. I encourage her to do this after every session.]

SESSION 4

We are now moving out of stabilization (Stage 1) into restructuring (Stage 2). Fern tells me that she wrote down in her narrative reflection on the last two sessions that perhaps she was "just seeking out some comfort when I allowed myself to have the affair. It was longing—that was the big carrot, the 'irresistible' thing for me." She also tells me that the voice of her inner judge is now softer, less "judgy." She understands now that she didn't just go off and decide to hurt people, "like I am a monster," and has put herself through hell for 6 years because of the "struggle in my head" about "whether I can forgive myself—not be so hard on me." We agree that, although she broke her own "rules about being faithful," she is starting to take her "pain and loneliness" into account. There is, in fact, a "common-sense Fern," who is starting to accept what happened, and that is "such a relief; it's like a huge weight off me." However, Fern comes into Session 4 upset because Dan has insisted that she attend a gathering with his family. She tells me, "This means I will be in the lion's den all alone. He says that I will probably just sit silently and not try to talk to them, so then, of course, I will feel alone. I am stuck here. I can't face them." Let us see, in distilled form, what the Tango looks like around this issue. First, I reflect, describe, and distill what she tells me, focusing on triggers, emotional experience, and attachment meanings.

EFT Tango Move 1: Mirroring Present Process

> SUE: (*Using a proxy voice, speaking directly as Fern.*) So help me here, it seems that you say to yourself, "I will be so 'exposed' here. Thirty people will be judging me as an 'unfaithful' person and a bad wife, as a 'failure.'" What happens to you as you say this to me?
>
> FERN: I don't know . . . it's the old judgment thing again. [She goes off into a long story about Dan's family and how some of them have had affairs and divorces, but for her, this doesn't count in terms of how she feels about her behavior.]

EFT Tango Move 2: Affect Assembly and Deepening

> SUE: (*Slow, soft—refocusing.*) Can we go back—stay with the feelings for a bit? This is your raw spot, to feel judged by others, and then this sets off the judge that sits in your own head. It is scary to be judged, to fear that you will never be accepted. Is this the hardest part? What does your body say right now?

[I outline the trigger element of the emotion here and want to move into the bodily sensation that goes with it.]

FERN: Even when I talk about this I feel sick. I feel so vulnerable. Dan is right, I do sit silently at those times, and then I leave as soon as possible. I try to put on my brave face, but I feel sick, almost dizzy. Like I can't do anything—get my thoughts together.

SUE: This is scary to stay with this feeling? Your body says, "This is dangerous"? You say to yourself, "They are judging me and I want to shut down or run"? (*Fern nods emphatically and weeps.*) What is it that is the most dangerous? Dan is not there with you, is he? [I voice the action tendency element of her emotional response and am also touching on the message here—the meaning Fern makes of this. Attachment tells us that danger and vulnerability faced alone are unbearable and disorganizing, hence the "dizziness."]

FERN: Yes. Worst of all is that he will always choose his family over me, and I will be all alone. This is just like my dad always choosing my sister, even though I tried so hard to please him. I can't do it. I freeze up.

SUE: [I repeat emotional handles and use images in a soft, slow voice—inviting deepening.] The aloneness is unbearable here—overwhelming. You expect a tidal wave of disapproval, one that fits with your own judge's voice—with your fears about who Fern might be, a failure. And you are always alone facing this, so alone. Aching. Dizzy. Feeling sick. Unseen. Like you don't exist. No one is there with you when you feel exposed. Part of you says that you must *deserve* this—otherwise it makes no sense? That is so so hard. [I am linking Fern's traumatic isolation to her negative model of self.]

FERN: I am shattered. No one gets it. It's like I am always deserted. The one who doesn't matter. So when Dan tells me now, "I do love you," it just kind of bounces off. [This captures the terrible irony of anxious attachment—when love is offered, it is not trusted, so it cannot be taken in. Fern's word "shattered" seems to me to perfectly capture her experience of hurt and her helplessness to tackle the hurt constructively, and is the kind of emotional handle that can be used to smoothly help her "change the channel" and enter this emotional realm in session.]

EFT Tango Move 3: Choreographing Engaged Encounters

SUE: Right. So can you close your eyes and see Dan. Can you see his face, telling you that you just sit silently at these gatherings, that perhaps if you tried harder? . . . What do you want to tell him right now?

FERN: (*Closes her eyes and weeps.*) But I hurt. I am afraid. You aren't there to support me. Like I don't matter. It's always the same. No matter how I try. You say you want to support me but . . .

SUE: (*Soft and slow—I touch her knee and leave my hand there.*) Yes. Your experience with the ones you love and depend on is that when it really matters no one sees your pain—no one is there for you. No one stands beside you. So when Dan says he wants to support you, you want to say, "I don't believe you. You don't help me with my pain—my fear." Can you tell him?

FERN: (*Closes her eyes.*) You leave me alone—facing all that disapproval, a tsunami of disapproval. It's scary, but it's so so sad. (*Weeps.*) There is nothing I can do.

SUE: A tsunami. Overwhelming. Terrifying. But you try to shut down this hurt, put on a "brave face" and try harder. *And* you end up blaming you. What do you need from him? How can he help you with these feelings? Can you try to tell him?

FERN: (*Face screwed up tight, very intently, in a soft voice.*) You say you are there, but I don't feel it. I want you to stand beside me, take my hand, and stand beside me. Show me I matter, so I don't have to be so sad.

We then process what it felt like to tell him this (Tango Move 4, processing the encounter), and we celebrate (Tango Move 5, integrating and validating) that she did something new; she didn't shut down, put on a façade, or even blame herself here. She risked and asserted her pain and asked for what she needed. I recognize with satisfaction that Fern is now able to move into the assertive, authentic statement of need that is part of constructive dependency. We also talk very briefly about how Dan may not know quite *how* to support her, rather than not caring to. Her ability to state her needs explicitly and from a place of vulnerability is the best way to help Dan respond. Ironically, the centered, regulated sense of self and emotional balance she is building here is also her best resource if Dan, in fact, cannot respond to her needs.

SESSION 5

The key process in Session 5 revolves around how Fern had met her older sister while visiting her mother in the hospital and how "everything was polite and pretend." She wanted to talk to Dan about this encounter but found that she could not bring it up. We explore together how she finds that she is now sick of the brave-face act. She realizes that even her mother does not "defend" or support her when she is "condemned" or ignored by her older sister. She had found the courage to tell her mom later that "this hurts." I suggest that it is her truth that no one came to help her when her marriage and her life fell apart, and no-one has ever reached out to help her in the years since or seen her pain at being judged for her mistakes. A key moment occurs when Fern asks a question.

FERN: So, if being excluded hurts, what do I do then? Do I apologize for being hurt or making a mistake? (*I ask her how she feels as she says this. Does she feel this is right, to apologize to the one who hurts her? Does she agree that she is at fault for being hurt and excluded? She is silent for quite a while, then she looks up at me.*) Maybe I am a terrible person. A person who doesn't deserve to be accepted.

SUE: Hm—you turn the hurt on you. It's so natural for you to decide it must be your fault? Then you can try harder and maybe change it? It's more manageable than just feeling the pain and the sadness and loss—the helplessness and aloneness? Shut out, excluded, less than, invisible, who can deal with that! [Bowlby suggests that a child will naturally decide that he or she is a bad child to maintain some sense of control, rather than deal with the overwhelming panic and grief of abandonment, and that this can be functional, at least in the short term. Fern's response makes sense, and I validate her way of coping, but now it leaves her trapped in narrow, negative frames of self and other, and limits her choice of action.] No one was there for you when your life fell apart—that is sad, scary. [When in doubt, I return to a focus on the pain. When clients feel safe enough to really allow themselves to feel their pain with the therapist, self-compassion and the ability to formulate and stand up for their needs naturally follows.]

FERN: It's overwhelming. I needed someone to be there. I could not ask Dan, who I had hurt. So I put on a mask and decided that it must be me—my fault—not deserving. If I am always invisible, judged, and alone, then . . .

SUE: Life is unbearable. You are so so strong to reach down and look this sadness and aloneness in the face, Fern. I am honored to work with you here. You are finding another way, right here. To open up and share here with me, to face your fears and hurts, and to begin couple therapy with Dan. You are amazing. [Authentic validation, given in a personal, heartfelt manner, is the most powerful response a therapist can offer to support an emerging sense of self in a client. Pinpointing a new response that has just occurred in session and use it to build a sense of efficacy are also an inherent part of Tango Move 5, integrating and validating. Success is something that is happening now— and the client is creating it, rather than being something that occurs in the future, perhaps at the end of therapy.]

SESSION 6

This session was dedicated mostly to an imagined encounter with Fern's father and processing Fern's responses in this encounter. The focus of the session was then on Tango Moves 3 and 4, which involve choreographing and processing more engaged encounters with significant others. In this kind of encounter in Stage 2, restructuring, I am constantly tracking and setting up the dialogue, repeating cues and images, and validating and deepening emotion to help Fern shape a new sense of self and new responses from the evolving dialogue. This dialogue is fostered by newly formulated and more coherent emotional music. For the sake of brevity, only part of this session is discussed here.

Fern comes into the session elated, reporting that she has told Dan that she would not go with him to a family gathering unless "he has my back, checks in with me lots, and holds my hand," and he had heard her and reassured her. She had also told him, "Not being close and heard started this whole cascade of me turning into this obsessed person who is always afraid I am somehow not good enough, so I need your help here." We celebrate this together. [From an attachment point of view, it is clear that being able to acknowledge vulnerability in this way and ask for what you need, rather than making constant attempts at self-regulation and self-soothing, is a positive sign of strength and growth. For Fern, asserting her needs occurs as an organic process based on new emotional experience rather than as the result of a "skill" she has been taught in therapy.

FERN: I don't want to suck it up and pretend any more. I want to listen to my feelings. I even told my mom, "I look like I don't care, but every day I hurt about everything that happened." She was shocked. I was a little shocked, too, that I said it.

SUE: (*I am impressed and delighted here.*) Wow. That is something. Amazing. You survived by pushing your hurt aside and trying to do what others expected, so that is risky—new. How does it feel?

FERN: Uncomfortable! (*We both laugh.*) My family is just all judgment about anything and everything with me, so . . . to come out into the open . . . to put down my mask . . .

SUE: Yes. And you took that judgment and learned to do it to yourself as well, to hide your hurt and turn the blame for your approval starvation back onto yourself. So this is new—to ask Dan for support and to tell mom, "I hurt." To say, "I deserve support!" But I think Dad is the linchpin here, isn't he?

FERN: Yes. I tried so hard to please him as a kid, and I excelled in school and in music, which is what he cared so much about. But I could never measure up to his standards. Never. He wasn't like that with my sister and brother. And mom was just kind of silent. He set the tone.

SUE: So, it got to be the norm. You got used to knocking yourself out trying to excel and please, but the message was that you don't deserve acceptance or approval. The onus was on you to find a way to please and if you couldn't, well—there was obviously something wrong with you!

FERN: (*Smiles.*) You always hit the nail on the head, don't you. I would always go into, "What is wrong with *me* that he is never pleased?" In my late teens I asked him—kind of—and he just said he always thought I could do better. This was always in my head, all those years, but I try not to let it bother me. It's in the past now, I guess.

SUE: Is it? Really? I can see the hurt and bewilderment on your face right now. You are still asking, "How come he was so hard on me, judged me?" Let's ask him. Let's have that conversation right now. Can you close your eyes? Can you see him, as he was when you were in your teens—you always trying so hard to please and masking your pain at his disapproval. What do you want to tell him?

FERN: (*Eyes closed; intently, softly.*) Why wasn't I good enough? I tried so hard. It hurts . . . (*Turns to me.*) But he is better now. He is old, and he is less demanding. I don't want to hurt him.

SUE: Hm—Perhaps it would be being a bad daughter to even let yourself imagine this? (*Fern nods slowly.*) And you always tried so hard to be good? (*Fern nods again.*) Can you tell him, right now, just for you, "I don't want to upset you, but I need to tell you that I hurt all the time—you hurt me. I spend my life hiding my fear that I am somehow flawed and pretending that I am fine—wearing a mask."

FERN: (*Closes her eyes, long silence.*) I always thought, no, I knew there was something wrong with me. You never knew it, but every day I obsessed about it, if only I could figure it out, maybe I could fix it, maybe. That hurt. (*Loudly.*)

SUE: (*Reflects and repeats the above.*) How does it feel to say this, right now?

FERN: It helps. It feels unburdened. But it's also scary—scary.

SUE: Right. It's stepping out of the familiar dance with him, isn't it, where you are always trying to please, worrying about how you are failing, hiding behind a mask. What will happen now—what is scary—what will he do?

FERN: I'm afraid he will get mad at me like when I was a kid. He'll say, "That is not accurate. I always loved you. You are my daughter," and I will feel even more disapproved of. (*I ask her what it is like to hear him dismiss her hurt and she weeps. She then spontaneously closes her eyes again to speak to him.*) But I have *always* felt that way. You made me feel that way, always telling me to improve, improve, improve. You know that is true! I just couldn't figure out how to please you, ever. I am over 40 years old and I have spent all this time in agony, trying to figure out what is wrong with me. [Fern now expresses the core of her pain at her perceived rejection by her father and how it has shaped her sense of who she is. She is open to her experience, responsive to its nuances, fully engaged in the experience, coherent and clear. From an attachment perspective, this is a regulated exploration of difficulty and fear typical of secure individuals. From an EFT perspective, this unburdening parallels the events studied in couple interventions labeled "softenings," in which fears and needs are expressed in a regulated fashion that leads to constructive action. Also, these softenings predict successful outcome and follow-up in EFT for couples.]

SUE: What do you want from him, Fern—what would help right now? Tell him.

FERN: (*Sets her jaw firmly.*) I want you to hear me and say you are sorry.

SUE: To tell you that he cares about all the pain you have been in for so long—that this pain matters—that you matter. That you deserved more than judgment. Tell him.

FERN: (*Eyes closed; in a quiet but intense voice.*) How could you do that to me? I longed for your approval—for you to be pleased with me. But you withheld it. You judged me to death. You starved me, Dad. I was excluded—everyone else had their flaws accepted. You never said anything when my sibs screwed up. I never ever felt like I fit in our family.

SUE: (*Softly, using a proxy voice to deepen emotion.*) Yes—"I was never accepted. You left me judged and starved. So I always doubted myself. I took all this on me. I decided that I was a screw up, unacceptable. And then it happened again with Dan, so I got stuck here again, desperately wanting approval and trying so hard, feeling empty and raw [these are her words from a previous session]—starving and unwanted. But trying to put on a brave face till my life just fell apart. And I was sure I was flawed and to blame, so I tortured myself for years going over and over this. But it started with you, Dad. You left me starving for love and caring." (*Fern is nodding and weeping all through this.*) How does it feel to hear me say this, Fern?

FERN: (*With tears.*) Sad, sad, sad. I have wasted so many years trying to figure this out. (*Closes her eyes again and talks to her dad.*) Everyone says you are a great guy, but to me you were a meanie. You were so mean to me. In fact, I feel pissed off at you. Maybe that is why I have always had such a hard time buying you a mushy Father's Day card. I don't want to be a bitch here but . . . you were *not* some kind of great dad to me, you just weren't. (*Opens her eyes and looks up at me.*) It's hard to say that! Feels like I am a bad daughter maybe, saying this.

SUE: (*Leaning forward, in a soft voice, occasionally placing my hand on her arm.*) Yes. You are *so* used to being careful to please him, trying to prove you are what he wants you to be, not risking his disapproval. It is hard to stand up and declare that he failed you. The only way you got anything from him, didn't lose hope of being loved altogether, was to suck up your pain, not protest. So you move back into that familiar place of, "I must be bad somehow." Hard to feel you have the right—the right to be mad at him? (*Fern nods.*) Hard to tell him, "You didn't give me what I needed, what a good dad would have given me. You didn't delight in me, show me I was valued."

FERN: (*Staring glumly at the carpet.*) That's right. That's right, but he would say I was ungrateful, that he pushed me for my own good. (*I ask her to use his voice and reply to Fern.*) He says, "You are exaggerating. You were fine."

SUE: So, can you tell him how it feels to be so dismissed—like your pain doesn't matter? That has you feeling even more alone and excluded, even more helpless? (*Fern nods emphatically.*)

FERN: (*Closes her eyes, speaks softly.*) *Don't,* just *don't*—don't dismiss me, Dad. This is scary, but whether you get mad or silent or not, I have to tell you this stuff. I don't want to live behind this façade feeling bad about myself my whole life. Listen to me! (*I ask her to tell him that again and she does so. Here Fern naturally shifts into an assertive, felt statement of need.*)

SUE: How does this feel now, to say this? To say, "I have the right to be mad at you. To demand that you hear me. I needed your acceptance—your approval so badly"?

FERN: (*Calmly and clearly.*) Yes, I do have the right. It feels good now. But I know he can't respond to me. He would just go silent. He doesn't know how, really. Funny, I see the pattern here, all of it. All of it. I am really good at judging myself. I have taken over from him.

SUE: (*Laughs.*) Yes. Yes. Indeed. You wanted to be a good daughter—to please your dad. You learned the lesson well. And maybe your dad can't really move from that. But you can, and you are. You are changing the pattern right here; taking the reins and deciding what your reality is and how to deal with it in a way that leaves you feeling strong. (*Fern squeezes her shoulders together and giggles in delight.*)

SESSION 7 (ABBREVIATED)

Fern emailed me in a panic before the session. She had met her ex-lover on the street and was shocked to find herself panicked and in tears. However, rather than go into her usual pit of shame, she had taken a huge leap of faith and called Dan and asked for his help. When he responded with comfort, she was able to take this in. She then called her best friend, who told her that the panic was understandable because she was a "victim" of this man who took clear advantage of her vulnerability. Fern found this response validating and a clear contrast to her previous and long-standing "I am the villain in this story" stance. However, she then reverted into questioning how she could have been such a fool as to be taken in by this man. She tells me, "He did use me but I should have said no." I became frustrated and pointed out in a rather mechanical way that judging herself harshly is a well-practiced skill, and indeed she had a choice, but none of us can live without approval, acceptance, and belonging forever; we all ache for this. We are programmed to reach for this loving connection. I then hear my tone and center myself again, and reignite my empathy, asking her to see the lonely, aching Fern in her mind's eye. *When in doubt or off balance, return to the client's pain; this is a good maxim.* When she can do this, I ask her to tell this Fern explicitly what she has always whispered to this part of herself: That she has to be infinitely strong and dismiss her lonely, aching heart. She is required to simply turn down the promise of love she saw in that ex-lover's face and starve. She begins, but then looks up at me and bursts into laughter. We laugh together at the now apparent outrageousness of this demand. She tells me that she gets that this is way too hard and that she can't do this to herself anymore. But then she becomes serious and tells me that in the background she does, in fact, hear the voice of her older and very religious sister, May, telling her this.

We then distill her feelings around her sister and set up an encounter with this sister in the session. Fern imagines May chanting "selfish, selfish, selfish" to her. We examine Fern's response, which is to feel suddenly totally "tired out." We are able to formulate together that she is simply tired of trying to meet the expectations of her sister (and formulate that behind her sister stands the chorus of her father, her husband's family, and the Judge within herself). In a quiet voice, she tells May, "Just let me be me." I expand that to, "Just let me be me. I am really not so bad. I am a good person who just needs love, to be safe, and to belong." Fern tells May her version of this, and amazingly the sister just "fades." This is a "big relief"; May and her judgments are not as powerful as before. Fern then adds that, if she is going to take the mask off and admit her vulnerability, this is new and a little scary and she doesn't want May to see this. I validate that her façade was like her armor; it kept her safe on one level but alone on another. Now she can choose whom to trust and with whom to take risks. Fern imagines herself telling May that she is afraid because May will see her vulnerability and have even more power to hurt her. She speaks to this image of her sister and she knows very well that May will never be able to really accept her. She identifies that it would be "crippling" to be open and to let in the reality that, indeed, May does not care about her pain at all. This sister demands perfection in others. I ask if the judgmental part of Fern stands with her sister in this.

FERN: No. No. That judgy part of me is softer, more compassionate now. I just don't want to show myself, unmasked and vulnerable to her and her rejection.

SUE: So, with her you may still need your guard up, but *you* don't demand that you are perfect anymore? (*Fern nods.*) So you can choose with whom you feel safe and whom to keep at a distance. You don't have to listen to your sister's demands to be "perfect"? You can maybe forgive yourself a little for your humanness? If you can accept you, maybe her approval doesn't matter so much *after all*?

FERN: (*Laughs a full belly laugh.*) I hear that. Well, I like that. That is surprising, isn't it? It is so simple. Not like some big bang moment. I am forgiving myself more and more so . . . if she can't give it . . . well . . . (*Laughs.*) This is a relief. This is one big relief.

SUE: You will survive just fine, I think. You are learning so much, so fast. You are so strong, so brave, and it sounds like you are dancing in new ways with your husband and learning to be more gentle with yourself, so . . . perhaps May cannot respond in the way you longed for. Maybe May needs to hold onto her judgments. The question is, do you feel crippled now? Remember, that is the word you used to describe how these judgments affected you?

FERN: No. No, I don't. That was just an old fear, maybe. Maybe she is just stuck in her righteousness.

SUE: Can you close your eyes and tell her, "Whether you can accept it or not, my pain matters to me. And I can accept the places I have gotten stuck, times when I have tried to find a way out of that pain—and done things I regret."

FERN: (*Excitedly.*) Yes. Yes. Yes. That really resonates with me, Sue. My pain matters to me, and I am not going to spend my life judging the hell out of myself so, you don't get to say . . . um . . .

SUE: Maybe, it's like, "You don't get to say who I am and if I am bad or not"?

FERN: Right. This feels really good to say this.

I now ask her to put it all together again, close her eyes, and speak to her sister in a way that's right for her, and she does this eloquently. I then ask her if she can do this a second time, and really hear herself say these words and make sure she feels them deep in her bones. She does this. I suggest that she can touch this place and now hear this message anytime she wants.

We then summarize the session and outline the risks taken and discoveries made (Tango Move 5, integrating and validating). We agree that Fern should now begin to focus more on doing couple therapy with Dan and that, for now, the next session will be our last.

FINAL SESSION (SESSION 8)

We discuss Fern's fears about couple therapy and how, when Dan gives her any validation and care, she has a hard time trusting it and taking it in. I validate this in the light of her vigilance for disapproval and how "strange" and "new" this sense of acceptance still is for her. We agree that it is hard to let go and bask in the light of someone's love when you have trained your brain to be ever ready to deal with a "tsunami of disapproval." She tells me that she likes my images and will keep them. (Note that she is telling me that, most often, evocative images work much better than cognitive insight-oriented statements.) She confides that she has taken a "big, big risk" and told Dan that she wants to move back in with him and that he responded positively, but both of them are still very "careful." She admits that inside she still sometimes struggles with feeling truly entitled to expect this acceptance. In general, she reports that she feels much more hopeful about her relationship with Dan, is connecting more with her mother, is planning to go to family gatherings with Dan, feels much calmer when meeting her sister, and is recognizing that she does not need to confront her father, who is now frail and more affectionate with her. She generally reports less depression and anxiety. She tells me, with a big smile, "I feel like I am doing great. I feel better about myself than I have in a long, long time."

I ask Fern, "So what happened to the 'tsunami' of disapproval"? She laughs, "It's not so front and center anymore. It's like, at a distance, or maybe I can swim!" She continues, "When that old music starts up, I think of our sessions and what stands out is 'my pain matters.' You always act like my pain matters, Sue! This really helps when I see my sister. Our family was all about competition, and she will always be judgmental but I don't have to bow to that. And, you know, it's her loss because I could be a good sister to her." I suggest that, when others discount her intentions and her emotional reality, she now knows that she doesn't have to accept that. She agrees.

I ask Fern how her inner Judge is doing, and she tells me, "That voice is not so loud now. It feels like I can breathe. It's been so suffocating. I am gentler with myself. And I hear your voice in my head sometimes, and that helps." She goes back to the "starving" image and says it really helps her forgive herself for her affair. I validate her for all the changes she has made and her bravery and openness. We go over the story of our sessions together and weave a coherent narrative of how Fern learned to "swim" and be gentle with herself.

> SUE: So, can you see that desperate Fern who came to see this therapist, who could not sleep and who felt so alone? What would you like to say to her now?

FERN: (*With eyes closed.*) I can tell her, "You don't need to pay for that affair for the rest of your life. You have paid. You have suffered enough now. And folks like your sister don't get to define you."

SUE: Aha. That is so right on. How does this feel, to say this? Can you tell her again? (*Fern does.*)

FERN: It feels peaceful—and like space. (*Smiles a big, wide smile at me.*)

SUE: So maybe she deserves some loving? She can even ask for what she needs and speak her hurts and not keep the mask on, hiding her hurt? (*Fern nods, so I ask her to tell her suffering self this, and she does.*) My sense is that you are proud of what this vulnerable part of you has done here? Is this right? (*Fern nods.*) Can you tell her?

FERN: Hm—that is a bit of a struggle, but yes. (*Closes her eyes.*) You have struggled and come out the other end. I am proud of you. (*Looks up at me.*) I have to practice this a bit. (*Giggles.*)

SUE: (*Leans in and touches Fern on the knee.*) Well, I am proud of you, Fern. You have been amazing to work with, to go on this journey with. (*Fern tears up.*) It feels like you have done what you came here to do?

FERN: Well, it feels like there has been a huge shift—I feel so different. I met this woman, you see, who is able to find those bits in my brain that help me see what was happening.

SUE: Oh—I don't think so. You did this, Fern. I would like you to take that in. You wept nearly every minute of the first sessions, and look at you now!!

FERN: Yes—we touched on lots of painful things, but I am so much better equipped to deal with so many things. Thank you.

SUE: Thank you, too—thank you for your trust.

At the end of this session, Fern completed the Beck Anxiety Scale, now scoring 4, and the Beck Depression Scale, now scoring 5. This is a dramatic change. I asked myself if there was a demand issue here; perhaps she was trying to please me or thank me—to be a good client. However, in retrospect, the reduction in scores did seem to reflect how she presented in sessions and the changes she had made. In particular, there was an apparent difference in her somatic symptoms, such as feeling "unsteady" and "shaky," which were visible in the first sessions when she was labile and wept copiously. Her endorsement of items, such as constantly feeling "fear of the worst happening," which shifted from a "moderately" designation (described in the test as "very unpleasant but I could stand it") to a "not at all" designation, also reflected her presentation during sessions. In the last two sessions she sometimes became upset about something, but she quickly recovered and presented as much less flooded and more centered, calm, and confident. This picture and these assessment measures also mirrored her less-negative, less self-critical sense of self and her shifts in her interpersonal relationships—her sense of others.

Fern was relatively easy to work with, in that her emotions were accessible, although she was very labile and disorganized in early sessions. It is interesting to note how she responded to my evocative images in session: she picked them up and actively used them. Such a response signals to me that a client will respond well to my interventions and progress will be rapid. If Fern had been less in touch with her emotions, the process would have been similar but slower, and I would have had to engage in more refocusing/redirection and use more affect assembly and deepening interventions. Fern did, indeed, do well after these sessions, engaging fully in couple therapy with her husband, selling her house and moving back in with him, as well as reuniting with his family and her own, including finding a way to reconcile with her older sister.

EXERCISES

1. Find two places in the transcript where you might have done something different. What would you have done? Formulate a rationale as to why I intervened the way I did.

2. Find three places where the interventions used here fit with or illustrate the principles of effective change laid out in Chapter 3 of this book.

3. If you had seen this woman for a consultation session, what do you think you would have found most difficult about working with her?

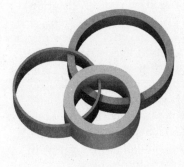

Chapter 6

Getting to Safe and Sound in Emotionally Focused Couple Therapy

How spouses respond to one another's every day disclosures and requests for support may be more consequential than how they negotiate differences of opinion. . . .
—K. T. Sullivan, L. A. Pasch, M. D. Johnson,
and T. N. Bradbury (2010, p. 640)

Love doesn't just sit there, like a stone, it has to be made, like bread, remade all the time, made new.
—Ursula K. Le Guin

A long-term pair bond is viewed widely as one of the most important goals in life (Roberts & Robins, 2000). It is not surprising then that couple therapy is now offered by almost two-thirds of practitioners in North America, or that relationship distress is one of the most common reasons for seeking therapy. However, practitioners often find that working with couples is an overwhelming enterprise (likened in one *New York Times* article to "flying a helicopter through a tornado") (*New York Times*, April 3, 2012). Love relationships are everywhere and in plain sight—but at the same time they are complex dramas that no one can ever entirely master. Couple therapists need a clear way to see and work with this complexity. The field has offered therapists different ideas about the core nature and defining factors in close relationships. We can view an intimate relationship as a contract in which negotiation skills are paramount; an inevitable and unconscious repetition of one's relationships with parents; or a companionate friendship based on respect. Relationships can also be seen in broad terms as simply social constructions, or as based in biology and biological imperatives. In this book we view intimate relationships in terms of (and thus base couple interventions on) the integrative and substantive science of adult attachment (Johnson, 2004, 2013). Romantic love is then seen as an attachment bond, which is a key survival strategy designed to keep significant others close and available for support and protection—so that the task of dealing with life's uncertainties and threats can be shared, and individuals can encounter the world in an open, exploratory manner, thriving and growing in relative safety. As Mozart said, "Love guards the heart from the abyss."

RESEARCH ON ATTACHMENT-ORIENTED EFT FOR COUPLES

The attachment perspective and the EFT approach to relationship repair echo all the key recent empirical findings on the essential nature of relationship distress (Gottman, Coan, Carrere, & Swanson, 1998). Both emphasize:

- The power of negative emotion, for example, as seen in facial expression, to predict long-term stability and satisfaction in relationships.

- The importance of process, or the nature of emotional engagement and how partners communicate (rather than the content or frequency of arguments).

- The toxicity of negative cycles of demand–withdraw and stonewalling behaviors.

- The need for cycles of mutual soothing for relationship stability.

- The power of positive emotion, termed positive-sentiment override in the behavioral literature, but referring to more secure connection in the EFT world.

EFT places all these factors in the context of attachment and explains such factors in attachment terms. For example, attachment offers a compelling explanation as to exactly why stonewalling behaviors are so corrosive in adult close relationships. Lack of emotional responsiveness shatters assumptions of secure connection and induces overwhelming separation distress. Attachment also explains why husbands in happy, secure relationships can accept attachment protests and complaints while staying engaged, showing less reactivity to perceived criticism, and being open to the implicit bids for contact in such behavior (Johnson, 2003).

In terms of outcome and process-of-change studies, EFT, more than any other approach, exemplifies the highest or ideal level of empirical validation as laid out by the American Psychological Association for couple and family therapy (Sexton et al., 2011). As required by this standard, EFT has been validated in a number of randomized control trials and demonstrated consistent positive outcomes with large effect sizes; has been studied in a direct comparison with another intervention (namely, traditional behavioral marital therapy); has been shown to have stable results over longer-term follow-up; has been validated in terms of the stated change mechanisms of the model (in nine process-of-change studies to date); and has been successfully used to address different problems in different populations and different problems within distressed relationships. The only significant gap in this body of research is that EFT has not been systematically tested in terms of outcomes across different cultural groups, although in clinical practice it has indeed been adapted to and used successfully with traditional and nontraditional couples, gay and straight couples, Muslim and Christian couples, Eastern European and Californian couples, military and civilian couples, monogamous and polyamorous couples, and low- and high-social-status couples (see Johnson, Lafontaine, & Dalgleish, 2015, for a summary of research, and *www.iceeft.com* for a complete list of studies and reviews).

Since relationship distress primes other mental health disorders, and vice versa, it is particularly relevant that EFT has been shown to be easily and effectively adapted to couples facing problems such as depression and PTSD (Dalton et al., 2013; Denton, Wittenborn, & Golden, 2012). Couple discord is associated with a wide range of mood, anxiety, and substance abuse disorders (Bhatia & Davila, 2017). As already stated, relationship discord increases depressive and anxiety symptoms over time; and as symptoms occur, satisfaction decreases (Whisman & Baucom, 2012). Higher levels of anxious attachment seem to increase the link between discord and depression (Scott & Cordova, 2002), and depressive episodes are predicted by negative relationship events, especially those associated with betrayal or humiliation, such as affairs (Cano & O'Leary, 2000). Simple lack of support from a partner also increases one's risk for a depressive episode (Wade & Kendler, 2000). Perhaps most telling of all is that perceived criticism from a partner predicts a relapse of numerous disorders (see Hooley, 2007, for a review). These findings speak to the pain that criticism from a partner inflicts, a pain that is perfectly logical given the principles of attachment science.

Process-of-Change Research

Although some changes in attachment models and styles resulting from individual therapy have been found, namely, longer-term psychodynamic therapy (Diamond et al., 2003; Fonagy et al., 1995), little or no research has examined changes in attachment security in couple and family therapy, even though key interactions with attachment figures are most accessible in these modalities, and patterns of attachment responses are most salient and open to potential modification. Our lab recently conducted a study showing that 20 sessions of EFT can increase attachment security in both anxious and avoidant partners, and this effect remained solid at a 2-year follow-up (Burgess Moser et al., 2015; Wiebe et al., 2016). The results of this study were also extended by a brain scan study that showed that the brains of female partners were more able to use the safety cue provided by holding their partner's hand to change their perception of the threat of electric shock after EFT sessions (Johnson et al., 2013). These results support the premises of attachment theory and also confirm the positive impact of EFT on a physiological level. Attachment science in general, and EFT in particular, links to and is supported by research studies of neuroscience processes in couple relationships (Greenman, Wiebe, & Johnson, 2017).

As a clinician oriented to decreasing emotional disconnection and shaping secure bonding events, and more specifically as an EFT therapist, what does this plethora of studies tell me to expect? First, it tells me that I can anticipate, once I am trained in EFT and understand attachment principles, that 70–73% of the couples I see will no longer be distressed at the end of 8–20 sessions of therapy and will make changes that last. Also that an even larger number, approximately 86% of distressed couples, will report significant improvements in their relationship even if they are not quite where they want to be when they decide to stop therapy. This body of research reassures me that even if partners struggle with mental health issues, such as depression and anxiety that especially result from traumatic experiences, I can work with these issues in a relational context and make a difference in relationship quality and the symptoms of emotional disorders. The research encourages me to work toward a truly collaborative alliance with both partners, gradually deepening emotion and shaping more open, engaged, and affiliative interactions, particularly mutually responsive interactions, termed *withdrawer re-engagement* or *blamer softening*, which occur in change events in EFT. In the EFT relationship education literature these are called Hold Me Tight conversations. The research gives me a solid, secure base to stand on. It gives me hope and direction when couples walk into my office.

ATTACHMENT AS A GUIDE TO THE PROBLEM
AND THE SOLUTION IN COUPLE THERAPY

What is the essential problem in distressed relationships? There are many candidates: Conflict itself; differing expectations and distorted communication; patterned responses that become automatic and constraining; and differences in temperament, goals, mental health, or commitment levels. Bowlby would have suggested that we look past corrosive disagreements and consider *deprivation* as the key—the loss or lack of attuned responsiveness. We can capture Tim and Sarah at one of their most difficult moments.

> TIM: I don't want to talk about this cause you exaggerate all the time, and I am always in the wrong. You make things appear bigger than they really are.
>
> SARAH: It's clear that you never believe what I say! I tell you my truth, and you dismiss it as somehow crazy. You don't hear me at all.
>
> TIM: I can't handle the constant complaints. There is no point. You are always focused on what I am doing wrong—in fact—I can't do anything right. I brought you flowers yesterday but that doesn't count, does it?
>
> SARAH: What about when I got sick. You didn't even care. I am overlooked. Not on the agenda. When I had sinus surgery and you came to the hospital, you were there for about 10 minutes is all. And you ate my popsicle! I woke up and you were gone, and the popsicle the nurse had brought me was gone!
>
> TIM: You told me I could have it. I don't want to talk about this. (*Turns away with a blank face.*)
>
> SARAH: You are so unsympathetic. Like when I left the hospital, you just stuffed me in the car and just dropped me off at home.
>
> TIM: (*Silence. Sighs.*) This is so pointless—frustrating. This story, like all the stories, starts changing and taking on another life. I am wrong. There is nothing I can say anyway. I have to go back to work.

An attachment-oriented EFT therapist sees this as a drama of emotional disconnection and unmet attachment needs that triggers alarm, specifically, deep fears of rejection and abandonment by the one person that each partner counts on the most. One partner deals with the alarm by shutting down and shutting the other out; the other deals with it by protesting her partner's lack of responsiveness with critical comments.

Both handle their vulnerability in a way that triggers the vulnerability of the other and maintains or exacerbates distress and isolation. Here, Sarah is trying to get Tim to respond to her terrifying sense that she does not matter to him, while expressing anger and indignation. Tim is trying to get away from his sense of failure and rejection by defending and discounting Sarah, and then withdrawing. *Both constantly confirm the other's worst attachment fears.* Later, when she has regained some of her emotional balance, Sarah can "change the channel," reach for Tim and say, "Feels like my pain doesn't matter to you, Tim. I call and no one is there, no one comes. I am alone. It hurts." But Tim is still caught in his own sense of helplessness and failure, and so rather than tune in to her vulnerability he says, "I try so hard but nothing works, so maybe I am not the one to help you here." The cycle begins again.

The emotions displayed here, specifically the threat that is the key thread in the plot line, are more than compelling, they are disorganizing. The longed-for safe haven other becomes instead a source of uncertainty, danger, and pain. Fear narrows down cognitive frames and response options. The partners lose control of their dance, generating a sense of helplessness. This process makes both partners more susceptible to mental health issues, such as depression and anxiety. From an attachment perspective any intervention that does not shift the emotional music significantly and directly address the attachment threat will, at best, be minimally effective and then only for a limited time. As Zajonc notes (1980, p. 152), "Affect dominates social interaction, and it is the major currency in which social interaction is transacted." However, if as until recently, emotion is seen in terms of ventilation and catharsis, it is not that useful a focus in terms of therapeutic change in couple therapy, and indeed, until the advent of EFT, it was generally avoided. In contrast, in EFT emotion is viewed as a key target and active agent of change capable of evoking core changes in the most potent organizing element in the partners' bond—the emotional responsiveness between partners. As stated frequently in the EFT literature, emotion is the great organizer of interactions—it is the music of the dance between intimates. It is almost impossible to change a dance unless you change the music.

The relationship problem here is framed for the couple in terms of *how* they dance together and how their emotional signals push each other off balance and into painful isolation. This sense of isolation is a danger cue to each partner's nervous system and tends to limit each person's response repertoire and maintain the couple's negative dance. The lack of safe connection also precludes their ability to change the channel when distressed and effectively reach for each other. The solution to this problem is, first, to help the partners view their relationship as an attachment dance, recognize their impact on each other, and begin to join together to limit their negative dance and the insecurity it breeds. Second, it is necessary to help partners move into a positive dance of reaching and responding to each other's attachment needs for safe connection. Research on EFT change events and the key elements of secure bonding as laid out by attachment science informs us that the core aspect of such positive bonding dances are Hold Me Tight conversations, as mentioned earlier. These interactions, wherein both partners become able to tolerate, name, and share their soft, vulnerable emotions, that is, they are emotionally accessible, responsive, and engaged with each other, are significant corrective emotional experiences. At such times, attachment fears are soothed, working models of self and other are transformed, and interactional behavioral repertoires expanded. These change events consistently predict success at the end of EFT and at follow-up (Greenman & Johnson, 2013). They also predict changes in attachment, particularly anxious attachment, and changes in key relationship factors, such as the forgiveness of injuries (Makinen & Johnson, 2006). The relationship is then redefined, for both partners, as a safe haven to go to and a secure base to go out from.

What would a Hold Me Tight conversation look like for Tim and Sarah? In Stage 1 of EFT, stabilization (called de-escalation in the couple therapy literature), the therapist helps them identify their negative dance, which they decide to call the Popsicle Dance. Here, Sarah feels abandoned and dismissed and so tries to reach her partner by "making a case against him." He hears her accusation and turns away since he is always "in the dock." In EFT sessions, they begin to grasp how they press each other's alarm bells and move into self-protection. The cycle begins to diminish in frequency, speed, and momentum. For example, Tim can now ask, "Is this one of those times when you feel like I am just leaving you high and dry, like I don't care? I don't want you to feel that way." The fact that he asks calms Sarah and opens a door into another kind of conversation. In the Hold Me Tight conversations, in Stage 2 (restructuring) both partners change the level and the channel of their communication. Tim is able to say, "I do turn away. I don't know what else to do. I am flooded with this horrible feeling of total failure, so I run. But I don't want to do this anymore. I love you and want you to be able to trust that. Perhaps I need your help. Can I blow it sometimes and still be enough?" Sarah reassures him, and then touches her own fears of never mattering to Tim or to anyone, something that has fueled her previous problems with depression. She tells him, in an explicit and evocative attachment reach, "I am never really sure someone else will care about my hurts and fears—whether I even have the right to expect that. I need to know that I can call, and you will do your best to be there. Is that okay?" Clear, distilled messages of fear and need naturally evoke caring and empathy in human beings, unless they are blocked by absorbing affect regulation tasks like regulating fear or dealing with rage. These kinds of events move a couple into a safe bonding dance that is coded as massively significant by our social- and attachment-oriented brains. These events change how partners see themselves and each other, and so their inner working models. They also shift their sense of competence and confidence about their relationship, and evoke new levels of the explicit responsiveness that are associated with long term happiness in relationships (Huston, Caughlin, Houts, Smith, & George, 2001). The attachment literature is clear that, as in these change events, secure adults can better acknowledge their needs, can give and ask for support more effectively, and are less likely to be verbally aggressive or withdrawn during conflict (Simpson, Rholes, & Phillips, 1996; Senchak & Leonard, 1992).

CASE FORMULATION AND ASSESSMENT

Assessment in EFT for couples has been outlined in previous literature (Johnson, 2004; Johnson et al., 2005) but will be briefly summarized here. In terms of self-report questionnaires of relationship satisfaction, most studies of EFT have used the DAS (Spanier, 1976) but more recently the CSI (Funk & Rogge, 2007) has been used. Other specific questionnaires, such as the Beck Depression and Anxiety Scales (Beck et al., 1996; Beck & Steer, 1993) and the attachment questionnaires described in Appendix 1 of this book, can be used at the therapist's discretion. Therapists are also using the A.R.E. Questionnaire from my book *Hold Me Tight* (Johnson, 2008a, p. 57) as a quick, impressionistic way to get a sense of how partners deal with attachment fears and needs.

BEGINNING THERAPY: THE PROCESS OF THE FIRST SESSIONS

The first task for any therapy is the creation of safety within the therapeutic alliance. In couple therapy the obvious complication is that this safety has to be created and maintained with two clients at the same time, in front of each other, when they live in different and often conflicting universes. The shaping of this safety is a crucial part of the process of getting to know a couple and fostering a climate of openness, honesty, and exploration. However, in the first sessions the therapist is also assessing the partners and their relationship, checking out contraindications for EFT that undermine the in-session emotional safety that is necessary for effective intervention. Contraindications include significant, ongoing violence between partners, ongoing untreated addictions that compete with attachment to the partner, or current affairs that will stymie the recreation of trust in the couple's relationship. The therapist also needs to determine whether he or she can join with the client's treatment goals and whether partners have compatible goals. When a client, Mary, agrees with my formulation that, for her, the sole focus of therapy appears to be changing her silent depressed husband's "defective personality," and she does not intend to explore anything about herself, I suggest that this is a goal that a couple therapist cannot agree to, or even pragmatically achieve. Her husband also does not in any way share this goal! The therapist then empathically reflects each client's position and clarifies what is possible in couple therapy and what he or she can authentically agree to work toward.

The assessment process itself is described in the EFT literature (Johnson, 2004; Johnson et al., 2005) and consists of two joint sessions and one separate session with each partner. This individual session is confidential; however, if issues come up that need to be addressed in a conjoint session in order for therapy to be effective, then clients are told that the therapist will help them share those issues in ways that advance their relationship goals. Such sessions are necessary if therapy is not to be undermined by secrets or unexplored issues of which the therapist is unaware. This individual session allows for the exploration of personal relationship history, including to whom a client turned and depended on as a child, and whether there is a history of violation, betrayal, or abandonment in childhood that may complicate the promotion of trust. It also allows for exploration of any intimidation or abuse that may be present in the relationship (see Bograd & Mederos, 1999, for a clear summary article that parallels the EFT stance on violence in couples). In the individual session, the therapist can also ask the client how he or she experiences the partner in general, as well as explore whether there are other competing attachments such as affairs, or sexual issues such as a compulsive use of pornography, that the client is finding hard to share with his or her mate.

Clinical wisdom tells us that the confiding of secrets that emerge in individual sessions is managed relatively easily and constructively by therapists with EFT skills. However, deception is hard to maintain over time and is clearly toxic to future secure connection. Assessment and treatment are not separate here; for example, outlining a couple's negative interactional cycle as it occurs in session is formally termed Step 2 in the EFT treatment guide, but often begins in the first session. Assessment may involve the use of questionnaires, but it is conducted in the same tenor and tone as the rest of EFT sessions. The process is collaborative and respectful, with an emphasis on clarifying and making coherent sense of each client's experience, relationship processes, and patterns. Given the almost complete dearth of relationship education in both developed and developing countries, at the outset of therapy the most basic need of most partners is to be heard and reassured that their stories make sense, that neither they nor their partner are mad or bad, and that relationships can be understood and intentionally shaped; in short, that there is hope. The EFT therapist has the perspective, skills, and research base to provide this reassurance.

Assessment typically addresses 12 questions:

1. How did the couple decide to come for therapy—what is the catalyst, and how does each partner feel about coming?

2. What are each partner's goals, and what changes would occur if therapy was successful?

3. How did the couple meet and become committed (if they are), and what was the relationship like at the beginning?

4. How did things begin to go wrong, and what does each partner see as the key factor in their distress?

5. How has each partner upset or wounded the other; are there specific injuries, such as abandonments at moments of high need, or affairs, or betrayals?

6. How do conflicts or periods of distance get triggered and maintained, and how do they end?

7. If partners cannot turn to and help each other with their emotions, how do they regulate them?

8. What are the strengths of the relationship from each person's point of view—are they still able to have fun, share activities, show affection, and make love?

9. Are there moments when their bond is apparent and "felt"—when they are able to be there for each other—or high points in the relationship that they hold onto from the past?

10. Are they still both committed to working on the relationship, and, if not, what is the main trigger for their ambivalence?

11. In a typical day, can they give you a picture of their interactions, schedules, and time together?

12. What are the couple struggling with in their lives—parenting issues; job problems; health issues; issues of depression, anxiety, addiction, or other mental health issues—and how do these affect their everyday interactions?

Couples' responses are explored in a down-to-earth, concrete way that offers the therapist and the couple a picture of how they interact, get stuck in conflict or distance, and try to solve relationship issues, and the manner in which each regulates their emotions at key moments. The attachment framework is inherent in the way the therapist comments on and integrates information with the couple. The therapist may make validating, normalizing comments such as, "Everyone gets stuck in their relationship dance; we are all so sensitive to any negative responses from our partners. This is because they are so important to us and because we depend on them," or "We all miss our partner's cues sometimes. And feeling alone in a relationship is so hard. It hurts everyone, even the strongest of us, just because that is the way humans are wired."

During the assessment phase, partners are invited to interact, so that the therapist may see patterns of interaction firsthand as they unfold. I might ask, "Do you think your partner really knows how difficult things are for you and how upset you are? Could you tell him, please? Help him understand." In general, the therapist assumes that separation distress and the inherent threat it presents create emotional and interactional chaos. Partners have no idea how much negative impact they have on each other, given that they are preoccupied with managing their own overwhelming emotions and trying to solve the no-win dilemmas they are caught in. Neither can truly reach for the other and speak her or his needs and fears coherently, and even if this does begin to happen, neither can access the trust or reliable empathy to respond positively. As stated previously, self-protection becomes a prison; in fact, it becomes solitary confinement!

Judging from research studies, EFT interventions are effective in building an alliance, and therapy dropouts, a key issue in the couple field, are generally not a problem. In a study of predictors of outcome in EFT (Johnson & Talitman, 1997), therapeutic alliance was found to account for 20% of the variance in outcome. This is double the variance in outcome usually accounted for by the alliance in individual therapy. Interestingly, if alliance is viewed as constituted by three factors—the bond with the therapist, agreement about goals, and the perceived relevance of the tasks the therapist sets up—it is the task element that has the greatest impact on outcome in EFT. This accords with the consistent feedback that clients share with EFT practitioners. As Paul tells me at the end of Session 5:

> "I don't know how you know this stuff, but the way you work is right on for us. It seems to capture our relationship and all our struggles so well. It makes everything clear, like you are going to the heart of things. So, I know in the beginning I was pretty uncooperative. I didn't want to turn to my wife and risk saying emotional stuff, but I did it 'cause inside I know you are getting us to hone in on what really matters. We are not messing around on the edges, just discussing everything and nothing. This stuff really moves me. I know this is where we need to go."

The integration of attachment and experiential interventions that shape the therapeutic alliance in EFT tells us that once we tune in to clients' emotional reality and really listen to their pain, especially the pain of not being seen and accepted by others, everything they do, no matter how apparently self-destructive, makes sense. There is a deep organic logic to how people put their emotions together and how they engage with others. All of us are overpowered at some point in our lives by the unforeseen consequences of how we have learned to both protect ourselves from and be with others. If we are attuned as therapists, the only possible response to these consequences is compassion. The key intervention used in building a stable, resilient alliance in EFT is the therapist's nonjudgmental reflection of the clients' inner and outer realities—together with constant validation and normalization. The therapist models secure attachment by intentionally working to be personally accessible, responsive, and engaged. He or she also openly discusses the process of therapy itself and any reactions a client may have to this process. As an example, I find myself saying, "June, can you help me here. It seems like whenever I ask you to linger a little and taste your feelings, you begin to talk about other topics and you seem irritated with me. Perhaps this is hard for you to do—something you are just not used to? Perhaps I need to help you a little more, or do you want to just tell me to stop asking?" The therapist is a surrogate attachment figure and, just like an attuned parent, tunes in to the client's vulnerable places, addressing this vulnerability and the dilemmas it presents directly.

It is also now standard practice to suggest to couples at the beginning of therapy that they read or listen to the audio version of the book *Hold Me Tight* (Johnson, 2008a). This book lays out and normalizes attachment processes and offers many images and stories of couples caught in insecurity and disconnection and then finding their way to a more secure bond.

The moves of the EFT Tango have already been examined in Chapters 3 and 4. The general process of the stages of EFT for couples has also been outlined many times in the couple therapy literature (in numerous entries on the *www.iceeft.com* list of publications and in basic texts on EFT, e.g., Johnson, 2004). So we will focus now on examining the core Tango metainterventions and associated change processes as they apply specifically to couples, and integrate them into descriptions of the different stages of therapy. How the Tango is applied will look a little different in different modalities. When implementing Tango Move 1, mirroring present process, for example, the couple therapist focuses particularly on outlining a couple's negative interaction cycle in its most essential elements and its attachment consequences. The therapist does this in a way that externalizes this dance so that partners can see how they help construct the dance, but also see it as a process that takes over their relationship and that, together, they can control.

STAGE 1: STABILIZATION— PROCESSES AND INTERVENTIONS

The first stage of couple intervention involves de-escalating the negative cycle or dance, usually one of complaint and criticism followed by distancing and stonewalling, that has taken over a couple's relationship and constantly primes insecurity and distress. The goal is to stabilize the relationship around renewed hope and a sense of agency. The main tasks in this stage are to outline the negative cycle in a couple's relationship and help partners come together to curtail it. The therapist then helps partners assemble their softer emotions in ways that lead to more positive affect regulation and engagement strategies. Once partners can achieve a metaperspective and frame the negative dance as their joint enemy, they begin to be more accepting of their partner, and the relationship becomes more positive. A blaming, agitated partner will be able to move from a stance of, "My wife is so cold. She is not my soulmate. In fact, she is impossible to live with and all her family are like that," to "I never understood how sensitive she is to my messages that I need more from her. I guess I sound pretty critical at times. The other night she said to me, 'Hey, slow down here. Are you feeling shut out right now? I can feel that pressure, that failure feeling starting. Our spiral dance thing is starting. Let's not freak each other out. We don't have to do this.' Now, is that different or what!" The couple here can see their dance and move into coregulation, helping each other to step into equilibrium and constructive joint action. If comorbidities, such as depression or anxiety, are part of the clinical picture, they are included in the description of the cycle. The ways in which they both trigger and are maintained by negative interactions are outlined. Negative relationship events trigger symptoms such as depression, and depression results in less social support for the other partner. Less support then triggers relationship distress and more symptomatic behavior, sometimes in both partners (Bhatia & Davila, 2017). Past traumatic relationship events, termed attachment injuries, that violate attachment expectations by abandonment or betrayal at a crucial moment of need, are also integrated into this description.

The Tango in Stage 1 of EFT

We can now integrate a description of the stages of treatment in EFT with the recurring processes and interventions laid out in the EFT Tango.

EFT Tango Move 1: Mirroring Present Process—
The Demon Dance Description

There are only so many key recurring patterns that characterize intimate interactions and define the quality of a couple's attachment. Four negative cycles can be identified in distressed relationships (Johnson, 2008):

1. The relatively short, sharp cycle of *attack–attack,* typified by escalating aggression and critical blaming, which EFT therapists call *Find The Bad Guy,* since the struggle is always about who is to blame for the relationship distress or who is the more unlovable of the two partners. To define the other as at fault offers an illusionary moment of control in the wave of distress that engulfs a couple's relationship.

2. The most common and often endlessly repeating *criticize–withdraw cycle.* This particular cycle has been found to predict relationship dissolution (Gottman, 1999); EFT therapists often call it the *Protest Polka,* since one person is explicitly protesting disconnection, albeit often in an aggressive way, that disguises his or her separation distress.

3. The *Freeze and Flee cycle,* wherein both partners, burnt out and discouraged, retreat and stonewall each other. For the previously pursuing partner, this is often the beginning of grieving the relationship and moving toward detachment.

4. The *Chaos and Ambivalence cycle,* wherein one partner may demand closeness, but then when it is offered, the threat involved in being vulnerable with a needed other triggers reactive defense and distance, which then pushes the other partner into frustrated withdrawal. This cycle most often reflects a fearful avoidant attachment style, in that the most active partner makes anxious bids for connection, but then switches into more avoidant mode and retreats.

These ambivalent responses are associated with a history of traumatic childhood attachments, in which closeness was longed for but always infused with threat and overwhelming pain. Partners, like past attachment figures, are then simultaneously a source of safety and a source of threat, and every interaction is a potentially impossible choice between isolation and dangerous connection. In general, the more complicated the tasks of emotion regulation and the more chaotic and overwhelming the nature of partners' attachment history, the more elements there are in the cycle and the faster and more compelling the triggers and emotional music in a couple's dance (Johnson, 2002).

What principles does the EFT therapist use when naming and so taming a couple's cycle as it unfolds in session? First the therapist has to carefully observe and find the key pattern in a couple's dialogue; often nonverbals are key here. Someone who mostly withdraws may explode when he can no longer suppress his emotions, but his habitual strategy is withdrawal and the trigger for this is often very clear. So, Neil tells me that when his wife pursues and begins to bring up relationship issues, he "wants out now." The microsteps in outlining a couple's cycle, which is part of Tango Move 1, mirroring present process, are as follows:

• The therapist notes the *specific steps* in a couple's dance and *describes them* in simple, neutral, concrete language—verbs are best.

"Fred, when you begin to talk in this quiet but intense voice about how 'out of whack' this relationship is and how Mary could change, I notice that you, Mary, turn your head, look away and go still and silent. Then you change the subject. Fred, you then express anger, and then point out all the ways you want Mary to change. Does this sound right?"

• The focus is on how the couple move in their dance, on their pattern of connection and disconnection. The therapist also *notes surface emotions* that accompany the steps, for example, observing that Mary seems to shut down, as if she feels nothing, when Fred talks with more and more intensity.

• The therapist explicitly *links each partner's moves to those of the other in a circular loop*. This demonstrates that the couple's dance is a self-sustaining feedback loop. The therapist *frames the cycle as the enemy,* rather than the other person or the differences between partners.

"Fred, it seems like the more you try to make your point and tell Mary how you want her to improve and how frustrated you are, the more you push her to hear you, the more, Mary, you turn away and shut down. You kind of shut him and his comments about how you are disappointing him out? Yes? And the more you shut down and shut him out, the more you, Fred, try to insist—to make your point. And Mary, you then see him as 'lecturing' you, and you shut down more, until, as Fred says, 'Everyone gets tired and gives up, and we don't talk for days.' You are both caught in this dreadful dance of lecture and are shut out. This dance has taken over your whole relationship, whether you are talking about the kids or sex or issues around time together."

• The therapist *adds a normalizing frame and attachment consequences* to this picture. Attachment and the EFT literature give the therapist a map to the interactional moves and strategies and how they link to the way in which inner emotions and working models of self and other are constructed so the therapist can conjecture with confidence and link all three together.

"Many couples get stuck in this kind of dance, and it's so hard to see when you are caught up in it. The dance does you in after a while. It becomes automatic. Often it feels like you are on different planets. This dance leaves you both alone, feeling either unheard and unimportant, no matter what you say, or criticized and like you are failing, and not a good partner, so it feels safer to hunker down to avoid more criticism. Does this fit for you? Help me if I am getting it wrong here."

• It is helpful to guide partners into giving their negative dance a name so that they can move into a metalevel and identify it when it is happening.

Once the cycle is clear, the therapist continually reflects it, as it occurs, as it is revealed in stories of the couple's fights or in past incidents, and as it is primed in therapy. Therapist inputs lessen as the couple themselves are able to see and address the cycle, though they are part of every EFT session and are often only referred to as background as therapy moves forward.

EFT Tango Move 2: Affect Assembly and Deepening

The most essential skill of the competent couple therapist is the ability to *change channels* from the big picture of a couple's dance, to the microcosm of the individual's construction of emotion and that person's inner world.

The therapist, as in the EFIT therapy process described in Chapter 4, moves into each person's inner world, which is constantly primed by interactions with her or his partner, and helps clients reach for the softer, deeper, attachment-oriented emotions beneath the surface of the interactional dance. These are the emotions that individuals often hide from their partners and from themselves and that render them vulnerable. As in EFIT, the therapist adopts a curious stance and asks evocative questions about the triggers, initial perceptions, body responses, thoughts and conclusions, and action tendencies that arise, describing and distilling the formation and expression of clarified and more-regulated emotions.

The therapist pinpoints the moments that constitute blocks to secure attachment processes, which are even more obvious in couple therapy than in individual sessions. So she or he tracks *how* partners talk about attachment vulnerabilities and needs, especially if these needs are deemed shameful or unacceptable, helps clients reframe them as simply a core part of being human and also listens for beliefs about the responsiveness of others in general. The therapist also tracks partners default affect regulation strategies and how they deal with separation distress, particularly noting extreme vigilance about responsiveness from the partner; ramped-up alarm-oriented aggression; numbing withdrawal and immobility; flooding, resulting in disorientation; and flipping between fight and flight. As these strategies play out, *the therapist notes how attachment messages become distorted or so ambiguous as to make attunement almost impossible.* After weeping at her emerging sense of loneliness in her marriage, Marjorie then shifts into a contemptuous tone and announces to her husband, Pete, "Even a retard would know that I need support at such times. But then, of course, you would have to also be listening!" She cannot clearly formulate her loneliness, and expresses only rage. The next block to attachment is easy to predict: When she does begin to touch on her aloneness, Pete does not trust this disclosure and responds with careful distance. The next block arises when he does, with some help, manage to summon his empathy and reaches for her; she cannot respond to this longed-for but strange stimulus and begins to shut him out. The easiest way to register these blocks, accept them, and bring partners through them is to be attuned to the affect regulation tasks inherent in the partners' interactions.

EFT Tango Move 3: Choreographing Engaged Encounters

As noted in Chapter 3, when shaping encounters, especially in couple's sessions, the therapist first intensifies the clients' core emotions into a clearly 'felt' reality, distills the core of this reality in simple terms, and then directs clients to share in a brief, cogent way with the other partner, refocusing and offering direction when necessary. If the other partner interrupts, the therapist holds space for the speaker to continue. So, in Session 4, I bypass Clyde's rationalizing responses to his wife's "coaching" behaviors and evocatively repeat and actively explore the "caught-in-the-headlights desperation" he has identified in previous sessions. We stay with this reality until he distills this experience into a core sense of "always less than" and a feeling of "not being wanted." I then ask him to share this with his partner. As he speaks this reality, it becomes clearer, and this disclosure is, in itself, an assertion of self.

The last two moves of the Tango—Move 4, processing the encounter, and Move 5, integrating and validating—are essentially the same in couple sessions as in EFIT. I might ask Clyde how it feels to risk telling his wife about his "always less than" reality, and help her stay engaged with this reality, rather than explaining that this is indeed his "neurotic inner child problem." I will then celebrate with them how they could manage this new kind of interaction.

In the restructuring attachment stage of EFT (discussed later), these encounters eventually become powerful bonding events, and so the therapist gradually builds the momentum—the gradual drama of sharing poignant fears and needs, and the sculpting of sensitive responsiveness from the listening partner—in such encounters.

The EFT Tango in Couple Therapy: Additional Notes

Although the modifications made to the Tango moves in the couple modality can be discussed separately, they come together in and are part of the cross-modality EFT Tango process. Again and again in couple therapy, the interactional cycle is reflected in the present as it occurs, as is each partner's spoken experience. This experience is assembled, deepened, and distilled, albeit at different levels and intensities, depending on the stage of therapy. Clarified messages based on the affect assembly process are outlined and used to shape new, more-engaged encounters or enactments between partners, and each person's experience of this dialogue is processed. In Tango Move 5, integrating and validating, the whole process is summarized and celebrated in a way that recognizes each person's potential for competence and efficacy. This integrating dialogue should begin to reduce partners' negative views of the relationship so they can create new narratives of their relationship problems, their partner, the potential for safe connection, and their sense of their own worth and abilities and come together as a team to solve pragmatic problems.

After the assembling emotion process (Tango Move 2) and as part of the engaged encounters process (Tango Move 3), Pete is able to tell Marjorie for the first time that he finds her "intimidating" and indeed does reflexively shut the door on her, not out of indifference, but out of a frantic desire to avoid the "judgment of incompetence" he expects her to deliver. Marjorie is shocked and confused and dismisses Pete's message, but the therapist helps her process this encounter further, and she begins to listen in a new way, gaining just a little distance from her "cast-iron" assumptions about Pete and about men in general. This is progress. The Tango becomes *more focused and more compelling* as the couple move through mirroring present process with a special emphasis on the demon dance description and on clarifying the insecurity and isolation this dance creates. The dance itself, rather than individual partner's behaviors, is framed as the couple's problem and one that they can defuse and change together. Marjorie is able to say to Pete, "I don't want to do our Wobbly Waltz right now, do you? If you are feeling criticized right now, I am sorry. I know I am coming on strong."

*Refinements on Techniques for EFT with Couples: Slice It Thinner,
Catch the Bullet, and Changing Channels*

The specific interventions we discussed in Chapter 3, such as the reflection of inner and interactional realities, validation, and asking evocative questions, are used constantly with couples. However, there are also a few interventions that are particularly pertinent and necessary when working with couples. When creating enactments in Stage 1, where "new" emotions are owned and expressed to attachment figures in session (rather than in imagined interactions as in individual therapy), the two interventions *slice it thinner* and *catch the bullet* are particularly important. Both of these interventions help the therapists manage interactions between partners effectively, exploring the process of risking opening up to a partner or the difficulties of responding to new messages from a partner.

When the therapist first asks Pete to share his newly accessed, panicked response to his wife's angry outbursts directly with her rather than talking to the therapist, he literally freezes in his chair. He points out that this is unnecessary since she has heard what he said, and that it is "stupid" to repeat it. The therapist helps him explore his reluctance to risk engaging with his wife while feeling vulnerable, and to focus on this process and then take a smaller risk—a risk that is sliced thinner. The smaller risk is to talk about the anxiety around sharing itself. With the therapist's help, Pete can tell Marjorie that he is "worried" about directly sharing these kinds of feelings because, "You will laugh at me and see me for a fool, and I will be even more crushed." The therapist validates his risk, and Pete grins widely. But then Marjorie, still caught in her frustration and feelings of abandonment, confirms Pete's fears. She says, "Well, perhaps it *is* foolish for a grown man to get wimped out by his wife getting irritated." The therapist catches the bullet here, turning to Marjorie, and asking, "What happens to you when Pete takes this kind of risk and opens up to you? My sense is some part of you has been wanting him to do just this, to open up and show you his heart, but it is hard for you to take in his message right now. It's hard for you to respond. You are not hearing that he becomes worried just because you are so important to him. [The therapist offers Marjorie a reassuring message here.] You don't see yourself as having the power to 'crush' him! What happens to you as I talk about this with you?" Marjorie begins to look puzzled and looks again at her partner's face. Then she says in a soft voice, "Are you really worried that I would laugh at you? I never see you as caring about what I think!" The therapist asks Marjorie to tell Pete, "I have a hard time hearing you right now—you are playing such different music—I can't quite take it in that what I say has such an impact." After she expresses this thought in her own words, the couple takes a step forward toward connection.

The ability of the therapist to keep his or her balance, to tune in, and to maintain focus and engage, that is, to provide a safe haven and a secure base for exploration, is crucial in all modalities of EFT. However, couple therapy is a modality in which it is particularly easy for the therapist to lose focus and become confused. The therapist has to *follow* both clients' experience, piece their joint experience together, and then *lead* partners systematically into new kinds of interactions. The technique used in this situation is simply called *changing channels,* and it is especially useful with escalated couples whose interactions shift rapidly in terms of content and levels of engagement. In fact, being able to occasionally stop the process of therapy (literally as in, "Stop. Can we stop for a moment? I would like to go back to/focus on . . . "), and change the channel to get back on track, is crucial in all sessions with individuals, couples, and families. An EFT therapist will typically change the channel in the following ways:

- Shift from past to present: "Yes, this happened many years ago, but right now as you talk about this, how do you feel?"

- Shift from individual to cycle/interpersonal context: "And you see yourself as 'lazy,' but it sounds like this dance that has taken over your relationship defeats you, makes it hard to try?"

- Shift from cognition, from exits into abstract discussion and simply talking about something, to engaged emotional exploration: "Yes, that is fascinating. But can we go back here. You used the word 'shattered' a few minutes ago; could you help me, what happens in your body when you say that word?"

- Shift from content to process: "Yes. This is important, but I would like to stop for a moment and go back to the way you guys dance together. It seems as if all these arguments about tasks and stories of incidents take up all the space here. But the dance—the way you guys move with each other, respond to each other—is always the same. You . . . and then you . . . , and it seems that there is no solution. You can never get together and help each other."

- Shift from diagnosis or label to describing behavior patterns: "You see her as 'crazy' and bring up the label the doctor used. What was it, 'borderline'? You just can't see why or how it would make sense that she would demand closeness from you and then, when you offer it, turn it down? Yes?"

Throughout each session, the therapist simultaneously holds in mind the interpersonal context, that is, the dance-cycle systemic perspective, the individual personal perspective, the overall attachment frame, and the therapeutic direction—moving toward the goals of EFT. This may seem complicated at first, but, like playing a musical instrument, it becomes part of muscle memory with time.

STAGE 2: RESTRUCTURING ATTACHMENT— SELF AND SYSTEM

All of the Tango moves apply to Stage 2 of EFT, and we can now simply describe how the change process in this stage unfolds and how these moves become part of this change process. While Stage 1 is about widening the couple's perspective in terms of the nature of their dance and changing the level of the dance's emotional music, Stage 2 is about deepening partners' awareness of their attachment fears and needs and shaping attuned, accessible, responsive, and engaged interactions. Stage 2 is all about shaping constructive dependency. The aim is for withdrawn partners to become more open and engaged, and for blaming partners to ask for their needs to be met in a soft, evocative manner. This stage culminates in specific and special engaged encounters or enactments in couple (EFT) and family (EFFT) therapy, called *re-engagements* and *softenings*, but also referred to as Hold Me Tight conversations. In these encounters, both partners are guided into offering a safe haven and secure base to one another and, ideally, both are able to reach for and respond to the other. These Hold Me Tight bonding conversations predict success at the end of EFT (Greenman & Johnson, 2013) and positive follow-up results, as well as reductions in anxious and avoidant attachment (Burgess Moser et al., 2015). The basic process of change involves three steps: Guided by the therapist, each partner discovers and distills his or her attachment fears and gradually takes the risk to share these fears with his or her partner in a coherent, evocative manner; this partner is guided into more and more accepting responses to these fears in a series of interactions; once this occurs, the vulnerable sharing partner is able to disclose and ask for his or her specific attachment needs to be met; and the other partner now responds with comfort, care, and reassurance. Such events are transformative on many levels. They shift individual existential realities, the definitions of self and of other encapsulated in "hot" cognitive working models, habitual affect regulation strategies, and each person's sense of relationship agency.

Pete is able to identify his deep fears of being found wanting, or as his father used to put it, "just not man enough." He can access his constant vigilance for signs that he is not "getting it right" with Marjorie and share how this fear "stops me dead in my tracks." Marjorie is now more able to hear him and respond with empathy. Pete then weeps and moves into sharing attachment needs, telling Marjorie that it is too hard to dance with her while she judges him so harshly, and that he longs for the reassurance that, even if he is never totally sure and strong, she accepts him and chooses him as her partner. As Pete becomes more present and engaged, Marjorie is also able to really touch and explore her "terror" of finding that she will never matter to anyone, that she will always be kept on the "outside" as "too difficult to love." Pete can now respond with attuned caring, and his wife moves into actively reaching and owning her attachment needs to be told she is "wanted, needed, that I belong to you." Clinical practice and research results tell us that these kinds of interactions, where vulnerability is shared and held, are classic corrective emotional experiences that move partners from insecure to secure connection and lead to stable changes in self and system.

Stage 2 Process in the Couple Modality

The Tango interventions as they are used in Stage 2 are pitched at a deeper level and require partners to take more significant personal risks. In particular, Tango Move 2, especially the *deepening* of emotional awareness and expression, is stressed here, as vulnerabilities are made concrete and specific. This deepening stage then results in more intense and transformative sharing in the engaged encounters set up in Tango Move 3. Experiential techniques, such as attuned process reflections, evocative questions, conjectures, reframes, and validations, continue to be used in Stage 2 of EFT with couples, albeit with more focus and intensity. The one technique that is almost exclusive to Stage 2 of EFT is *seeding attachment* (Johnson, 2004), which is usually employed as a prelude to or to address blocks to choreographing more engaged interactions in Tango Move 3. Here a partner's reluctance to risk reaching for the other is at once validated and challenged by a simple image of possible secure interactions. This technique is particularly useful when partners do not seem to have ever experienced this security, either in their families of origin or in their romantic relationships, and have no image of what secure interactions look like. The therapist conjectures what a secure interaction might look like at a certain moment, so as to present a foreign, but potentially positive, image. The therapist might say:

"Yes, I understand that it seems strange to you to even think of turning toward your partner when you feel vulnerable. You have never experienced how this might turn out. You could never imagine, right now, turning to your partner and telling her, 'I am scared and my instinct is to hide, but really I want you to help me with this fear so I am not so alone with it.' To say that would seem weird and strange. You can't imagine your partner being touched by this and wanting to comfort you. All your images are of others despising you and turning away. So this is hard—to even let her in a little—yes? What happens to you as I say this to you?"

This seeding intervention seems to prime attachment longings and also to expand clients' sense of what is possible.

As stated earlier, the emotional exploration of core themes and triggers is now deepened and emotions take on a more existential tone in Stage 2. The therapist stays longer with the process of really engaging emotions such as fear, shame, and sadness that have been previously outlined and assembled. In the service of deepening emotional experience, the therapist typically uses repetition and images, and the emotional "handles" the client has already identified, to *hold* clients in their experience and distill the meaning of this experience. The goal is to stay at the cutting edge of clients' awareness and their ability to tolerate a felt sense of vulnerability. This vulnerability usually involves contacting attachment longings and catastrophic fears of isolation and loss of belonging. Again, as noted earlier, core definitions of self and other are discovered and explored here, and core attachment experiences are more fully engaged with. At this point, clients can also see the significance of and tolerate the therapist working with their partner for longer periods in session.

This deeper engagement with emotion allows for the more authentic and intimate disclosures that characterize Hold Me Tight conversations. Generally the therapist begins by working most actively with the more withdrawn partner and helping him or her to gradually disclose attachment fears and needs to his or her partner, who is then guided to take in, accept, and begin to respond to these messages. The therapist asks the withdrawn partner to begin this process of reaching for secure connection before asking the more blaming partner to take the same risks. This prevents a relapse triggering scenario whereby the blaming partner moves into vulnerable risking and reaching only to be met with more stonewalling or lack of response. Both partners need to be on the dance floor to shape a new kind of dance.

This process of discovering softer core emotions, distilling them, and then disclosing both fears and needs is then repeated with the more blaming partner. Once this process is complete, mutual accessibility, responsiveness, and engagement elicit transformational, full-blown bonding sequences and responses. These responses are heightened by the therapist, and their significance for each partner and for the connection in the relationship are outlined. These are termed *softenings* in the literature, because both partners have moved into vulnerable emotions; blaming partners have "softened" their more aggressive stance, and withdrawn partners have taken down their rigid walls. The more intense and more structured enactments, in which withdrawn partners open up and actively define the relationship they want and blaming partners ask for what they need from a position of vulnerability, shape new dances, that is, new cycles of positive attachment interactions that create secure connection, sometimes for the first time in clients' lives. Tango Moves 2 and 3 are at the heart of these Hold Me Tight softening change events. Deeper experience of attachment emotions leads to direct reaching for the other and invites compassion and connection from the other. The essence of bonding is vulnerability felt and responded to.

Tango Move 5, validation, often has a different quality in Stage 2 of EFT and EFFT. As a therapist, I am often powerfully moved by partners or by a parent and child finding each other, perhaps for the first time. Of course, it is also moving in EFIT to see how an imaginary encounter with a loved one plays out into a more profound level of connection. But to be part of this drama as it unfolds between intimates in session, as they both stumble toward connection, has a unique ability to grab the heart of the attuned therapist. I am even more likely to validate with tears in my eyes here and to feel thankful to my clients for teaching me in a concrete and immediate way about my own humanity.

So how can we capture the unfolding of Stage 2 of EFT with a couple? Pete is encouraged at the beginning of Stage 2 to really move into and engage with his fear that he will "never be man enough for Marjorie." He begins to not just name, but to feel and be able to tolerate and walk around in, this fear of always being found unworthy by others. On an existential level, this triggers deep hopelessness and helplessness. He shares this helplessness as the therapist helps him step into Tango Move 3—a more engaged interaction. The therapist then helps Marjorie hear this and tell Pete that she never understood how her comments might trigger these feelings in him and how she does not want him to be caught in this pain. The therapist then asks Pete how Marjorie could help him with this painful place that he spends so much of his energy trying to push aside. (Note how the EFT therapist actively encourages the coregulation of difficult emotions, rather than containment or self-soothing.) Pete tells the therapist, and then is able to tell his wife, that he needs to hear the message that he is special and valued by her; that he can make mistakes and still be seen this way. Marjorie responds with empathy and caring, and her husband weeps with relief and amazement. As this process has unfolded, the therapist has also been supporting Marjorie to slowly get in touch with her fear (in the deepening process that is part of Tango Move 3). She is able to articulate that if she risks really reaching for Pete, she will find that her needs are judged as "irrelevant," and she will know that she is forever alone. Now the therapist normalizes these fears and supports Marjorie to stay with her softer emotions, rather than trying to tell her husband how to solve their marital issues. She is guided into a series of structured enactments in which she touches and deepens her awareness and then shares this with Pete, who is now responsive and engaged. She is able to tell him of her need for reassurance when she accesses her pain at never being able to count on others to be there for her. Both partners provide an antidote bonding experience for the other where models of self and other are revised and emotional repertoires expanded. Hold Me Tight conversations change our world into a safer place where we can trust others to be there for us.

In this creation of positive cycles of accessibility and responsiveness, it helps the therapist to be generally aware of the blocks to the attachment process I have outlined. In particular, in Stage 2, attachment injuries, best described as moments when violations of attachment assumptions at moments of intense need have occurred, have to be dealt with. These injuries have most often been described in attachment terms and placed into the couple's cycle in Stage 1 sessions, but now have to be directly addressed and healed for new levels of accessibility and responsiveness to occur. The forgiveness conversation and the healing of such injuries constitute a specific form of Hold Me Tight conversation. For example, Marjorie, when exploring her fears of reaching for Pete, returns to an injury that she referred to in early sessions when she needed him to go with her to a medical procedure and, from her point of view, he dismissed her need as immature and left her to deal with the procedure on her own. The steps of this conversation, including stating the pain of the injury, having the other partner hear this pain and take responsibility for the fact that it occurred, helping the injured one understand the other's frame of mind when it occurred, having the hurt one openly express this pain in coherent attachment terms, and helping the other respond with remorse and caring in a way that heals this injury, are outlined in detail in the EFT literature (Johnson, 2004; Zuccarini, Johnson, Dalgleish, & Makinen, 2013).

From the EFT point of view, extramarital affairs, a common issue in couple therapy, are viewed as attachment injuries. There is usually one moment of acute pain that is viewed as epitomizing the pain of the affair. As already stated, the EFT therapist places events in an attachment frame and helps the wounded client move into this pain and regulate and share it in a way that fosters empathy, remorse, and reassurance from the injuring partner (MacIntosh, Hall, & Johnson, 2007; Johnson, 2005). The nature of such injuries and of the forgiveness and reconciliation process are clarified and kept on track by seeing these phenomena in an attachment frame.

STAGE 3: CONSOLIDATION

The goals of the third stage of EFT with couples are to stabilize, reinforce, and celebrate the changes, both within and between partners, that have been made in previous sessions and to help partners come together as a team to deal with pragmatic problems. Previous sessions have focused mainly on the process of affect regulation and engagement with others, rather than the content of issues and problems. Now, the newfound safety with one's own emotional life and with close others fosters tolerance of differences, effective cooperation, and coordination of responses and empathy, so that previously impossible problems can be addressed and solved relatively easily. The therapist can simply facilitate a goal-oriented conversation between partners, mostly using mirroring—Tango Move 1—to keep them on track. For example, as Pete and Marjorie openly discuss their parenting problems, they find that their parenting goals are actually almost identical, but that Pete is more comfortable with a more collaborative style with their teenage daughter, whereas Marjorie is more anxious for her daughter's safety and becomes more dictatorial. When Pete can listen to Marjorie and calm some of her fears around her daughter, they can come up with parenting plans that suit them both. The therapist encourages the couple to look at content issues and to deal with them, using their newfound openness and responsiveness. Security increases flexibility and the ability to explore options, and the therapist validates this new found collaborative stance. The couple also literally seem to have more energy to dedicate to this process, given that they do not spend so much of it being vigilant for threatening and defensive maneuvers. The teaching of communication or problem-solving skills, a large part of many couple interventions, does not seem to add anything to the effectiveness of EFT (James, 1991). Rather, the couple experience new emotional balance and learn new ways to engage each other organically, from the inside out.

The therapist also reflects, validates, and celebrates the couple's new dance of positive responsiveness (a more-than-usually intense Tango Move 5) and helps partners create a new integrative narrative of how they have transformed their relationship and moved from helplessness to agency. This narrative acts as a reference point for the future and empowers the couple to deal with future difficulties (Johnson, 2004). EFT therapists expect their clients to continue to grow their relationship and grow in their relationship; there is evidence of this continued growth after EFT in follow-up studies.

Clinical observation and attachment science suggest that the lack of relapse associated with EFT is associated with five factors:

1. The compelling and inherently rewarding power of positive bonding interactions that continue to resonate and offer the couple a

safe haven and secure base. The human brain is designed to hold onto this crucial, survival-oriented information.

2. The new ability on the part of partners to maintain inner coherence and order in the face of vulnerability that is associated with better affect regulation and more secure connection.

3. The shifts in sexual and caregiving connection that accompany more secure interactions.

4. The potent memory of risks shared and responded to, and trust rewarded, that offset hurts and misattunements when they do arise.

5. The redefinition of close relationships as understandable and manageable and the self as a competent interactional partner.

At the end of EFT, partners know the music, understand why it is so compelling, and grasp how to dance together in harmony and also how to reset music and steps when the dance goes wrong.

All of these stages tend to take more time and require more repetition when mental health problems complicate relationship distress (see EFT adapted to PTSD issues in Johnson, 2002). Among these problems are extreme withdrawal, including Asperger syndrome; limited ability to use language (Stiell & Gailey, 2011); and extremely escalated interactions. These issues are all placed within the context of default-option affect regulation strategies and interpersonal cycles of disconnection and connection with attachment figures. Highly escalated couples tend to alarm and overwhelm therapists. The EFT therapist sees such escalation mostly in terms of desperate attempts to gain a sense of control when the threats of rejection and abandonment take over, and so is able to reach below the explicit aggression for the vulnerability that is triggered and use reflections and reframes. The therapist also becomes more directive and takes control of the interactions between the couple, slowing them down and reflecting the dance, as it catches both partners up in its rhythms. So the therapist tells Pete and Marjorie at one point:

"I want you to stop right here. Stop. You are both getting caught in this Find the Bad Guy conversation, where each of you proves to the other that they are a bad partner and almost unlovable! You are both labeling and triggering each other, smacking each other's raw spots, and fanning the flames. Everyone is getting burned here. This began when, Marjorie, you were talking about Pete letting you down by not coming to the hospital, and, Pete, you defended yourself by calling your wife out as a tyrant who gives orders. I would like to go back. . . . "

The therapist then reflects and empathizes with both partners' softer underlying hurts and fears and moves the conversation onto a safer level.

NEW DIRECTIONS FOR ATTACHMENT-ORIENTED COUPLE INTERVENTIONS

The new vision offered by attachment science opens up new pathways for clinicians, who help couples create more positive and lasting relationships, to explore new ways to use couple interventions in the service of health and happiness.

Educational Programs

Once we understand love and attachment, we can educate couples more effectively and prevent relationship problems. The integration of the attachment view of love and couple intervention has resulted in a new, preventative educational program called Hold Me Tight®: Conversations for Connection (Johnson, 2010). This program is based on *Hold Me Tight: Seven Conversations for a Lifetime of Love* (Johnson, 2008a), a book for the general public that, in turn, is based on many years of research and practice in EFT and on the science of attachment that underlies that practice. This positive outcome of this educational program has recently been replicated (Kennedy, Johnson, Wiebe, & Tasca, in press; Conradi, Dingemanse, Noordhof, Finkehauer, & Kamphuis, 2017) in several studies in community settings with more novice and experienced leaders. This program is now offered in many different languages across the globe. It has also been adapted for use with Christian couples and educational groups offered by churches (Johnson & Sanderfer, 2017) based on a Christian adaption of *Hold Me Tight,* entitled *Created for Connection* (Johnson & Sanderfer, 2016). It is interesting to note that the stories of Christ's actions in scripture provide an exemplar of accessibility, responsiveness, and engagement, and there is now a fascinating literature on God as an attachment figure. Hold Me Tight® is the first relationship educational program that is based on a clear, substantiated understanding of romantic love and on an extensively researched method of relationship repair and maintenance. This program reflects the ability of attachment science to change our cultural awareness of the nature of adult love relationships, just as the science has already changed our awareness of the needs of children and our parenting practices.

Physical Health Interventions

A clear link has emerged in the last few years between physiological functioning and health and the quality of social support and close connection with others, so it makes sense that couple-based interventions for medical problems are becoming more common (Baucom, Porter, Kirby, & Hudepohl, 2012). Positive close relationships have an impact on specific indicators of health; for example, interactions with attachment figures (family members and partners) have been found to be associated with lower rates of ambulatory blood pressure compared to other social interactions (Gump, Polk, Kamarck, & Shiffman, 2001; Holt-Lunstad, Uchino, Smith, Olson-Cerny, & Nealey-Moore, 2003). *Attachment interactions regulate physiology, and partners become internalized as representations of safety or danger, that is at the level of emotional and physiological realities.* Specific links between health conditions and attachment have been found; for example, chronic pain has been linked to insecurity, and anxious attachment seems to be especially associated with cardiovascular disease (McWilliams & Bailey, 2010). Specifically, links have been outlined between heart disease, immune function, and chronic stress responses and relationship factors, such as hostile criticism, or positive factors, such as a calming, felt sense of security (Pietromonaco & Collins, 2017; Uchino, Smith, & Berg, 2014). The shaping of interpersonal support has now begun to be seen as an essential element in health promotion and positive coping with illness. It makes sense then that the Hold Me Tight® educational program is now used as part of the treatment protocol for recovery from heart attack and the ongoing management of cardiac disease. This program, entitled Healing Hearts Together (Tulloch, Greenman, Demidenko, & Johnson, 2017), is now routinely implemented in a large cardiac hospital in Ottawa, Canada, and positive preliminary outcomes have been collected (Tulloch, Johnson, Greenman, Demidenko, & Clyde, 2016). As Mike, who has a new heart in his chest, tells me:

> "Just when my world fell apart and I was most vulnerable, Lise and I started fighting about how much wine I should drink and me taking my meds. I knew this put my heart rate through the roof, and it got me so agitated that I would forget my meds altogether, and she was getting depressed. We needed some help here. I need her with me and supporting me if my new heart is going to keep going, and my anxiety is going to be manageable."

Different versions of this educational program have also been adapted for couples facing Parkinson's disease, cancer, and diabetes. As the famous study by House, Landis, and Umberson (1988) delivered many years ago, emotional isolation is more disastrous for health than smoking, obesity, or lack of exercise. Attachment science, by integrating biology and social connection, offers us targeted prevention and health-enhancing interventions to promote the antidote to such toxic isolation.

Effectively Addressing Caregiving and Sexuality

Attachment realities shape the other two key elements of adult relationships, caregiving and sexuality. The map provided by attachment here, as in every other area, helps the therapist understand and deal with issues in an on-target manner.

Caregiving that is colored by high levels of anxious attachment tends to lack attunement and be less effective. Caregiving strategies then become compulsive and controlling and less accurate in terms of interpreting a partner's needs. Highly avoidant partners tend to be dismissing of their own and their partner's needs, less empathic, and less likely to see others as deserving of care (Feeney & Collins, 2001). This seems to be equally true in same-sex couple relationships (Bouaziz, Lafontaine, Gabbay, & Caron, 2013). Significantly for the couple therapist, subliminal priming procedures aimed at enhancing a sense of security effectively elicit compassionate and supportive behavior (Milkulincer et al., 2001, 2005). This priming effect parallels clinical experience in EFT, where it is rarely the case that a partner, even an avoidant one, when supported by the therapist, cannot begin to respond to the other partner's expressed vulnerability in key bonding interactions. Consider Andrew, the epitome of silent nonresponsiveness at the beginning of therapy. Ten weeks later, when his wife, Louise, expresses pain at the loss of her dreams of closeness with him, Andrew is able to say, "When you cry, I get all confused. Part of me just wants to run. But then I remember the things you have said in these sessions and my body feels warmer. I don't want you to hurt, and I don't want to hurt you. I want to comfort you. I am just not sure how to do this. Can you help me?"

The literature on sexuality and attachment has exploded in the last few years (see Mikulincer & Shaver, 2016, for a review; Johnson, 2017). Conceptually and clinically it makes sense that the qualities that define a secure bond, that is, accessibility/openness, responsiveness, and attuned engagement with others, also enhance the ability to read intentions, coordinate cues, and come together in the bedroom. Security shapes confidence and comfort and the ability to explore sensuality, as well as the ability to let go and play in sexual interactions (Birnbaum, Reis, Mikulincer, Gillath, & Orpaz, 2006). Casual, detached sex, an exclusive focus on performance and sensation with low levels of intimacy, and less sexual satisfaction are more common in avoidant partners; while a focus on sex as a barometer of love and on closeness with one's partner is more common in those who are anxiously attached. Insecurity lends itself to lower sexual self-esteem and higher anxiety, especially in women. In general, a secure, connected, positive relationship appears to be the best recipe for sexual fulfillment (Johnson & Zuccarini, 2010). This is reflected in the fact that a much improved sex life in terms of frequency and satisfaction is routinely reported by couples at the end of EFT (Wiebe et al., in press). This echoes a recent finding that levels of closeness and sensitivity, which may be expected to rise in EFT, are the main factors linking insecure attachment and lower sexual satisfaction in both distressed and nondistressed couples (Peloquin, Brassard, Delisle, & Bedard, 2013; Peloquin, Brassard, Lafontaine, & Shaver, 2014).

Attachment then offers a bridge that allows us to integrate sexuality and relatedness in a specific and concise way that integrates couple- and sex-therapy interventions (Johnson, 2017). Just as Hawton, Catalin, and Fagg (1991) found years ago, it is the EFT experience that communication patterns at the beginning of therapy predict partners reports of sexual satisfaction, and additionally, that as these patterns change, they positively impact sexual connection. This may be especially crucial in terms of women's satisfaction, since all the evidence on female arousal suggests that women monitor the level of safe connection in a relationship before allowing their physical arousal to be experienced as actual desire, and that this desire is also often in response to feeling desired by the other, rather than to spontaneous lust (Gillath, Milkulincer, Birnbaum, & Shaver, 2008; Basson, 2000).

The EFT therapist helps couples outline cycles of sexual interaction, whether they mirror a couple's main patterns or provide a contrast to those patterns. More avoidant, withdrawn men do reach out in their sexual dance, but are often rebuffed, since they do not offer safe emotional connection elsewhere. If the therapist aids these partners in moving into their emotions and helps them to share the need to feel desired, doing so can shift the other partner's perception that he or she is just an instrument to achieve orgasm, and so create a new climate in the bedroom. New perspectives that tie attachment realities to sexual behavior shape new and targeted interventions. The EFT therapist is more likely to work from the organic base—the within, bottom-up base of emotions and how they are expressed by the body—to shape new positive sexual cycles, rather than rely on top-down, skill- or technique-oriented interventions. Such interventions become irrelevant when they do not jibe with a partner's emotional reality. When Terry is able to express the deep fear of failure that triggers his erectile dysfunction and receive comfort from his wife, while also hearing that for her the best part of lovemaking is tender touch from him, he catastrophizes less. He and his wife can become a team dealing together with the occasional wilting of his erection.

When working with same-sex couples (Allan & Johnson, 2016; Johnson & Zuccarini, 2011), all the principles and techniques we have discussed apply. It is a fascinating irony that just as heterosexual couples seem to be turning toward more detached, less-committed relationships in hookups or open relationships, the group of people associated with promiscuity in most people's minds, young gay males, are now turning toward monogamy and commitment. This makes sense. It is hard to hope for and believe in secure attachment and commitment when your relationships are outlawed. Research documents that some 82% of this gay male population now aspire to committed long term relationships (Gotta et al., 2011). The attachment-oriented therapist accepts the evidence of attachment science, that human beings are naturally wired for romantic love and what Bowlby called hierarchical attachments. We can be attached to a few precious others at the same time, but we usually have a central and primary attachment figure, and we will fight to hold onto and protect this relationship. Secure attachment is a primary and supremely functional life strategy, and extremely hard to create and sustain in more detached, less-committed relationships. Attachment actively challenges us to revise some of the old myths and conventions around sexuality, for example, that long-term commitment to one person naturally results in a dull familiarity that kills eroticism, and that constant novelty is the main ingredient in passion. This view confuses the alive, active engagement that typifies secure connection with constrained lack of intimacy and responsiveness. In a loving bond, in which disconnection naturally occurs, but is followed by reattunement and re-engagement, partners fall in love again and again over the lifespan of their relationship.

CONCLUSION

Acevedo and Aron (2009), completed a brain scan study showing that physiological responses to a partner in a certain proportion of recent and long-term lovers were identical, suggesting that romantic love is much more than an ephemeral response and can last over time. In another study, these researchers and other colleagues (O'Leary, Acevedo, Aron, Huddy, & Mashek, 2012) found that 40% of those married more than 10 years reported being "very intensely in love." They have then directly challenged couple therapists to focus on intentionally shaping the responses that we call love, rather than addressing everything but these responses, and hoping that love returns as a result of other, less-central changes. Obviously, to respond to this challenge, the therapist has to have a detailed, explicit understanding of love itself. Attachment science offers us this understanding. The central bonding question, "Are you there for me?" is implicit (and at times explicit, indeed) in all chronic relationship distress; however, partners may not know how to formulate their distress in these terms. The consistent reports of couples in clinical practice, the lack of dropouts in research studies and practice, and the results of EFT in general point to the perceived *relevance* of this focus on love and emotional connection for clients, who very often tell EFT therapists, "You are getting to the heart of the matter here. This bonding stuff really hits the nail on the head. For the first time things make sense." Attachment science and practice based on this science offer couple therapists a safe haven and secure base on which to stand and find their confidence and creativity. Standing on the solid ground of attachment science, the field of couple intervention can move forward on a whole new level.

A HOMEPLAY EXERCISE

For You Personally

Can you pinpoint a pattern or negative cycle that you become stuck in with a partner or someone you love? In the simplest terms possible can you outline the steps in this negative dance? Do this as if you were watching what each person does—how each one moves. Try doing this from a distance, with no judgments, and also note how each person's actions trigger the other's in a recurring feedback loop ("The more you . . . , the more I then . . . , and the more I . . . ").

How do you deal with your most vulnerable emotions in this drama? What signals would you be sending to the other—what would the partner see? How might an empathic therapist summarize the dance the two of you do in a way that felt safe and seen? How might this therapist then reflect the surface feelings you were showing and begin to introduce the underlying, more vulnerable feelings you are feeling in this situation, especially any attachment fears that arise.

See if you can write down what this therapist might say.

For You Professionally

A couple, Zena and Ted, become stuck in their usual negative cycle which looks like this:

> ZENA: (*Very calm, reasonable tone and writing notes on a pad.*) I really don't think this is a useful discussion, Ted. We can simply pay the bills any way you prefer. There are many ways to do it. (*Lists three complicated alternatives.*) I don't see the point in getting emotional about pragmatic issues like bill paying. (*Begins to outline how her sister and her husband deal with this issue.*)

> TED: (*Agitated and angry.*) How did we get here? I was talking about how we never talk about anything about us! When is it okay to get emotional—can you tell me, Miss always cool as a cucumber? I was talking about how worried I get about money. I don't need a damned lecture on what your sister does. (*Slams his hand on his*

knee.) If I want a chartered accountant for a wife, I will go out and find one. You are like a ticker tape machine just spewing out advice all the time. (*Covers his eyes with his hands.*) I don't even feel like we are a couple any more.

ZENA: (*Blinks rapidly, takes a deep breath, and leans back in her chair.*) I would like you to be reasonable here. I really don't understand why you get so upset. It seems that you are always upset. Some men would appreciate a wife who helps with problems like this. But it seems that no matter what I try to do these days . . . (*Long pause; runs one hand over the other a number of times.*) This is one of these moments when, if we were at home, I would usually just give up and go up to my study to wait until you calm down. You do not appreciate my . . . efforts.

TED: (*Turning to the therapist.*) She doesn't get why I am upset. Maybe I don't even get why I am so upset! Am I a nutcase? Do you get why I am so upset here?

How would you, in the simplest terms, reflect this couple's cycle to them as it occurs here, include its apparent attachment consequences, and end with one statement that frames this dance as the problem in this relationship?

How would you reply to Ted's question using an attachment frame, without invalidating or criticizing his partner?

Try writing out what you would say. (This is play, so again, there are no wrong answers.)

 TAKE IT HOME AND TO HEART

- Couple therapy, if it is to be on target and effective, requires a map outlining the essential nature of love relationships, of what goes wrong, and what exactly is needed to put it right.

- Emotional disconnection and deprivation—unmet attachment needs for comfort, support, and care—are at the heart of relationship distress. The solution is the shaping of emotional accessibility, responsiveness, and engagement (A.R.E.—as in "Are you there for me?").

- EFT for couples meets the criteria for the highest level of empirical validation as set out by the American Psychological Association's couple and family division and has been found to change the quality of attachment in couple relationships.

- The stages of therapy—stabilization, restructuring attachment, and consolidation—and the key therapeutic change process and interventions are the same for EFT and EFIT. The essential moves of the Tango are the same across modalities, except for some modifications that arise from the fact that two, often warring, parties are in the session with the therapist, rather than just the therapist and an individual client. For example, outlining the negative cycle—the "demon" dialogue in the mirroring present process Move of the EFT Tango—is more elaborate, and some interventions, such as *catch the bullet* and *seeding attachment,* are more relevant and frequent.

- The four cycles found in distressed relationships, in which partners flip between pursuing and fleeing, are *Find the Bad Guy, Criticize and Withdraw, Freeze and Flee,* and *Chaos and Ambivalence.*

- The couple therapist has to know how to change channels with clients to keep a focus on the present, on the cycle rather than on one partner's flaws, on emotion rather than on abstract discussion, on process rather than on content, and on concrete behavior rather than on labels or diagnoses.

- As always, blocks to the shaping of constructive dependency, such as past injuries that prevent risk taking in session, are targeted. The EFT therapist approaches such blocks with the client and "softens" them. Bonding events—Hold Me Tight® conversations—that change relationship security and partners' working models of self can then take place. In bonding events, Tango Moves 2–4 are intensified and used until new levels of safe engagement are attained.

- Understanding love relationships and the crucial nature of emotional responsiveness allows us to craft new relationship-education programs, such as the Hold Me Tight® program, to use this kind of program to address physical health problems that challenge relationships, and to understand other aspects of love relationships, like sex and caregiving, in new ways.

- What you understand, you can shape. Attachment science is taking us into a new era of conceptualizing romantic relationships and creating effective couple interventions.

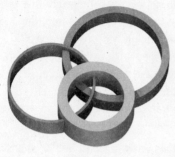

Chapter 7

Emotionally Focused Couple Therapy in Action

There are many case examples and transcripts of successful EFT change processes in the couple therapy literature, as well as training DVDs of these processes at different stages of therapy and with different kinds of couples (see lists of chapters, articles, and training DVDs at *www.iceeft. com*). Rather than presenting another such case, in this chapter I present a consultation session with a challenging couple, who are chronically distressed and have issues that block relationship repair.

SARAH AND GALEN: THE BACK STORY

This couple have been in EFT therapy on and off for several years. According to their therapist, they have struggled through to the end of the stabilization stage. At this point, their negative cycle of distress is now de-escalated, and a secure base has been established for the growth of positive bonding cycles. But now, the therapist is stuck, and progress seems to be stymied.

Sarah came to North America as an immigrant in her 20s from what appears to have been a very abusive background. As a child she was physically, sexually, and emotionally bullied and demeaned constantly, especially by an older relative. She then met Galen, married him, and quickly had two children. From the beginning their relationship has consisted of "decades of violent fighting," with Sarah pursuing Galen for the first few years but then moving into rage, constant threats to leave, and stonewalling. Galen then shifted into pursuing her. Sarah admits that her habitual "defense" is to hurl "vicious insults" at Galen and "spray him with bullets."

In one incident of violence years ago Galen spent the night in jail but was not charged. Physical violence was not a concern at the time they entered therapy or at the time of this session. Before this consultation, Sarah had engaged an army of lawyers, but agreed to one more try at changing the relationship. Neither partner seems to have ever experienced secure attachment in their childhood or with each other. Galen reports that he has never known love and acceptance, and Sarah seems to be dealing with complex trauma, as identified by trauma expert Judith Herman (1992); that is, she is someone who experienced a "violation of human connection" as a child. Other people are then, at the same time, an active source of fear and a much needed solution to fear. As I listen to the therapist's presentation of this case, it occurs to me that if Sarah had been seen in my hospital clinic years ago, she would have undoubtedly have already been labeled borderline. As I go into the session, I say to myself, "This is then a 'trauma couple' (Johnson, 2002; Greenman & Johnson, 2012), whose attachment panic and vigilance for danger and injury are always primed, and this sensitivity has been exacerbated by more than 20 years of chronic conflict. So, tread softly, then."

The goal of the session, set by the therapist who is bringing the couple in, is to reinforce de-escalation and to work through one of the key blocks to progress in Stage 2 of EFT—the ability of one partner, in this case the female partner, to see and take in the vulnerable reaching of the other, that is, to begin to trust these new signals, so that a corrective experience of safe connection can begin. The therapist tells me that the couple know their negative cycle and the impact they have on each other and that Galen is now taking a risk and reaching for his partner, but continually comes up against a wall of suspicion and sarcasm from Sarah. She sees herself as either in her "turtle shell" or as a "warrior," always ready to go into "battle mode."

In the few minutes before the session begins, Sarah turns to me and asks, "Do people really hope for love? Really?" I do not get a chance to answer her before the session begins.

CONSULTATION SESSION

After introductions and small talk, we begin.

> SARAH: (*To me.*) So, I think this stuff works but . . . what happens if two people aren't right for each other then, just grow differently?

SUE: Oh. Not sure any two people are really ever "right" for each other over the long haul. Most of us don't know how to dance close—together—but hopefully we can teach each other. If we are precious to each other we stay, and struggle and learn. There is no perfect person waiting out there. But some relationships are easier. I hear that you two didn't have a huge bank account of trust and safety to draw on when you met. But it sounds like you have already grown lots here—shown lots of courage fighting for your relationship!

GALEN: We have never gotten to the place where we stand and hold hands and look at the sunset together! (*Laughs.*) It's almost like I am used to our relationship being a battle!

SARAH: (*To me.*) But now I just stay quiet—say nothing. We've had quite a battle. Fight like cats and dogs.

GALEN: But now she never dances with me at all! We have reached some place of . . .

SARAH: Comfort . . . more peaceful . . .

GALEN: But I wish it could go further; it's difficult you know. . . . What's the next step?

SUE: Aha. Now you would like to know how to create the standing-in-the-sunset place together part?—Yes? You want to be more together with Sarah? (*Galen nods.*)

GALEN: But I don't want to say anything that might cause . . .

SUE: An argument. (*Galen nods.*) So you tell yourself that you need to be careful, cautious? Maybe waiting for a sign from her that she is ready to let you in?

GALEN: Exactly. Exactly. But I don't get it.

SUE: So things are calmer—less dangerous. And you are standing outside the door waiting—saying, "Here I am—wanting to be closer. Are you going to let me in?" [Reflect present process—beginning to shift into Tango Move 1—capturing the most essential elements of his position.]

GALEN: I am waiting. I am waiting. (*Looking at Sarah.*)

SUE: (*Turning to Sarah.*) What happens to you when this man says, "Sarah, I am waiting at the door"?

SARAH: (*Smiles.*) Well, I like to be chased. I don't pursue anymore. I did that for years and years. But sometimes I want to get into a fight to actually have action in the house. If I withdraw . . . , I still feel rejected somehow. Loss of power. But, if you don't want to pursue me, that is fine. I don't care.

SUE: Hm. Even though they were bad, there was connection in the fights? Now you can withdraw, but it somehow feels like a loss—not so powerful—you still hurt. It's almost like some part of you is saying, "I need you to come and walk through the door and tell me you want me 'cause deep inside I still feel rejected?"—Do I have it?

SARAH: Kind of. He wasn't honest with me when we got married. I checked and found out stuff about his family that he hadn't told me.

SUE: And that rang alarm bells for you. (*Sarah nods.*) You have very good reasons for being vigilant. Those who came close to you when you were young were dangerous, so the alarm bells rang. And then you got into this long battle with Galen and hurt each other badly. (*Sarah nods again.*) [Validating her wariness] And, Galen, you are scared of making a mistake here so you wait . . . for her signal. (*To Sarah.*) But it's like you are saying to him, "Aren't you going to come and get me then? I don't want to risk or reach. I don't even know how to open the door."

SARAH: When he sleeps downstairs, I leave him there. But I am pissed off he hasn't come to bed. And then when he does come, I am still pissed off. It's like—"Oh now you are here are you!" [Here we see a set of classic no solution binds; she cannot risk or reach, but she is still deprived, and when he does come close, she resents and rejects him. The road to healing connection is closed.]

SUE: Hm. So you are refusing to chase him but are still kind of mad that he isn't chasing you. (*Sarah laughs.*) He is waiting for you to show you want him, is that okay, Galen? (*Galen nods.*) Neither of you has what you want. You have a truce but . . . and it seems like neither of you really knows what a good relationship would even look like here? It's foreign territory—strange. So no one really knows how to move. But it's like you are saying, Sarah, "I still feel rejected. I have a raw place where I hurt. I need you to show me you want me—to come and get me— invite me in"? [Heighten attachment message—clarify her signal. Setting the stage for the work of the session—focusing on her block to responding to his overtures.]

SARAH: Yes. I would say so. Yes . . . I don't know how to lean forward. I have to go on the gondola. I can't climb anymore. And then, there were those times . . . (*Turning to Galen.*) you weren't there for me. My sister had to come to pick me up at the hospital when I had our second child. Times like that.

SUE: Yes. Those memories still ache, yes? (*She nods assent.*) And they remind you of how dangerous it is to need him—to want to count on him—to open up to him. So you need help from him. After all the struggle, you can't be climbing mountains to try to get to him. [Galen is watching and listening to this intently. Maybe I am presenting a different image of his wife from the one he usually holds.] You need his help with this. You have been so hurt—and you still ache with rejection. You can't reach—not sure even how to give him this message—how to open the door? Even this takes huge courage to be open and say this? [Generally I stay with, reflect, and validate her block—her reluctance to trust. This is also part of Tango Move 1—mirroring her present emotional process.]

SARAH: Yes. I have learned to be independent. So I come across as The Boss. But—it would be nice if he took care of things sometimes. We have hurt each other dreadfully. I was let down and alone for years, and he had his own pain. [This framing tells me they are indeed de-escalated. She can acknowledge his pain.]

SUE: If he took care of things—if he took care of *you*—especially in this. This reaching for a new connection that is kind of unknown, but that you still know you want—because you hurt, you ache when it's not there. Fighting was a terrible way to grab at connection, but . . . withdrawal isn't so good either.

SARAH: If he would take care of the VISA bill—I asked him to reconcile the figures the other day. (*Exits into less intensity.*) He said, "No—don't ask me to do that."

SUE: You need his help now, with moving into this new emotional territory. And it doesn't seem to work to ask for help—even with simple tasks? You are saying something profound here, Sarah. You wanted him to be with you, and he didn't know how to do that, so you went into spraying bullets and lock down. But there is still an ache—a desire to be wanted—reached for— 'cause you are a human being (Tango Move 2—assembling her bodily feeling and meaning making in her present narrative, reaching for the deeper emotion underneath the protective aggression.]

SARAH: (*Fast and in a high voice.*) I don't let him take care of me 'cause he has never done it. I don't lock the door!

SUE: Right. Some part of you wants him to reach in and get you— help you move toward him. But you can't open the door— even though you are still longing—in spite of your anger and decision not to need, to be independent. You are still longing for connection with Galen. (*Sarah smiles at me and nods her head.*) Can you tell him—the door isn't locked but I can't open it? I can't risk being hurt again.

SARAH: I hate this bit—this is the part I hate.

SUE: (*Quietly and gently.*) Everybody hates this bit. It feels risky. Can you tell him—I don't know how to open the door now. It's not safe, too risky. [Tango Move 3—take clarified emotional response and use as music to set up new dance move—a more engaged encounter.]

SARAH: (*With her shoulder turned to Galen.*) I don't know how. I don't know how. How to let you in.

GALEN: (*Looking at me.*) And so I take that as rejection—get confused. So I just try to deal with it on my own.

SUE: Yes. That is so normal, so natural. You guys came into this dance knowing that needing someone was fraught with danger—never having seen what a safe, in-tune dance looks like. So naturally, when you lost your balance and hurt each other, you flayed around, picked up your weapons, put on your armor. But look at you now. You are learning to be open and working so hard here. Listening to the ache that tells you to try to give each other a chance to learn how to love—that is amazing. [Tango Move 5—Validate.] The irony is, Galen, if you didn't love this lady the way you do, you wouldn't feel so threatened—rejected. You would just see her, and respond maybe like you would to a child who needs your help, but you are scared of getting stuck in all those battles and hurts again. So you stand still—unsure.

GALEN: I do love her. I don't want to hurt her.

SUE: Yes. I believe you. What happens to you when she says, "I don't know how to let you in"? [Evocative question technique—part of Tango Move 4—processing the choreographed encounter.]

GALEN: I feel rejected. Not part of a couple.

SUE: Some part of you says, "Maybe she doesn't want me"? That would be scary!

GALEN: Yeah. Scary. And she used to say that in our fights. So I just try to keep the peace . . . but she takes that in a different way.

SUE: Right. So let's stay right here. This is a key moment. You guys get stuck in distance when you could be moving in a whole new direction. Lots of us get stuck here. Your lady is in a strange, scary place—a place she doesn't know—worried about trusting you, and reminding herself of the times when she got hurt—let down—all the aching hurts. Scared to open the door to you. (*I look at Sarah, lean forward, she nods. I put my hand on her knee.*) You know you want more, but you freeze at the idea of another fight—unsure. And you wait for a clear signal from her that she wants to risk coming closer. But there is no clear signal, so you tell yourself, "She doesn't want me anyway." Then she decides that you won't reach for her, so the ache comes up again in her. You both end up feeling rejected—alone and stuck. That is hard, hard. [Return to Tango Move 1—reflect or mirror the presently occurring core relationship-defining emotional dance in attachment terms. The therapist is also outlining the block—the essential stuck place in this couple's relationship.]

GALEN: Exactly. Yes. Exactly. I don't know she is waiting for a signal from me! I don't want to do it wrong.

SUE: Right. You are being careful here—careful. You don't get that she needs your help—that she can't open the door—that she needs you to walk in and pick her up—show her how to be close? (*He looks at Sarah now like he doesn't know who she is.*) But Sarah, you have a hard time sending a clear signal here—yes? You can't really send out a "Come and get me—help me" signal? [This is one of the quintessential blocks to attachment repair and reconnection—she cannot ask for what she needs.]

SARAH: (*Softly.*) I don't do that—I don't want to let him—let him—take care of me.

SUE: (*Leaning forward, in a soft, slow voice.*) Yes. Maybe you have never felt held, soothed, taken care of, and comforted, and learned to let go and relax within that closeness—never had that. So your brain says, "Are you kidding? . . . Watch out. . . . The only real thing is the battle . . . It's not safe." (*Sarah tears.*) But then you are all by yourself. And you have this ache. Because when you met Galen you let yourself long for that safe connection—yes? But you have been so hurt, hurt. It seems safer to just live with the ache—to give up the longing? [Tango Move 2—deepening the emotional conflict between the longing and the fear of hurt.]

SARAH: I can't let go of the hurt from the past. I cannot forget.

SUE: You don't have to forget, Sarah. Those hurts matter. But you and Galen can help each other with them and step past them. I think you have already done some of that in therapy. But right now seems like you are saying to Galen, "I can't risk here. I need your help—can't open the door. I don't even know what being loved really feels like—can't imagine taking that in." Hm . . .

SARAH: (*Softly and full of hesitation.*) I just can't talk about it. I don't know how to do this. (*To Galen.*) I don't know how to ask for your help—to rely on you. [Sarah does Tango Move 3 by herself.]

SUE: (*Softly.*) And it feels dangerous I think. You learned to take care of yourself—watch your back—and fight. And with Galen this happened too. So you're telling him, "I don't know how to open the door so we can learn to dance together in a new way—a safer, closer way." But you are taking a step—right here—sharing this—saying how hard it is. [A brief shift into Tango Moves 4 and 5—processing the encounter and validating/integrating.]

SARAH: Yes. That is encouraging. (*Smiles a little smile.*)

SUE: But Galen—I hear that you are careful. You don't want to go back to the war again. (*Galen nods.*) But do you know how to court her—help her move toward you? Did you court her, way back?

GALEN: (*Smiles.*) Yes. I did. And it helps me a lot to know that she needs my help here. I would like to be here for her. [This confirms their therapist's assessment and statements in his introduction to this case before the session. Galen is re-engaging and trying to be present for his wife.] To know that she needs me! (*He turns to her.*) I need to hear that. Really.

SUE: (*Heightening his message.*) You're saying, "It's scary for me, too, to come close after all our battles and wounds. But if I know you need me . . . , maybe I can figure out how to help. Maybe I can help you feel safe enough to move closer? But it's scary for me too." Can you tell her?

GALEN: (*To me.*) What if I do the wrong step and step on her toes? There is the uncertainty. I might do it wrong. But—if she needs me—then it's like, I have found the answer!

SUE: Aha—That helps so much to know you matter to her—then you have a way forward. So you have been caught in being so careful. Caught in, "I mustn't put one step wrong here." But now, when you hear that underneath this distance, this guardedness, that Sarah still aches with rejection, that she needs some help from you, that she is in foreign territory, that she doesn't know what it really feels like to feel safe and loved and taken care of—so she can't reach for you, can't risk. Then, this feels better, clearer maybe. (*Galen nods.*) [Repetition to help him consolidate this image of his wife and to continue to engage her around this frame.] How does this feel in your body, to hear that she is kind of frozen—waiting for you to court her—to help her move toward you? [Tango Move 4—processing the encounter Galen and Sarah are creating here.]

GALEN: (*Laughs.*) It gives me goosebumps. (*I motion with my hand for him to tell her this. He turns toward her.*) To find out that you need me to help you—to step up and court you. Woooooo! (*Sarah bursts into giggles.*)

SUE: Can you take this in, Sarah? Can you see how he wants to know how to find a way to you?

SARAH: Well . . . I'll try. But the dragon comes up. The part of me that wants to protect me.

SUE: And what does this dragon say to you? (*Sarah is silent.*) Maybe it says that he will let you down again? [Interpretation at the leading edge of her experience in the service of furthering the process of Tango Move 2—deepening the emotion that shapes how she dances with Galen.]

SARAH: That's right on. It says he is going to let me down again.

SUE: Yes. And we do let each other down in love. We can't dance together and always tune in. We can't never step on each other's toes. But you are learning to understand and heal these slips— these misses. And I understand that this is not what you have lived in your life before and with Galen. You got terribly hurt. How does it feel to hear him say he gets goosebumps when he hears that there is a way to get closer to you?

SARAH: Feels good. Good. It's a leap of faith though. It will be a leap of faith. (*Turns to Galen.*) When I have tried to do that, we end up in a fight. You yell at me. [Again Sarah moves into a more engaged encounter with her partner—Tango Move 3— without therapist urging. As therapy progresses, the process of the Tango flows naturally, with the couple taking over from the therapist and shaping the process.]

SUE: How do you feel as you say this? It's a leap. It has been so bad before—you have been so hurt. When you hear that he wants you to risk opening up . . .

SARAH: (*Her face is soft here.*) Scared. How do I know what will happen? I don't feel safe.

SUE: (*Leans forward and touches Sarah's arm.*) Yes. You are saying this is a hard place to be—a scary place—to think of risking, taking a leap of faith, letting in the hope that Galen might be there. It's like, "I will be letting myself long for your love—letting myself hope—following the ache. I will be . . . " [Tango Move 2—deepening emotion—exploring the catastrophic fear that keeps Sarah stuck.]

SARAH: Naked somehow. It's scary just being here now!

SUE: Yes. (*Honoring her ambivalence.*) Some part of you must just be saying don't don't (*Sarah nods and nods.*) that you will be hurt again. But here you are—talking about this leap of faith. You didn't just refuse. You said, "It *will be* a leap of faith." And you are right. He could hurt you—for a moment you won't have your gun and your armor. You asked me that question in the beginning, before the session, about love. Part of you is still struggling here, asking, "Can I hope for this?" You are risking just by being here. And you need his help—to calm the protective dragon part of you? (*Sarah nods.*) You guys scare the hell out of each other. Sounds like you know how to find the soft places and strike or shut the other out in the cold. But here you are—in strange territory. And you are asking, Sarah, "Can there be someone to really take care of me? What happens when I am open and naked with someone—can I make a leap of faith?" So hard. What is happening, Sarah, as we talk? It's such a risk to open up and give him the chance to hold you—court you? [At this kind of moment in EFT the existential significance of a partner's struggle becomes vividly apparent—the themes of isolation, conflict, choice, and the fear of helplessness are clear.]

SARAH: (*Softly.*) Do people do this? Can people do this? I am asking you? Maybe love never works. [This is the kind of question that breaks the therapist's heart, and it is one for which the therapist must have an authentic answer!]

SUE: Yes. People do this. And it's scary for all of us. But it's especially scary when the people you counted on when you were really small wounded you—betrayed you—taught you that closeness was dangerous, and when you and your partner don't know how to create a safe place. You and Galen got so caught in your battles. But people do it. We want something—something really important.

SARAH: Yeah—I want the connection. I want to experience that. I don't think I ever had that at all, not at all. (*She weeps.*)

SUE: Hm—hard to live without that—yes? (*Sarah nods.*) Even if we never had it, we know there is something we are longing for—an ache when it is missing. That is sad—to never have had that—so painful. And the longing is still there. Can you tell him? [Direct priming of innate attachment longing. Tango Move 3, after deepening her emotion, choreographing an engaged encounter in tune with this deepened emotion.]

SARAH: (*To me.*) I never even had that connection with my own mother! No one to protect me—to come for me! I don't know how to do this . . . this connection stuff. (*She weeps.*)

SUE: Aha—So it's so risky even to hope—to sit here and tell Galen, "I need your help. I need you to come and get me, help me open the door. It's sad and scary—and I still want that connection." (*Deepening emotion with proxy voice.*) Can you tell him? (*Motions to Galen.*)

GALEN: (*Breaks in.*) I will show you how to do that. I want to show you. I will help you. I may not be any expert, but I think I can do it—I want to. I learned stuff from being a dad, and my uncle told me . . .

SUE: (*Breaking in—refocusing.*) Galen, you want to be there for her—to stop the ache—to help her feel safe—yes—tell her.

GALEN: (*To Sarah.*) I can't bear to see you sit and cry like this. I will show you how to do it. I will be there. I will make mistakes sometimes, but . . . if I know you need help . . . the mistakes might be hard . . . (*Losing his focus.*)

SUE: You don't want her to hurt? You want to be there for her? To help her feel safe and not have to spend her life getting ready to pick up her gun—that is so lonely. But it's hard for her to risk—to trust. Can you tell her again? [Refocusing and keeping him in Tango Move 3.]

GALEN: (*To Sarah, leaning forward, softly with intensity.*) I just want to be there for you. (*Sarah is staring at Galen.*)

SUE: (*Softly.*) Can you hear him, Sarah? Can you begin to let that in?

SARAH: I am struggling to let it in. My mind is racing—to trust it?

SUE: Yes, it's so hard. To risk in the face of all your hurt. How can he help you? Right here, right now, how can he help you?

GALEN: (*Compellingly.*) Tell me. Tell me. What do you need me to do?

SARAH: (*Changes channel, exits into humor.*) Right here. Nothing—too many people watching!

SUE: (*She has exited, so I work to intensify his invitation.*) Wow, Galen. You are reaching for her right now. It's almost like you are saying, "I just needed the signal to be clear—to know you needed me. I want to help you—not to hurt you." What I see and hear is that you are really with her right now. This feeling is urgent; seeing her caught in her fear and knowing she still wants connection just fires you up! You really want to take care of her, don't you? [Heightening his message and its attachment significance.]

GALEN: Yeah. It's like I wake up—*wow*. I don't know just how to say it—to get through to her. I don't know how to have her feel this—believe me, trust me, give me a chance.

SARAH: (*To me, she changes channel—uses an intellectual tone.*) Yes—how do you build trust anyway?

SUE: This way. You are doing it. From what I was told, Sarah, even before you met Galen, you had no earthly reason to ever trust a man again—to put yourself in a man's hands. But you have struggled along with Galen, neither of you knowing how to create a safe, loving space, and here you are. And you are here asking these huge, hard questions. You are taking tiny risks with him, and asking him to help you with your fear. Amazing. Brave. And, Galen, you are reaching past your fears too—fears of getting caught in the battle—and of making a wrong move and disappointing Sarah. You are reaching for her—right. [Tango Moves 4 and 5, processing the encounter and validating and integrating the ongoing process here.]

GALEN: (*To Sarah.*) Yes. Yes, I am. I am reaching for you. I want you to make a leap of faith.

SARAH: (*Suddenly looks small and shy.*) I . . . I don't know what to say. That makes me feel very . . . awkward.

SUE: You're not used to this. (*Sarah shakes her head.*) This is an awkward place for you. When we are scared and the music is new, we don't usually leap like a ballerina—we are off balance. Afraid the other person will let us fall. (*Sarah giggles.*) You said you wanted the connection with Galen, but when he is right here, it's awkward. Different. Here he is, full of energy, asking you to risk opening up to him, to start a new kind of dance. [Returning to Tango Move 1 and the intervention of reflecting present process.]

SARAH: Yes, I see it. But I am fighting it, too. I do want the connection. But I am not sure I want to go there—does this make sense?

SUE: You bet it does. Yes, it does. You want to be close, but my sense is that some part of your brain tells you, "Are you insane? Stay guarded; just stay with what you know, which is to fight or wall him out. Just silence that hope, that longing, and wait for the enemy to show up! You know this one." [Using proxy voice to keep her engaged with her emotion and validating her fear and the necessity for her to be vigilant.]

SARAH: Until now the enemy has always shown up. I had a father and five brothers. And then we got into our war. So . . .

SUE: You are a fighter—fierce. Can you tell him, "It's so hard for me to put my weapons down and ask for your help—to show you I need help here. Hard to admit I do want connection and I can't reach, 'cause it's too scary. It's terrifying." Is that okay? (*She nods empathetically.*) [Attunement and empathic interpretation are relatively simple here given the EFT map of emotion and attachment meanings.] It is like jumping into space to say, "I need your help with this fear." If this is right, can you tell him?

SARAH: (*To me, smiling through tears.*) You are so good! [Potential exit—diversion.]

SUE: *No!* I just know this dance. It is *you* who are good, brave. You are taking a new step here. I just created a little direction, a little safety. Can you tell him? [If the therapist knows she is on target, she can persist while holding space for resistance and ambivalence.]

SARAH: (*To Galen.*) Can you pick up the signals if I ask? I make jokes sometimes, and you don't get them!

SUE: (*To Sarah.*) Oh. Do I understand? You kind of give a signal about this—needing connection—but in disguise, as a joke. The signal is disguised. It's less risky that way. (*She laughs and agrees.*) But then he doesn't get it! And your warrior self says, "This is stupid—you think he is going to respond. He just let you down again! Go to hell with the whole risk thing."

SARAH: Exactly. Yes—

SUE: Yes. I think we all do that when we don't feel safe, don't we? We try to hide and call out at the same time. We don't want to be seen—seen in our soft places. I do that too with my husband. I call out in Greek, and then get angry that he doesn't understand my message. (*We all laugh.*) I expect him to decipher my message without me taking the risk to be clear, to know that I am scared behind all my words. But he doesn't get the message. [Disciplined self-disclosure to normalize and prevent shame is part of EFT.] It's so hard to risk—ask—be seen— come out and take a leap of faith. . . . We can get so hurt. We want the connection without the risk. Me too! (*Shifting tone.*) But Galen is here (*He is indeed—intensely engaged, leaning forward.*), and he wants to hear you. (*Slowly.*) Sarah, when he really hears—he is here! (*Sarah looks across at him, studying his face.*) It must be hard to take that in, Sarah, to believe that this connection—that has always been out of reach—is being offered. He wants to take care of you. [His message can prime her longing, soothe her fear, and offer her the solution to her existential dilemma. I simply repeat it.]

SARAH: (*Breaks down, weeping.*) I want it. I long for it. So alone. But now I don't know how to let it in. I don't know what it is like. . . . How do I know if it is real? (*Looking at the floor.*)

GALEN: (*Softly.*) I want to help you, Sarah. I want you to feel . . . feel . . . well . . . loved.

SUE: Sarah, can you look at Galen please. Did you hear him? (*She looks up at him.*) Galen, can you say that again, please. (*He does. Sarah looks confused. She is at the leading edge of her known experience and breaking all her rules.*) You have such courage, Sarah, to be trying to let this in, to say, "I need connection, Galen." That must be so scary for you, to let yourself feel that need and admit that you need help here. The only way you survived has been to pick up a weapon or wall others off—to see them as enemies. This is a new kind of struggle—yes? But you are taking a leap—a leap away from battling alone—showing Galen where you are, so he can come and get you!! What happens to you as he says this—"I want you to feel loved"? [Tango Move 4—processing the encounter.]

SARAH: (*Looking from me to Galen again and again. Speaking in a quiet intense voice.*) I don't want to be alone. I feel like I am alone all the time, and I have been alone for . . . forever.

SUE: Yes. Yes. (*Softly.*) You are telling him, "I am struggling to make this leap of faith, to take this risk—it just hurts so much to be alone. I don't want to be alone. I can't be alone anymore. I need your help." [Reflecting her existential dilemma that is the essence of all complex trauma, the choice between the danger of isolation or the danger of potential connection and retraumatization. Attachment longing is stronger than fear here.] Can you hear her, Galen? What happens to you as she says this?

GALEN: (*Smiling and reaching for Sarah with his hand.*) I hear her—I hear you. I just want to hug. To hug you. (*Sarah nods and smiles.*) It's been so tough—all the fighting—messing up our lives—our kid's lives.

SUE: Can you hear him, Sarah—let that in?

SARAH: (*Smiling and crying.*) I hear him. I hear him. It feels good.

SUE: (*Suddenly aware that we are over time.*) Hm—but if your kids could see you now! Staying with these difficult feelings, being so honest, facing huge fears, risking—learning to trust! Wow. This is the start of a different kind of struggle, one you can continue with your therapist, taking little risks, learning to help each other. It is a struggle to come home to each other. No one ever showed either of you how to do this—you had never seen safe connection—didn't know how to make it happen, and you got trapped in a dance that just kept confirming all your worse fears. But look at what you can do!! After all the hurts, after all the places you have been. This is special. This is huge. Galen, you said, "I am just standing, waiting for her signal, stuck in careful, afraid of doing it wrong, so I don't reach." Sarah, you said, "I can't turn toward him. It's too scary. A leap of faith. I don't want to be alone but . . . I need your help to move closer. To risk. Come and help me out of my protection, my prison. I need your help." Look what you did! [Tango Move 5.] That is amazing, guys. I am honored to be here with you.

The session then raps up. After a short break, the feedback from the group of externs who have watched this session on video is given to the couple. This feedback is framed in megavalidating messages of support and encouragement. The intention is to give the couple an experience of being seen, held, understood, and supported—of having a secure base—and encourage further progress in therapy.

COMMENTARY ON THE SESSION

This transcript is fundamentally accurate but somewhat distilled, in that in the actual session, I reflected and repeated myself more in order to deepen the partner's emotional engagement with the experiential process. When people are processing threat in an unfamiliar emotional place, experience tells me they need to hear a cue, a new frame, at least five to six times to actually begin to take it in. I like to think of this repetition in terms of amygdala whispering. Just as when calming a desperate horse, the therapist helps the client move from attention consumed by flooded alarm, to blocking any new element or resistance, to gradual relaxation and a miniscule curiosity about the new element, to slow engagement with this element, to taking in the new element with soothing and the down regulation of threat, which then begins to alter existing patterns of how a client's inner life is organized.

This session is particularly interesting, in that we can see how blocks to the bonding process arise and prevent the creation of moments of constructive dependency. This is how insecurity plays out and recreates itself. These blocks, which feed on each other in a cascade of disorganization and distress, can be seen in the original Strange Situation research with mothers and children and in sessions of EFT and can be summarized as:

- A loss of emotional balance at moments of separation distress, to the point of reactive flooding or numbing. Organized connection with self and with core emotional experience is lost. Attunement to one's own attachment emotions is then very difficult. It is interesting to note here that in attachment science, accurate, coherent communication on the part of the main caretaker regarding attachment-related emotions is deemed the major determinant of a child's later attachment style (Shaver, Collins, & Clarke, 1996). This person helps a child detect, reflect on, and act on feelings in a coherent way, modeling a theory of mind for the child. The child then finds himself in the other.

Example

This attachment issue may show up in the therapist's office in the following manner: A client says, "All right. So I am angry all the time. All these small things set me on fire. But . . . I don't even really know why I am so angry." Or, "I am fine. This is what happens. What do you mean, how do I feel about it? Wow, see that car going by—it was so fast."

- An inability to formulate clear, coherent emotional messages to the attachment figure and so prime this figure's attachment responses. Clear signals are obviously hard to shape if we are flooded or numbed out or if we are caught in fight or flight.

Example

In the therapist's office, a client might say, in an empty voice, "I don't know what I need. I feel sad a lot. But I sure as hell didn't get married to be left alone all the time. You blow it all the time." Or, "I shouldn't have to tell you how I feel. If you loved me, you would know." Bids for more connection are then often colored with shifting emotions or conflicting messages. The inherent threat scrambles the other's ability to decipher messages. As my client tells me, "I want him to respond, get me. But to be seen, really seen as vulnerable, I would rather not."

- An inability to take in a positive response and be soothed. We see in session that some partners demand soothing and reassurance, but when they are offered, they are not recognized, trusted, or integrated, and so are pushed aside.

Example

In the therapist's office, Cory requests and is offered reassurance from Steve, but then discounts it. He tells him, "If you can do this now, then where have you been all our years together. You are just saying what you think I want to hear!" Steve is then in a true double bind.

- An inability to attune to and reciprocate care with a partner. The aforementioned processing blocks to bonding occur within an individual, but of course some individuals block offering any empathy or care to their partner.

Example

In session, Joan tells me, "Yes, I see Bill's 'hurt' as you call it. But for me to respond to that—well that would just negate all the bad things he has done to me. He just wants to get off the hook." Avoidantly attached partners shut down precisely when they or their partner become vulnerable.

- An inability to integrate a safe haven and secure base into new meanings regarding models of self and others, and so be able to begin to trust others as a resource. Revising a working model implies the ability to generalize from a specific new experience; sometimes this is hard for people to do.

Example

In session, Jim discounts his partner's new responsiveness. He tells me, "Yes, she is telling me right now that she cares and I hear it. And it does help. But in the end I just don't believe that you can trust anyone. She says that now, but what about tomorrow and the next day. She will turn on me when it suits her."

Sarah seems to be aware on some level in our session that she can, at times, be exceptionally reactive and easily triggered in interactions with her husband. She sends messages that disguise her attachment vulnerabilities and needs in aggression and apparent detachment, which prime Galen's fear of rejection and foster his distancing. However, it is the block concerning her inability to open up to his caring message that we work on extensively. As with all blocks, in EFT we tune in to the process, identify the block, make it apparent, validate it, and massage it, much as a masseuse does with a stuck or spasmodic muscle that has no flow in it.

After this session, Sarah and Galen returned to therapy with their EFT therapist and continued to work on Galen staying emotionally engaged, being able to see Sarah's fear and respond to her needs (and vice versa), and helping her set aside her survival-oriented distrust enough to allow many more corrective experiences of safe connection with him. Sarah gradually was able to focus more on her struggle to trust Galen and less on his flaws. She is a trauma survivor who has been seared by chronic insecurity and traumatic attachment experiences, so she needs to go slow and take her time to develop a basic sense of trust in her husband, just as he needs time to do the same and to foster his confidence with his wife. An issue with Sarah turning to alcohol for comfort emerged and also had to be dealt with. Her trauma was also somewhat rekindled when her father died and she returned home for his funeral. As is typical in EFT practice with couples dealing with complex trauma (MacIntosh & Johnson, 2008), over time positive bonding interactions between Sarah and Galen increased and became more stable and integrated. Both became more positive in terms of their sense of self and being able to support each other, helping each other find balance when they were triggered into rejection or abandonment. Galen was increasingly able to help Sarah heal from the results of her abuse as a child and develop the basic sense of trust that is the cornerstone of attachment security.

A felt sense of security fosters communication competence (Anders & Tucker, 2000). It is not surprising then that a central reality of so many trauma survivor's adult relationships is that it is often exceedingly difficult for a partner to properly read a survivor's attachment signals and so to respond in a caring way. These signals are mostly distorted by defensive aggression or numbing and so are continually missed. This response then induces more panic and despair in the survivor, as well as alienation and distress in the other partner. *A survivor needs more support from a partner and is also less able to ask for it in an effective way.* Survivors of childhood abuse are much more likely to exhibit a fearful avoidant attachment style (Shaver & Clarke, 1994; Alexander, 1993). The emotional switches from extreme vulnerability and need to extreme avoidance and cutoff typical of this style are experienced as crazy making by partners, who then lose the ability to be empathic. As Goleman remarks (1995, p. 112), "Attunement to others demands a modicum of calm in oneself."

To intervene and address this and similar blocks that perpetuate the effects of trauma is to break the destructive cycle we so often see in couple therapy, where insecure connection and relationship distress exacerbate anxiety and depression and other symptoms associated with trauma, and then these symptoms consolidate insecurity and relationship breakdown. In working with trauma clients across modalities, therapists need to keep certain issues in mind. These include the fact that there are generally more difficulties in the client's alliance with the therapist; that specific education about the effects of trauma is needed; that there is more violence and escalation in relationships; that substance abuse issues are more common; that emotional storms must be weathered, and emotional containment must be provided (see Johnson & Williams-Keeler [1998] for an example of an EFT therapist dealing with a flashback in a couple session); that relapses and steps backward are inevitable; and that emotional risks must be titrated, sliced thinner, and supported at every step. Nevertheless, the power of an emotionally focused and attachment-oriented therapy to go to the existential heart of traumatic injuries is clear in the session with Sarah and Galen. The most obvious and natural place to heal wounds is in the arms of someone we love. As noted in the trauma literature (van der Kolk, 2014, p. 354), "More than anything else, being able to feel safe with other people defines mental health." Attachment science takes this a step further, suggesting that for us to heal, grow, and thrive, we need to be able to call on a valued, trusted other when we feel vulnerable and know that we will be heard and responded to.

EXERCISES

1. Find two places in the transcript where you might have done something different. What would you have done? Formulate a rationale as to why I intervened the way I did.

2. Find three places where the interventions used here fit with or illustrate the principles of effective change laid out in Chapter 3.

3. If you had seen this couple for a consultation session, what do you think you would have found most difficult about working with them?

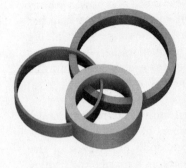

Chapter 8

Restoring Family Bonds in Emotionally Focused Family Therapy

There are, in fact, no more important communications between one human being and another than those expressed emotionally and no information more vital for constructing and reconstructing working models of self and other than information about how each feels toward the other.
—JOHN BOWLBY (1988, pp. 156–157).

The value of attachment theory lies in making the attachment needs that underlie "problem behavior visible. . . . Attachment theory enhances a systemic perspective on intervention because it helps clinicians understand the unique meaning of disruptive behavior within the context of the child–parent relationship."
—MARLENE M. MORETTI AND ROY HOLLAND
(2003, pp. 245–246)

Bowlby was arguably the first family therapist (1944) and the first clinician to adopt systems theory (Bertalanffy, 1968), and to grasp the enormous developmental and clinical implications of cycles of self-sustaining, negative patterns of interaction between intimates. As with individual and couple therapy, the attachment perspective offers a potent paradigm shift that allows for on-target interventions that transform individual family members, as well as the family as a whole. As Louis tells me in our last family session:

"Things have changed. I feel like I have my daughter, my Emma, back. I guess it wasn't so much about 'defiance' and 'rules' as about despair. Life is hard for young people these days, and now, with my wife's help, I maybe know how to stand with my kid and help her with those feelings. We are having our family suppers again. We never had conversations anything like the ones we had here. Heart to heart. We can kind of be a safe harbor for each other again. It's helped me and my wife too." (His wife smiles at him.)

Particular attachment strategies between individuals, for example, between a father and son, impact other members of a family synergistically, shaping other relationships and each person's experience of the family and the family culture. Insecure partners, in a number of studies (e.g., Finzi-Dottan, Cohen, Iwaniec, Sapir, & Weisman, 2003), report a less-positive family climate, and score lower on the dimensions of family cohesion (the extent of emotional bonding between family members), and family adaptability (the extent to which a family is able to adjust its rules in response to change). In family therapy, the lens widens beyond attachment in a particular relationship to take in the whole family drama. Patricia and her mother have a problematic relationship wherein Patricia anxiously tries to get her distant, rule-oriented mother to respond. Patricia resorts to dramatic suicidal gestures, which terrify Patricia's father into silent withdrawal. Patricia and her mother are caught in a tight cycle of criticism and wild protest. This cycle only changes when she can reach for her father, and he can hear her vulnerability, respond lovingly, and also protect Patricia from her mother's critical judgments. Just as with individuals and couples, the attachment frame offers the family therapist a clear way to see and shape relationships and bring the most vulnerable members, children and adolescents, home to a safe haven. Secure connection also fosters children's ability to expand their horizons and move out into the world as confident adults.

To set the stage for moving beyond the individual and the dyad, let us revisit the essence of systems theory. First, both Bowlby and Bertalanffy emphasized the power of linked sequences of interaction (Bowlby, 1969), whereby participants evoke predictable responses from others that form stable feedback loops, shaping homeostasis and limiting deviation (Johnson & Best, 2003). To grasp a living behavioral system, it is necessary to see the whole, not just the parts. So a withdrawn parent primes attention-seeking, acting-out behavior from a child. To try to treat the child without attending to the withdrawing, unresponsive parent is futile. The stability of the system can become constricting and rigid. A healthy system is an open and flexible one, ready to adapt to new circumstances.

Second, causality is never a straight line; it is never static or linear. Process, *how* things happen, determines outcome. Many beginnings can

lead to the same outcome. Tracking two-way and reciprocally determining evolving processes then becomes a priority. This principle suggests that systems theory is nonpathologizing in practice. People simply
become caught in narrow dysfunctional patterns that evolve for many
"good" reasons, and then are hard to change.

Third, there is nothing in systems theory per se that precludes an
inner emotional focus. However, the way it has been implemented in the
family therapy field excluded emotion, in spite of Bertalanffy's recom-
mendation that the best route to change was to find and alter the *defining
elements* of a system, which surely, in families, has to include the nature
of emotional communication. There was also little emphasis on inner
motivations (rather structural factors, such as hierarchy and boundaries,
were stressed), except that luminaries like Minuchin and Fishman (1981)
did recognize the power of belonging in the family dance.

Finally, systems theory supports the focus on the present that is
found in EFT. As attachment theorists have suggested (Shaver & Hazan,
1993), it is the constant *process of confirmation in present interactions*
rather than existing models simply biasing perception, that maintains
and confirms rigid personal realities and responses.

DIFFERENCES BETWEEN EFFT AND EFT

The key difference between couple and family EFT in terms of goals concerns mutuality. Whereas with couples the therapist is working to create
mutual accessibility, responsiveness, and engagement between partners
(even if this process sometimes has to temporarily focus on one partner
more than on the other), in EFFT, the therapist works primarily to help
parents understand their children's attachment vulnerabilities and prime
a nurturing, attuned responsiveness on their part, and the acceptance
of this care by the child. The parent is helped to become a safe haven
and secure base for the child, who is then able to act as more securely
attached children naturally do. That is, they are able to stay regulated
and nonreactive when attachment figures are momentarily unavailable;
to formulate their emotions and needs coherently so they can unambigu-
ously reach for their parent figure; and to take in caring and concern
when it is offered and use it to regulate difficult feelings. This process
results in confidence and a sense of competence in dealing with inner
and outer worlds and positive working models of self and other. In
EFFT, the relationship between parent and child is transformed in a way
that fosters resilience and growth in the child or adolescent and a sense
of positive agency in the parent.

Due to the nature of the parent–child bond, there is also less emphasis in EFFT on the fostering of equality and intimacy than in couple

therapy. In the case study described in Chapter 9, the father is supported in his need to have his son respect his guidance and limit setting, and the intimate connection that is developed is one that is appropriate in level and intensity to that of parent and adolescent son. The father is encouraged to offer caretaking and support to the son, but to turn to his wife to get his needs for emotional support met.

DIFFERENCES BETWEEN EFFT AND OTHER CURRENT FAMILY THERAPY MODELS

What does an attachment-based approach, as exemplified in EFFT, offer that is new or different from family therapy as currently practiced? When we look at EFFT compared to other approaches, the following differences in practice and focus emerge:

1. EFFT is systemic in nature, focusing on tracking and shifting interactional patterns that define the family dance. Many current approaches, particularly more behavioral models, seem to emphasize instead coaching parents in parenting or communication skills as their main change strategy, in the belief that this strategy will positively alter emotionally loaded negative interactions between family members as a whole (Morris, Miklowitz, & Waxmonsky, 2007). In a similar but perhaps more relevant manner, John Gottman also teaches parents how to coach their children specifically about emotions and emotion regulation (Gottman, Katz, & Hooven, 1997).

2. Other systems approaches traditionally set up new kinds of encounters in order to challenge the habitual patterns of power and control and the coalitions in a family (Minuchin & Fishman, 1981), whereas attachment approaches, and EFFT in particular, attend specifically to patterns of distance and disconnection that disrupt effective caretaking and the creation of nurturance and moments of secure bonding.

3. Many approaches typically see the whole family together as a group and mostly use cognitive reframes to shift alliances with everyone present (Minuchin & Fishman, 1981). EFFT, on the other hand, begins and ends with the family unit as a whole, but usually incorporates sessions conducted with a series of family subsystems: Parents only, the child or adolescent who is having problems together with one parent, both parents and this child, or the sibling group in a family.

4. The most outstanding and unique feature of EFFT is its focus on the emotions that *organize* the dance in the family, and the process

of evoking, distilling, deepening, and regulating these emotions, so that newly accessed emotions emerge in a way that moves the family conversation toward accessibility, responsiveness, and safe, empathic engagement. Systemic family therapies have instead tended to target patterns of interaction, positions in these interactions and how they become constraining, rather than on the lived experience of the dancers in the dance (Merkel & Searight, 1992). (Notably, this is not true of the work of Virginia Satir, 1967, who focused on emotional growth and communication.) Minuchin, perhaps the most recognized trailblazer in the field of family interventions, now acknowledges that "ignoring emotion was the greatest mistake we made in family therapy," and that in hindsight he found it easy to recognize the value of working actively with emotional experience—the music of the dance of intimate interactions (presentation at a Networker Symposium in Washington, DC, March 2017).

5. Enactments, the shaping of interactions between family members, are different in an attachment-oriented therapy model compared to other family models. They will be more emotionally loaded and more oriented toward shaping secure engagement. This orientation differs from that of therapists, such as Bowen (1978), who studied schizophrenic families and popularized the concept of symbiosis, leading many family therapists to highlight the differentiation of self from other and the creation of boundaries as a core goal of family interventions. In attachment terms, differentiation is a developmental process that occurs *with* others rather than *from* others, and is a natural result of secure bonding, in which a child is attuned to, accepted, and allowed to explore and be different from his or her parents.

ATTACHMENT MODELS OF FAMILY THERAPY

EFFT shares many features with other attachment-oriented models of family intervention, such as Daniel Hughes's (2007) dyadic developmental psychotherapy (DDP) and Guy Diamond's (2005) attachment-based family therapy (ABFT). All assume that adolescents who enter therapy need to reconnect with parents in order to achieve more confident autonomy, and that a new level of coherent, responsive emotional communication is necessary for this to occur. They address a wide range of symptoms, both internalizing (such as depression) and externalizing (such as conduct disorder). All assume that attachment issues such as rejection, neglect, and abandonment are often obscured by conflicts related to behavioral problems (e.g., neglecting chores or homework), and that therapy must foster empathic, attuned conversations about relationship ruptures and attachment injuries.

All of these models elucidate interaction patterns in ways that clarify the attachment needs that underlie problematic behaviors. They stress being emotionally present and attuned to family members and attempt to deal with emotion and emotional issues more than is customary in the family therapy field. In practice, the DDP model shares the experiential framework with EFFT and in many ways parallels the core elements of EFFT (Hughes, 2004, 2006). DDP stresses the creation of a sensitive, reflective, and emotionally attuned connection between therapist and child, between caregiver and child, and between therapist and caregiver. It emphasizes, in ways that directly parallel EFFT, the joint organization of emotional experience and shaping new corrective emotional experiences of bonding in the session. Hughes stresses four so-called PACE elements—playfulness, acceptance, curiosity, and empathy—in ways that any EFFT therapist will recognize and resonate with. Both EFFT and DDP therapists are emotionally present and use nonverbal cues, such as voice tone, pacing, and repetition, as well as speaking in proxy voice (that is speaking with the voice of the child for a moment) to evoke the child or adolescent's emotional reality. Both might reflect and describe in an evocative manner how it makes sense for an adopted child to freeze out and defy his parents as a natural reaction to his fear that they are not committed to him and will abandon him.

In general, the key differences between these models are that ABFT seems to be considerably more cognitively and symptom oriented in application than either DDP or EFFT, and that DDP is extensively implemented with younger children and most often with children in foster care or adoptive situations. At this time, the ABFT model has more validation in outcome research than either DDP or EFFT models (Diamond, Russon, & Levy, 2016).

EMOTIONALLY FOCUSED FAMILY THERAPY

Before discussing EFFT in more detail, it is important to stress one aspect of this therapy that seems to be largely missing in traditional family therapy models. In EFFT, there is a clear recognition that, while a parent is more responsible than a child or adolescent for the organization of the relationship, nevertheless *both* parent and child are deeply impacted in their emotions and core sense of self by their interactions in attachment-oriented dramas. Good parenting is a moving target. Parents are often caught between anxious protection and concern for their child and a need for their child to take responsibility and grow. When parents perceive that connection with the child is lost, they often deal with this pain by moving into reactive criticism and control; they then become increasingly more unsafe in their child's eyes. Partners also often have differing perspectives on how the child should be handled, and so stressful rifts in the parenting alliance and the bond between the parents occur. Each parent also has to deal with the influence of their own models of attachment as they bias or constrain their responsiveness to their child. Parents are then caught in their own frustration, permeated by fear and a sense of helplessness, and also often deeply ashamed of their perceived inadequacies as a parent. The assumption in EFFT is that *parents need support to grasp and regulate their own emotions around their parenting roles and to find their balance, so that they can help their child do the same.* The EFFT therapist will not just support parents in a one-on-one session around the family problem (as usually occurs in DDP), but also will actively work in a couple session to process the pain associated with their parenting role, helping partners work together to regulate this distress so that they can be better caretakers and attachment figures for their children. The therapist will also validate that no parent can be perfect, that good-enough parenting is indeed good enough, and that it is always a challenge to stand alongside someone as he or she grows. Rather than teach parenting skills as cognitive skills per se, new corrective experiences of connection and new perspectives are created that evoke new responses to a child. As in EFT for couples, our experience is that in the final sessions of family therapy, parents join together and, in open communication with their child, formulate more skillful and effective ways of parenting. A therapist's empathy for parents' dilemmas offers a safe place for parents to regulate their emotions and become more accepting of themselves as parents and of the child who triggers their pain.

With this recognition in mind, the goals of EFFT are to modify the distressing cycles of interaction that amplify conflict and undermine secure connection between parents and children, and to shape positive cycles of accessibility and responsiveness that offer the developing adolescent a safe haven and secure base (Johnson, 2004; Furrow et al., in press). As outlined in previous chapters, therapy takes place in three stages: Stabilization, which involves the de-escalation of negative cycles of interaction; restructuring attachment by means of safer, more engaged interactions that address attachment triggers, fears, wounds, and needs; and consolidation, in which changes are integrated and new narratives of family problems and repair are constructed. This family therapy process usually occurs across 10–12 sessions. The first two sessions typically include the entire family. Once the network of alliances has been mapped out, the family members' views of the problem have been grasped, and the child or adolescent's problematic behavior have been placed in the context of family attachment patterns, sessions may be conducted with any combination of family members, including any one member seeing the therapist alone for a session.

The therapist concentrates on two tasks: The elucidation and repro-cessing of attachment-related emotions and emotional responses and the gradual revision of key patterns of interaction in order to create potent bonding moments that result in a more secure connection. As in EFIT and EFT, the therapist focuses on emotion as the organizing element in interactions and discovers and distills clients' experience with them rather acting as a coach. *The EFFT therapist relies on the power of new emotional signals and interactions to evoke new behaviors and revise expectations, perceptions, and models of relationships in both parents and children, rather than using formal instruction in skill sequences or the expert reframing or manipulation of boundaries and hierarchies.* The recognition, validation, and expression of attachment needs is a key part of EFFT, as is addressing the child or adolescent's frustration and despair over disconnection. Explicit vulnerability in a child also tends to prime a parent's protective, caring responses. Therapy also proceeds in the same manner as EFT for couples, with the therapist going through the steps of the EFT Tango with different family members in different sessions.

ASSESSMENT IN EFFT

To get a snapshot of family functioning, EFFT therapists may use a self-report measure, such as the Inventory of Parent and Peer Attachment (IPPA; Armsden & Greenberg, 1987). The IPPA provides the therapist an initial understanding of an adolescent's current perception of their family and peer relationships in terms of trust, communication, and alienation. This measure poses questions such as, "My mother expects too much from me," and "I can count on my mother when I need to get something off my chest" (rated on a 5-point scale). Research sug-gests that the trust and communication scales load primarily on attach-ment anxiety, while alienation loads highly on both attachment anxiety and avoidance (Brennen, Clarke, & Shaver, 1998). Another measure is the McMaster Family Assessment Device (FAD; Epstein, Baldwin, & Bishop, 1983). The FAD consists of seven subscales: Affective Respon-siveness, Affective Involvement, Behavior Control, Communication, Problem Solving, Roles, and General Family Functioning. Here family members are asked to respond to statements such as, "Planning activities is difficult because we misunderstand each other." Of particular interest to the EFFT therapist are the first two subscales, in which family mem-bers rate statements such as, "We don't show our love for each other," or, "You only get the interest of others when something is important to them."

However, in general, as discussed in previous chapters, the therapist assesses the family as an attachment environment and each person's experience of that environment by listening to and engaging with the family and by watching interactions as they unfold live in session. The therapist focuses on A.R.E. aspects of interaction: How open or *accessible,* sensitive and *responsive,* and *emotionally engaged* are family members? Can members collaborate to create a safe haven and, most important in adolescence, a secure base from which the adolescent can *transform* from a child to a young adult, who can take risks and explore his or her world but who can also turn to and use family resources when needed? As Daniel Seigel (2013) points out in his book *Brainstorm: The Power and Purpose of the Teenage Brain,* a healthy adolescent moves into interdependence, not "do-it-yourself" isolation. The adolescent brain naturally turns toward more novelty seeking, more engagement with and reliance on peers, and increased emotional intensity and more creative thinking, but it is also dealing with disorientating and often disturbing new realities. Exploratory and attachment safe haven systems often compete for primacy at this time of life, and so parents struggle to adapt to their child's alternating demands to be held and to be let go. In the process of finding a balance and as part of the adolescent's growing perspective-taking skills, parents also often suddenly find their child's new reflections on and evaluation of the attachment relationship uncomfortable and difficult. In an attachment-based therapy the focus is less on "whether an adolescent can establish autonomy in a disagreement, than on the autonomy challenge as a backdrop against which relationships are either actively maintained or significantly threatened" (Allen, 2008, p. 425). *Sustained connection potentiates individuation.* So the therapist watches not only to see if the adolescent can reach for his parents and use the relationship to regulate difficult feelings, but also whether the adolescent can safely differ from and distance from his parents, and also turn to peer relationships to get some of his needs for security met.

As noted in Johnson, 2004, Chapter 11, the EFFT therapist assesses family problems in the following manner:

• The therapist tracks the organization of the family patterns of interaction or dance. For example, who supports and allies with whom, how predictable, rigid, and negative are the family's interactions, and who responds to distress and offers comfort? In the case presented in the next chapter, the main family dance goes like this: The son expresses defiance and anger to his father; the father reasons and insists; the son completely withdraws into humming and looking away, but shows agitated nonverbal behaviors, like hitting his leg continuously. The mother then berates the father for never being home and confesses to being totally flooded by her son's behavior; the father reasons that he can do nothing to change anything at work or at home, and then withdraws. The mother weeps—a short pause occurs—and the cycle begins again. If we look at the interaction between the parents, the mother is in frantic, anxious pursuit and extremely distressed, while the father is distant and emotionally absent, working for some 12–14 hours every day. The conflict in their relationship fuels the out-of-control drama with their angry son. If we look at the interaction between each parent and the son, the son is aggressively threatening, which we see as his protest at his father's distance and disengagement. He receives reasoned rules and distancing in return. The mother is trying to be responsive to her son, but dissolves into her own pain and agitation, to which her son responds with temper tantrums and threats of suicide.

• The therapist tunes in to the emotional tone of the family—the music of the dance. The strongest negative emotional charges in the family depicted in Chapter 9 are between father and son and between father and mother. Son and mother appear to be in considerable distress, flipping between anger and anxiety, but the father stays relatively unemotional and sees his son and wife as unreasonable and out of control. The more in control he seems, the more angry and anxious his son and wife become. The son reports being able to go to his mother for comfort, but expresses this need in extremely incongruent ways, waving his hands and changing the subject continually. It is useful to formulate from observation exactly what each family member's usual affect regulation strategies are and the likely impact of these strategies on the quality of the attachment with others in the family. (For a general summary of how family context, for example, parental modeling of emotion regulation, affects the development of emotion regulation in children, see Morris, Steinberg, & Silk, 2007.)

• The therapist listens to the family's story, including the main events in their history, recent crises and how each person perceives them, and their understanding of the present problem. How is responsibility for the problem assigned by different members? The therapist probes with evocative questions, for example, asking what happens when the son has a violent temper tantrum and how each parent deals with it.

• The therapist observes and asks directly about the accessibility, responsiveness, and engagement in the family: Who turns to whom and is this reaching effective? A key question is always, how are the parents, as caregivers and attachment figures, blocking or remaining unresponsive to the child's pain and needs, and how do they see their child and understand his or her negative behavior? Have the parents ever experienced secure attachment as individuals in their families of origin or as partners (or is it completely foreign territory?), and have secure interactions occurred in parent–child interactions recently or in the past?

  • The therapist examines and explores the nature of the initial therapeutic alliance and the intended goal of therapy for each person and for the family as a whole. The therapist notes how open family members are to his or her questions and interventions and how easy each person is to connect with.

As this process unfolds, the therapist better understands the most problematic cycles of interaction and how they trigger and maintain the symptoms that brought the family into therapy. It also becomes clear in attachment terms what interactions have to change to create any kind of safe connection and a calmer and safer family climate. A focus on the dance, using the attachment lens and the emotional music, gives the therapist a calm place to stand no matter how chaotic or dysregulated the family.

The research on secure attachment in adolescence also helps the assessment process in that it tells the therapist what to look for and what to set up as a goal for the therapy process. In one study, securely attached boys, when becoming disconnected and or conflictual with their mothers, expressed less anger, maintained assertiveness, and moved into a metaprocessing form of communication (such as commenting on the interaction, as in, "We are both trying to be heard here but it's not working"). This capacity allows for relationship repair and reconnection (Kobak, Cole, Ferenz-Gilles, Fleming, & Gamble, 1993). Secure attachment has been linked to open and effective communication with both parents and close peers; conversely, difficulties communicating internal states accurately to others seems to be a robust marker of insecurity.

Dismissing adolescents are more likely to exhibit conduct disorders and substance abuse, but anxiously attached teens, who are highly sensitive to their social environment, often act out to protest a sense of rejection or abandonment and engage parental attention.

Considering the Parenting Alliance in EFFT Assessment

It is always possible, if the parents' relationship is in obvious distress, to include elements of the couple's assessment procedure as described in Chapter 6. However, it is important to remember that in EFFT the goal regarding the couple's relationship is to create enough equilibrium and safe connection between partners to potentiate effective coparenting and allow the caretaking system to operate smoothly, rather than to create or restore secure attachment for the couple per se. The main question in assessment is then how the present relationship between partners supports or interferes with each parent's ability to be there for the child and to create a consistent caretaking strategy. Spouses with higher attachment anxiety and avoidance report lower levels of marital adjustment, less coparenting cooperation, and more coparenting conflict. Moreover, it is marital adjustment that mediates the relationship between insecure attachment in parents and these aspects of coparenting (Young, Riggs, & Kaminski, 2017). It will be no surprise to family therapists that couple conflict is inherently traumatizing for children; what they may not know is that researchers are now actively suggesting that couple therapy alone can be used to reduce or prevent behavior problems in children (Zemp, Bodenmann, & Cummings, 2016). This makes sense in the light of new findings that document just how sensitive children are to conflict between parents, how they make self-blaming attributions for this conflict, and how withdrawal by parents from each other is often a more powerful predictor of child maladjustment than overt hostility. Children do not seem to habituate to this conflict, but rather become more and more sensitized to it. Young children seem to express their distress at parental conflict in externalizing behaviors (aggression and noncompliance), whereas in adolescents internalizing symptoms, such as depression, are more prevalent. Notably, more constructive conflict communication between parents fosters children's emotional security and enhances their prosocial behavior longitudinally (McCoy, Cummings, & Davis, 2009). Of course, attachment style also affects a partner's attitude to the tasks of parenting that are a frequent source of conflict between partners. Parents with more secure attachment styles perceive parenthood as less threatening and concerning and more rewarding (Jones, Cassidy, & Shaver, 2015). Attachment avoidance (especially in men) has been found to shape the reactions of new parents to child care—to the division of labor over the first 2 years of parenthood. More avoidant parents seem to view child care as more restricting to their autonomy and as blocking their other life goals (Fillo, Simpson, Roles, & Kohn, 2015).

The Adverse Childhood Experiences (ACE) study, with 18,000 participants (Felitti et al., 1998), shows potent correlations between early adverse experiences, such as loss and abuse, and later adult mental and physical health, as well as major causes of adult mortality in the United States. These and similar findings reinforce the idea that therapists should pay close attention to and address the impact of parental conflict and alienation on their children. In many versions of traditional family therapy, the relationship between parents was often overlooked. But the research generally implies that, for optimal development and functioning of children, the first concern is not, in fact, the creation of a "village," but the creation of a team of engaged and collaborating parents. The EFFT therapist, who most often also practices EFT for couples, will ideally be attuned to connection and disconnection between parenting partners, and thus will be able to explore how responsiveness in this relationship impacts the family as a whole, as well as the child presenting with problems. In practice it is not unusual as EFFT comes to a close, to recommend that the couples consider some sessions of couple therapy to strengthen their bond and their parental partnership.

STAGES OF EFFT

In the first stage of EFFT, stabilization, the therapist focuses on the presenting problem and assesses the dynamics between relevant family members, while validating each family member's perception of this problem and identifying and reflecting the family's negative interaction pattern (or dance). The therapist explores the impact of the negative family patterns on individuals and on different family subsystems (e.g., parental or sibling subsystem, or each parent's relationship with the adolescent). The therapist then reframes the family problem as one arising from negative patterns of disconnection that block collaborative problem solving and focuses on creating a safe emotional climate and normalizing family difficulties without blaming anyone (Palmer & Efron, 2007). As the steps in the main negative cycles of interaction become clear, the emotions that prime these steps are discovered, distilled, and disclosed (this is the process set up in Tango Moves 1 and 2). Most often both parents and children are unaware of the effect they have on each other and are caught in an arc of shame and blame. They either interpret the other's behavior in the worst possible light and attribute bad intentions to each other or sink into disempowering shame responses to their perceived failure as a parent or as a child.

It is especially important to regulate and process the parents' emotions in this stage, so that they can become grounded and begin to have the psychic space to empathize with their child. From an attachment point of view, it is terrifying to encounter the storms of childhood transitions or adolescence without a reliable parent figure at your side. However, it is also terrifying to face failure and helplessness as a parent and feel the fear that one cannot protect, guide, or connect with one's child. One of the early criticisms of Bowlby's work was that it placed too heavy a load on mothers, in terms of being constantly responsive to children. Later commentators have clarified this misconception. For example, Tronick (2007) makes it clear that the best of mothers, with securely attached young children, miss attuning to their children's bids for closeness much of the time. However, these mothers are also more likely to notice a child's distress and initiate repair and reconnection. A relationship is a constant flow of attuned connection, miscues and misses, and repair. Once the overall tone is one of security, then misses and mistakes are simply glitches in the dance, rather than signals of rejection or catastrophic abandonment. Both the parents' and the child's vulnerability must be seen and honored. From the EFFT point of view, the responses labeled as "enmeshment" that were often part of the diagnosis of family therapists, and invariably applied to mothers, can be seen as a natural response to the threat of not being able to protect or effectively engage with a precious child and to the pressure of facing this threat alone, without a safe coparenting alliance with a partner.

At the end of Stage 1, the therapist reframes individual, reactive, and surface emotional responses as part of a broader interactional dance fueled by underlying primary emotions (e.g., fear, hurt, sadness, and feelings of failure or loss) and unmet attachment needs. Accessing the primary emotions and sharing them (Tango Move 3) most often creates empathy and responsiveness among family members, and helps the family de-escalate (Johnson et al., 2005).

The second stage of EFFT, restructuring attachment, uses the basic Tango processes, interventions, and experiential techniques as in Stage 1, except that now the family have a more secure base and are less caught in reactive negative cycles and attributions. The goal in Stage 2 is to facilitate positive bonding experiences between parents and child or adolescent. The therapist evokes a more explicit and deeply felt articulation of attachment fears on the part of the young client and choreographs his or her reaching for parental connection and support. The therapist empathically addresses blocks to this reaching, such as fear of rejection on the part of the child. Similarly, the therapist addresses blocks to open, inviting responsiveness on the part of the parents, such as fear of vulnerability, in general, or fear of failing to "perform" as a perfect parent. The therapist helps each parent stay attuned and engaged and respond to their child's reaching with reassurance, authenticity, and caring. (This process is captured in Tango Move 3—choreographing engaged encounters.)

This interaction constitutes a *bonding event* that parallels the shaping of secure connection process in EFT for couples, except for two factors. First, in EFFT the process is less reciprocal than it is in EFT. The parent is supported by the therapist to be the stronger and wiser one, who is able to help the child acknowledge and share underlying attachment emotions and needs. Parents are supported to turn to each other for emotional support and closeness. Single parents are encouraged to seek help from supportive others, both imagined and actual, or to be open to the therapist's support in the session. Therapists often work with parents to discover and acknowledge their own vulnerabilities as they explore their parenting behaviors in session for the purpose of helping them to be more present and more attuned as a caregiver to their child.

So, a therapist may help a mother, who is frantic with worry about her daughter and her risk-taking behaviors, contact the underlining feelings that prime her obsessional problem solving and advice giving, which the adolescent simply dismisses and withdraws from. The mother accesses the helplessness and fear underneath her frustration that keeps her constantly "nagging" her daughter. When the mother and daughter come together with the therapist, the mother can then coherently, and in a more regulated way, disclose the fear and helplessness that arises when her daughter rejects her guidance and protection. The mother offers an image formulated with the therapist, and says, "I see you standing in the middle of the road with your eyes closed, not moving, while big trucks are cruising toward you. So I yell louder and louder at you from the side of the road. I get frantic. But you hear put downs and turn away from me and hide. There is nothing I can do. I don't want to be mad and nagging all the time. How can I help you see how scared I am for you, and maybe help you ask me for what you need? I want to be there for you." An effective bonding conversation in EFFT occurs when a parent can regulate her emotion effectively and become accessible, responsive, and engaged with her child or adolescent. The child can then, with the therapist's help, share fears and needs, reaching for connection to a parent who can then offer a safe haven and a secure base.

Second, the intensity of emotion in these Stage 2 bonding conversations is often less sustained than when it occurs between adult partners in EFT. Parents' urge to respond to and protect their children is usually easier to access and more compelling than is their openness to soothing a partner who has hurt them over many years. Also, once defensive strategies are less engaged, adolescents are more open to a shift in responsiveness on the part of the parent. The therapist is more careful about titrating emotional intensity with young clients, especially those who are younger in age and/or more fragile. As I suggested earlier, the therapist is careful about pacing, often alternating between helping an adolescent client touch difficult feelings and moving into more cognitive reflection or play in order to better pair the emotional tenor of the session to this person's ability to tolerate and process it.

The positive kind of encounters structured in such sessions is clearly a prototypical example of the responsive interactions that define secure attachment in hundreds of studies of attachment between parent and child. When these encounters occur in session between adult partners in EFT, they have been shown to significantly impact attachment security in both avoidant and anxious individuals (Burgess Moser et al., 2015). These kinds of events are coded as so significant by the human brain that their affect is *disproportionately impactful* on the quality of family relationships, just as family connection is *disproportionately important* in healthy development. *This kind of on-target systematic sculpting or choreographing of core defining attachment interactions is a crucial advance in the practice of family therapy.*

The therapist also continually frames and normalizes the unmet attachment needs of young clients and processes the pain of former failed attachment bids. So Amy sits in her numbed-out silence, punctuated with flashes of belligerence at her mother. But after many slow and softly spoken empathic reflections and evocative questions as to what exactly is happening in the moments when she again decides to steal her mother's pills and alcohol, she is able to pinpoint and weep for the loss she felt when her mother's new boyfriend moved into the house. The therapist helps Amy distill her fears that she has been replaced and validates her need for reassurance. The therapist helps her coherently share a key specific moment of abandonment by her mother and guides the mother past her pronouncements about how 16-year-olds should be "independent" into a new level of resonance and empathic connection. Key moments of transformation occur when a parent's new responsiveness to a child's vulnerability results in the child feeling a secure connection. The therapist helps the child "take in" this felt sense and integrate it with his or her sense of self (this process is captured in Tango Move 4—processing new encounters). These events have a cascade effect on all family members. When a mother watches a father respond to her child with caring, this response models similar responses for the mother. It also alters her view of her mate and her "problem" child.

In the final stage of EFFT, the therapist focuses on consolidating the changes family members have made in Stage 2. At this stage, the family is able to integrate the new ways of exploring difficulties and make family decisions characterized by openness, responsiveness, and engagement among all members. The family can create a narrative of rift and repair and a joint vision of how members want their family to function in the future. They can also create new family rituals to support this vision (in Tango Move 5). The therapist helps them formulate this narrative in terms of a safe haven and secure base that support growth and exploration for the child and realistic expectations as to how parents can provide this security. Positive emotion and positive cycles are highlighted and celebrated. The family's new sense of connection can then translate into everyday cooperation and problem solving. So an adolescent's refusal to get up for school on time dissolves when his mother, now less anxious about her parenting and her son's "performance," calmly tells him that she will not nag him and start into their "dance" or drive him to school as before. He will then miss class as a consequence and have to deal with the teacher himself. More flexible authoritative parenting seems to emerge naturally when parents have an engaged coparenting alliance, can accept their child's attachment needs, and can stay grounded and regulated in emotional or frustrating situations.

EFFECTIVENESS OF EFFT

Outcome studies of the EFT model have concentrated almost exclusively on the couple therapy modality. One might surmise that interventions that were found to be so potently effective in one form of attachment dyad would logically be expected to have similar effects in another. However, there is, as yet, only one preliminary study on the effectiveness of EFFT. This study, which indeed found EFFT to be effective, examined outcomes in a small sample of 13 young women diagnosed with bulimia nervosa at an outpatient hospital clinic (Johnson, Maddeaux, & Blouin, 1998). Most also met criteria for clinical depression, and several had attempted suicide. All subjects, except one, rated themselves as having either an anxious or a fearfully avoidant attachment, as assessed with the Relationship Questionnaire (Bartholomew & Horowitz, 1991). The effects of a cognitive-behavioral educational group were compared with the effects of EFFT. Both treatments (of 10 sessions) were supervised by experts in these interventions, and implementation checks were conducted. Both treatments were found to result in a decreased severity of bulimic symptoms, lower scores on the Beck Depression Inventory, and reduced general psychiatric symptomatology. Remission rates for bingeing and vomiting were better in EFFT than those reported for individual therapy. Case studies have provided some support for the efficacy of EFFT as a therapeutic intervention with families in which adolescents are struggling with symptomatic behaviors (Bloch & Guillory, 2011; Palmer & Efron, 2007) and interventions with stepfamilies facing adjustment issues (Furrow & Palmer, 2007). Future research by the International Centre for Excellence in EFT (ICEEFT) will focus on documenting the outcomes of EFFT.

THE EFFT TANGO WITH A FATHER AND SON: TIM AND JAMES

Perhaps the best way to elucidate EFFT is to outline what the core change processes of the EFT model, the sequence of interventions called the EFT Tango, and a softening or bonding conversation look like with a father–son dyad. This case has been described before in a different format in the clinical literature (Johnson, 2008b).

James was a tall, strapping 16-year-old. He had been expelled from school for aggressive behavior toward teachers and students. He was particularly oppositional and defiant with his father, Tim, and was repeatedly caught bullying and becoming abusive with his four much-younger siblings. James's mother, Moira, was clinically depressed and suffering from chronic pain, as well as preoccupied with her younger children. Most of the negative interaction in the family was now between the father and son, and that interaction was becoming dangerously hostile and explosive. Tim had managed to persuade his son to see me in an effort to try to "sort things out," since, years before, I had helped him and Moira repair their relationship. This made Tim hopeful that he might be able to repair his connection with his son. His son did not share this sentiment! Tim admitted that, until 4 years ago, when he gave up drinking, he had been "very hard" on his firstborn son, but was now trying to "make up for this." James dismissed Tim's efforts to be supportive, belligerently stating that he did not need anyone, that he hated his father, and that everyone was "against" him anyway. James had come to therapy reluctantly and refused to talk at all for most of the first session, swearing at me and determinedly staring at the floor.

In the first two sessions, the constant self-generating cycle of disconnection between father and son was clear. Tim was busy reasoning with his son, cajoling and pursuing, while James dismissed his father and curled his lip in contempt, openly defying Tim's attempts to discuss or set standards for their interaction. Tim finally became angry, making critical remarks and then withdrawing, triggering a sneering accusation from his son about his lack of caring. James saw his father's anger as "proof" that Tim was always looking to find ways to "accuse" his son for his failings. The cycle appeared to be constant and rigidly invariant. Difficult! But, for the therapist, the cycle was relatively simple to discover, describe and distill in terms of attachment meanings and action triggers. The other pattern discussed in the session, and outlined by me in narrative form with Tim as James listened, was that James's only tenuous positive connection in the family was with his mother, but this was now undermined by her need to protect her younger son from James's bullying. So she too had now withdrawn from James (and refused to come to therapy with him). In spite of his belligerence, it was clear to me that James felt desperate and alone in this family, but could find no way to begin to engage or trust his father, even when Tim tried to reach out for him. James reminded me of Bowlby's (1944) cogent description of the delinquents of London: "Behind the mask of indifference is bottomless misery and behind apparent callousness, despair." He went on to describe how he saw these young clients as frozen in a stance of "I will never be hurt again," and paralyzed by their isolation and rage.

In an individual session with James, his depression was clear. He told me that he was "useless" and had "no future." He spoke longingly about past moments when he felt connected to his mother or played with his young sister, but expressed only cold hostility for his father. We mapped out together the patterns of connection and disconnection, his feeling of aloneness, and how this *family* problem (not James's inherent inadequacy issues) had occurred. We outlined the options that he saw—to "show them," to "shut them out," and to "not care anyway," and how all these responses helped for a moment, but ultimately left him alone and hopeless. A tentative therapeutic alliance was made with James. The tipping point of this therapy process, however, was a session with James and his father. A father's current frame of mind concerning attachment is a powerful predictor of his child's externalizing behaviors (Cowan, Cowan, Cohn, & Pearson, 1996). Modifying Tim's attachment responses to his son was an obvious route to changing James's aggressive behavior.

The generic EFT Tango with Tim and James, which at its most intense moment also turns into a bonding conversation, can be distilled in the following terms:

- *EFT Tango Move 1: Mirroring present process.* The attachment dance of tentative reaching by Tim, followed by dismissal from James and mounting critical remarks and insistence from Tim, is laid out. The therapist then also discovers with James the inner emotional cycle that underlies these interactions, that is, how Tim's responses "confirm" James's sense of not belonging, and of being useless and unwanted, and so trigger his reactive rage. Both end up cycling through discouragement, rejection, urgent frustration, and numbing. Both are caught and helpless in this dance. The dance defines their relationship and James's sense of self.

- *EFT Tango Move 2: Affect assembly and deepening.* We focus on how Tim gets caught in his concern for James, in shame at his earlier treatment of James when he was drinking, and his feelings of failure as a parent. With my help, mostly using reflection and evocative questions, Tim assembles the specific elements of his emotional response. He describes moments when he is "smacked" by James's defiance but also by the pain he sees in James's face (triggers); and moments when his body goes hot and he tells himself, "It is your fault he is lashing out. You failed him. You are a shit parent" (body response—felt sense and meaning attributions). Then he feels compelled to try to take control or, overwhelmed by helplessness, turns away (action tendency). As we stay here, Tim begins to sob, touching his deep sorrow at his "failure to be the dad that James needed" and his sense that he has now irretrievably hurt and lost his connection with his son.

- *EFT Tango Move 3: Choreographing engaged encounters.* I distill Tim's emotions with him and ask him to share them with his son. Tim does this with authenticity and openness, telling James that he is right not to trust, because he has failed him as a father. He also apologizes to his son. I encourage Tim to share his fear that he has damaged his son and pushed him into not being able to trust at all—into seeing everyone as dangerous. James struggles to feign indifference for a few minutes, but then, in an amazing shift, actually starts trying to comfort Tim and tell him everything is all right. I gently reflect and *validate* this response, but encourage him to listen and let Tim say what he has to say; his Dad is offering his heart and his care as a father, and James does not need to take care of him. As Tim continues to apologize, both for his former aggressiveness and his absence as a supportive parent, both son and father weep.

• *EFT Tango Move 4: Processing the new encounter.* James begins to let his father's message in and to share how Tim's message soothes his fears about himself. He then recounts one episode in particular when he had decided to give up and try to shut down his longing for Tim's approval. At this point he also decided that there was "probably something wrong with me." Tim stays engaged and responds with empathy.

• *EFT Tango Move 5: Integrating and validating.* I reflect all of this interaction, validating their caring for each other and their courage to open up and risk sharing with one another. We talk about how this process offers them both hope for a different kind of connection. For the first time, James turns to me and gives a huge, open smile. We distill the positive "delight" Tim feels at having "found" his son again and James's amazement at having been seen and accepted. We spend time in the frame of how father and son became "stuck," Tim drowning in his own problems and unable to "hold up" his son. This frame is an antidote to James's perspective that he was somehow unlovable.

At the end of this session James was also able, with some help from me, to stay engaged with and distill his emotions, particularly the pain of feeling "outside" of the family and abandoned by his father. He shares how his anger and despair are "poisoning" him and turning everything "dark." Having first pinpointed his fear of being rejected, he is then able to express his buried longings for his father's acceptance and love. Tim is able to respond with caring and describe the kind of parent he wants to be for his child, asking James for the chance to learn to be this parent.

This corrective experience of secure connection constitutes a classic bonding conversation, the results of which are clear at a follow-up session some months later. James tells me he is learning to trust people more and doesn't have to "play the tough guy" so much. He is also back in school, mentoring rather than bullying his younger brother, and able to engage with me and family members with openness and positive emotion. The family demonstrate that they can now problem solve pragmatic issues and differences collaboratively. A more flexible, open system wherein family members are responsive to each other simply promotes effective problem solving. The process described above beautifully illustrates the megawatt power of tapping into, regulating, and using attachment emotions to improve family relationships and how family members define themselves in this context. This process is also very efficient, taking only a few sessions, and has staying power. The learning occurs in the very interactional context in which future, more positive responses must be accessible and enacted. This is different than coaching a family to use "skills" that are often not available (wrong level, wrong channel) in moments of problematic family interaction when they are most needed.

EXPERIENTIAL TECHNIQUES IN EFFT

What did I, as an EFFT therapist, actually do in the sessions with Tim and James in terms of using experiential techniques? In the sessions, I keep all of the change processes on track and heighten them by the constant reflection of interactions and emotional processes. Empathic reflection soothes and scaffolds Tim's and James's experience, as do validation and normalization. We normalize Tim's fumbling attempts at parenting in terms of his own upbringing and his "losing" himself in a maze of drinking to cope with his own insecurities when James was a child. I ask evocative questions to access emotion and to structure enactments. I ask James, "What happens to you when your father tries to talk to you about his regrets—the way he has been doing here with you?" I catch the bullet when James replies, "He can shove his regrets. They don't help me much." I say, "Right. It's hard to tune into his sadness, his hurt over hurting you and his loss of connection with you. Hard to believe he cares that much—that anything he says could really help you. You don't see anyone coming to help you—is that it? [James nods but shrugs.] That must be hard." A little later I set up an enactment by asking, "Tim, your son is saying—and James, please correct me if I am wrong—that he sees you as dangerous—as someone who will judge him and find him wanting. Can you help him with that right now?" The word "dangerous" is a conjecture here. It intensifies James's words and goes just one step deeper into his fear than he has acknowledged or articulated. Heightening is shaped by staying with the most powerful attachment-significant emotions and statements and by blocking detours and exits. I redirect and change channel when Tim tells a long, winding content-oriented story of how he lost his job when James was born, by reflecting his words, and then saying, "I would like to go back to when you told James, 'I am so afraid that I have failed you.' Can you tell him that again?" We use images that capture and heighten emotional realities. I suggest that James, just because he was a kid (and all kids need this), needed to be held to feel safe and special to his dad, but that Tim himself was losing his balance and was not grounded, so could not "hold" his son. Then James was falling through space, and that was scary because he was just a small boy in a big world; it also made him want to shout (attachment protest) and lash out—after all, it seemed like no one was going to listen to him and see how small he felt.

We stay with the emotional process, rather than focusing on goals or solutions, especially when attempting to shape new, more engaged interactions. When Tim first tries to open up to his son, and I ask James for his reaction, he only rolls his eyes and turns away. I say, "Your dad is reaching out here but, could you help me, it's almost like you are saying to him, 'Go to hell, Dad. I am not going to let my wall down and really listen to you. It's better to stay mad and keep you out, out, out.'" James nods at me with a half-smile and tells me I am not quite as stupid as I look! I tell him that this is reassuring. I also constantly use the two reframes: namely, that the family problems are about the dance that leaves James alone and Tim feeling like a bad parent, not James's defects, and that his behaviors are his way of expressing his desperation—a natural response to feeling alone and rejected. The sessions with James and Tim are a good example of going to the heart of the matter—to emotion, which "dominates social interaction and is the major currency in which it is transacted" (Zajonc, 1980), and staying in the attachment channel. Tim's and James's less-functional behaviors are placed in the context of attachment terrors and unmet needs and our limited strategies for coping with them without a safe connection.

Like James, many of the young people who come to family therapy sessions show signs of depression and anxiety. Some will also be dealing with trauma and loss, and the family may be responding in ways that inadvertently exacerbate the negative impact of this experience. Family therapy can address these issues as part of family intervention or a general treatment package that can involve other interventions, such as groups focused on depression or social anxiety. Bowlby (1973) was the first to contend that attachment insecurities can prime anxiety disorders. *Emotional isolation exacerbates every difficulty.* It is clear that, no matter how security is measured, attachment styles are linked to specific symptomatology, especially for those who are coded as or report anxious attachment. In avoidant attachment, anxiety symptoms link to the fearful aspects rather than to the more dismissing aspects of avoidance (Ein-Dor & Doron, 2015). The Minnesota Study (Sroufe, Egeland, Carlson, & Collins, 2005), designed to trace the developmental trajectory of early attachment orientations from before birth into adulthood and old age, shows that when infants are classified as anxious resistant (sometimes called preoccupied) they are more likely than their secure counterparts to endorse anxiety disorders at age 17 (Warren, Huston, Egeland, & Sroufe, 1997). The picture is even clearer in terms of depression. More

than 100 studies have outlined the link between attachment dispositions and the general severity of depressive symptoms. The Minnesota
prospective study found that both avoidant and anxious attachment is
linked to depression in adolescence (Duggal, Carlson, Sroufe, & Egland,
2001).

A so-called *dark triad* of processes that link insecurity to dysfunction has been identified. The elements of this triad are:

1. Difficulties with the regulation of emotions.
2. Greater vigilance for threat.
3. Lower levels of perceived responsiveness from others.

All of these elements can easily be seen in many family therapy sessions (Ein-Dor & Doron, 2015). Family factors also predict treatment
response among depressed youth (Asarnow, Goldstein, Tompson, &
Guthrie, 1993; Birmaher et al., 2000). As James tells Tim in a follow-up
session, "It was just easier to be angry and act like I didn't feel anything
but 'mad.' But inside it was dark. So lonely, to feel like no one cared. I
was just a screw up anyway, so why try. But for you to come here, Dad,
and say those things, that made everything different. I had to matter to
you for you to do that." The antidote to the dark triad is also a triad: The
accessibility, responsiveness, and engagement of an attachment figure.

CONCLUSION

Pinsof and Wynne (2000) suggest that although outcome research can
offer direction for practice in psychotherapy in broad, general terms, it
seems to have influenced most couple and family therapists only minimally. It has then failed to offer a substantive integrating base for the
discipline of family therapy. They suggest that more qualitative research
studies will address this need. Perhaps the issue is that the language and
mode of outcome studies are not well attuned to the therapist's dance
with a group of distressed family members caught in the vise of fear and
helplessness. Attachment research, however, offers a rich empirical and
conceptual base that translates very well into everyday practice with families. The solution here is for therapists to become aware of the advances
in developmental and social science research, which offer them a substantive map of family relationships and a clear picture of family health and
resilience to aim for. The huge wave of innovative family perspectives and
interventions that originally inspired so many clinicians in the heyday of
family therapy interventions seems to have receded to a trickle. There is
obviously a place for parent training and education in any mental health

discipline, and attachment science has given rise to wonderful parenting programs for the parents of young children, such as Circle of Security (Powell, Cooper, Hoffman, & Marvin, 2014; Hoffman, Cooper, & Powell, 2017), and the more recent Hold Me Tight®: Let Me Go program (Aikin & Aikin, 2017) for families with adolescents developed by my own colleagues. In addition, focused family interventions, explicating the present process of interactions using an attachment lens and shaping emotional signals to shift key interactional patterns, offer a potent multidimensional intervention. Here levels and elements of change in self and system spin off and enhance each other in a way that shapes core corrective emotional experiences in a predictable and efficient manner. It simply makes sense to see the problems of the identified "patient" in a family as a reflection of security—of attachment connections—and disconnections, and the relevance of this perspective is easy for family members to tune in to and accept. In terms of relevance, one research result that has always stayed with me is from a study published in 1985 (Lutkenhaus, Grossman, & Grossman), which found that children as young as 3 years of age, who were previously assessed as securely attached, responded to potential failure with increased effort, whereas insecurely attached children did the opposite. As Bowlby (1988, p. 168) noted, children in this study already demonstrated the "confidence and hope" for success that typifies secure attachment, in contrast to the "helplessness and defeatism" of less secure children. Surely, confidence and hope are what all parents wish to give their child as they move out into life.

The battle waging in a distressed family resonates in the nervous system of family members as a life-and-death contest. So much is at stake. An attachment-oriented family therapist can take this sense of urgency and offer safety and a way of ordering this experience that can bring the family back into balance and to a sense of mastery again.

A HOMEPLAY EXERCISE

For You Personally

Can you imagine a typical difficult moment, that is, a moment where people lost their balance in your family when you were an adolescent? Who would have been the most "dangerous" person in that interaction for you? How would you typically be dealing with your emotions at this moment? What signals would you have been sending? If a therapist had walked into the room at that moment, how could he or she have summarized your feelings in an attachment frame and supported you to share with this potentially threatening person? See if you can write down what this therapist might have said.

For You Professionally

A father tells you:

> "So, he is having a hard time at school. So what. I had a hard time too. I went and got him those practice books, and he doesn't even look at them! And he lies to me and lies to me. I know he is on drugs. How stupid does he think I am? He reminds me of my brother, who threw away everything my parents gave him. He destroyed my mother. Who does this kid think he is? The solution here is not to 'talk.' We have done too much of that. The solution is for him to just move out and disappear and for us to accept that we have a damned junkie for a kid. He is never going to finish school. It doesn't make a damned bit of difference what we do."

How would you, in simple terms, reflect this parent's thoughts in a way that validates his experience but helps him begin to regulate his rage, and then help him begin to see his child's responses and needs in terms of vulnerabilities and in attachment terms? Try writing out what you would say. (*Hint—One place to start might be to reflect how upset he is that his son appears to be throwing away his caring.*)

 TAKE IT HOME AND TO HEART

- The goal of EFFT is to shape a safe haven and secure base bond between parent and child, where blocks to this bonding process are systematically addressed and the parent can respond to the child's attachment needs.

- The attachment dramas in a family group all play into and reflect each other, so multiple relationships have to be considered and how they affect the child who is becoming dysfunctional.

- Systems theory helps therapists grasp the entire relational system and how this system is organized in ways that prevent positive connection. This perspective states that significant change calls for a shift in the organizing elements of an interactional dance; in attachment relationships, this involves changing the nature of emotional communication and moving the dance, not just to homeostasis but also to safe connection.

- In EFFT the parent is supported to redefine the relationship and offer secure connection to a child. The therapist supports parents to find emotional balance, stepping through their own hurt, fear of failure, fear of loss of the child, and anger, to 'see' their child's vulnerability and become responsive attachment figures who can provide comfort and set clear and caring limits. Each child is helped to tune in to attachment needs, to reach out and take in the care now offered. The child's model of self is on line and available for redefinition in this process.

• Attachment science offers a clear map of the defining factors in the complex family dance and a clear road home to better family and child functioning. Securely attached kids are healthier and more resilient. They are on a different developmental pathway when they discover how to shape a loving relationship with a needed parent, and can deal with depression and anxiety more effectively.

• The vast majority of parents who seek family therapy are in touch with the compelling drive to protect and care for their young; the power of this biological imperative, when given direction and honed by the therapist, is a potent force for change. Parents' fear of failure in this regard has to be held and regulated by the therapist and then transformed into a new sense of confidence and competence.

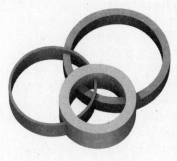

Chapter 9

Emotionally Focused Family Therapy in Action

This chapter depicts two family sessions that describe the EFFT process and outline interventions as they occur.

JOSH AND HIS FAMILY: THE BACK STORY

Josh, an 11-year-old who has his teachers, the local children's hospital workers, and his family totally alarmed at his aggressive behavior, comes to see me for our second session of EFFT. In the first session three family members were present: Sam, his father; Emma, his mother; and John, his older brother. In that session we outlined the key patterns of interaction in the family and Josh's part in them (these patterns are also summarized in the last chapter). Josh was agitated and tangential in this session: Interrupting, changing the subject, and making jokes. A picture emerged of an extremely distressed family in which the father, Sam, was under enormous pressure to work some 12–14 hours each day, but also admitted that he had turned to work to get away from the stress of his home life and the marital conflict with Emma. The oldest boy, John, was distant and uninvolved in the family drama, and told me that he spent his life outside the home and consumed with sports. Emma was extremely anxious and stressed, relaying in a high, fast voice with occasional tears how she dealt with her boys all by herself, and now had a small baby to care for, as well as her professional job. She responded to my empathic reflection that she was overwhelmed and scared with floods of tears.

The family tell me that Josh is bullied at school; does not sleep; has rashes all over his body, which doctors agree are the result of his high anxiety; and has tantrums where he smashes furniture, threatens to kill his father with a knife, and tells his mother that he will commit suicide by running out and throwing himself under the bus that stops just in front of his house. His explosions have twice resulted in the police coming to the house and removing Josh for a few days. In spite of his high IQ, Josh is also failing in school. Josh and I form a tentative alliance in this first session, mostly with playful, short encounters. He told me, "*I am not going to be here. I am going to be Peter Pan.*" When I shared that I would rather be in my garden on such a sunny afternoon, but perhaps it would be okay to be here at the hospital with him if he would allow me to be Tinkerbell, he gave me a broad grin and sat down beside me. But I could feel his agitation vibrating across the space between us. The patterns the family identify are that Josh and Sam are caught in constant conflict, with Josh taking an oppositional stance to every request made by his father and exploding when Sam repeats his requests; that Josh does talk to his mother and is less reactive with her, but when she tries to talk about family issues, terrifies her with threats of self-harm; that Emma and Sam have a constant complain/pursue followed by a dismiss/ withdraw cycle in their "always unhappy" relationship; and that John occasionally fights with Josh, but mostly remains outside the circle of anxiety and conflict the family is in.

The key blocks to secure interactions—the triggers for panic and spiraling chaos—appeared to be between Emma and Sam as a couple and between Emma and Josh, but most dramatically between Sam and his son. A little while after this initial session, Sam called to inform me that Josh refused to come to any more sessions.

In the next two sessions with Sam and Emma, we outline their negative cycle and how it contributes to Emma's spiraling anxiety and Sam's distancing and feeling of "hopelessness" in their relationship and in the family. We spoke about how this cycle undermines their ability to stay balanced and support each other as parents, setting Emma up for turning to her son as a confidant. The lack of a secure base parenting team also clearly contributed to Sam feeling trapped in his interactions with his son and becoming dictatorial, which Josh then met with more opposition. We set up a time once a day when Sam and Emma can just share any hard moments that have arisen that day with Josh and help each other with the feelings these moments evoke (they both feel like failures as parents), whether or not they are caught in their own negative couple cycle. We agree that I will work next with Josh and Sam. I constantly frame Josh as highly sensitive and anxious, vibrating with the tension in the family that emanates from his parents' marital issues and Sam's absence due to his long work hours, and as also facing the transition to adolescence and desperate for the secure belonging that his parents can provide. We revisit a poignant moment from the first session where, when I asked Josh what he would like from Sam (he had only expressed anger up to this point), he had suddenly turned and silently stretched out his open arms to his dad. Sam had then gone into freeze mode and, after a few minutes of still silence, had responded to my question about what was happening to him by commenting blankly, "I don't know what to do." I validated this. Sam had casually shared in the first session that in his family of origin you did what you were told and were immediately sent to your room if you were in any way upset or got "soppy" about anything. I framed this as Sam growing up all alone with no one to comfort or help him when he was scared or needed reassurance. He had shut his feelings down, whereas other kids decide instead to yell and scream and protest. He heard me.

Part of both Sam and Emma's difficulty in keeping their emotional balance and responding to their son in a coherent and sensitive way was the sense of failure and inadequacy they both felt as parents. This is a key issue, and one that seems to me is often bypassed in family therapy. The EFT therapist actively helps parents regulate and address these emotions, normalizing the fact that we all learn to parent on the run, as life happens, as our kids trigger us, as we are consumed by wanting to be perfect responsible parents, and as we realize that often we have no map for the dance that is occurring between us and our kids.

WORKING WITH JOSH AND SAM

Josh agreed to come to see me with his dad after I sent him an email saying that I was impressed to hear that he is so kind and helpful with his friend who is disabled (reported by Emma to me), that he seems to be good at seeing what is going on with others, and that I saw him as being able to help his family by pointing out the family's problems.

So, Josh walks into the session wearing a shirt he made, which says, "I am a hug dealer." I join with him in the positive, playful alliance that we began to set up in the first session. He seems calmer, makes more eye contact with me, and is a little more focused, but I remind myself to constantly monitor his ability to tolerate emotionally charged moments. His window of tolerance here is small; his attention span seems to be about 10 seconds or so. We chat about his and the family's summer plans. Sam bemoans how hard he has to work and his long hours. He has little time off to be with his family, and he knows this is hard on his wife and on Josh. Josh nods vigorously.

The atmosphere between father and son seems a little less volatile in this session than it was in the first session.

SUE: So how is the relationship between you guys? There seems to be a little less tension between you right now?

SAM: Yes. Things are basically better right now. But there are those times when we get into a yelling match and we can't talk at all. Then there are other times when I try to talk, when he seems upset, and I just get stonewalled—isn't that what you call it when someone just acts like you don't exist?. . . (*Long silence.*) I'm losing him. Can't reach him—can't help him.

SUE: So the yelling is when the old issue comes up of you asking Josh to do something and Josh refusing—yes? (*Sam nods.*) And then there are other times when you try to reach out to him and he shuts you out—yes? (*Sam nods again.*) [Reflect/describe the present reoccurring stuck places in Josh and Sam's relationship—Tango Move 1.]

SAM: I give a direction, like please turn off the TV, it's time to do your homework, and all hell breaks loose.

SUE: So in the first place, where you and Josh get stuck is when you are trying to do your job as a parent and give Josh some direction and Josh refuses—resists—gets very angry. In the second place, you want to help Josh feel better, and it's like he refuses your help? So as a parent you are pretty stuck. So what happens? You basically just get more directive or reach less? (*Sam nods.*) [Reflect cycle and reframe—we know from previous sessions that Josh does not see his father's care or reach.]

JOSH: I just need to cool down—to . . . (*He flaps his hands in the air—then looks out the window.*) is all.

SAM: (*To Josh.*) Well, my job is to help you grow up—to say stuff like, "I think you should clean your room tonight." But I can't tell you to do anything, anything at all. It's better than when we first came to see Sue but . . . I ask as nicely as I can. (*Josh starts to shake his head vehemently from side to side.*)

SUE: That is not how you experience this?

JOSH: (*To Sam, but looking the other way.*) You just say, "Do it." Like you are ordering me around, like a drill sergeant. And you say it about a hundred times. A hundred hundred times. (*He raises his arms into a circle about his head for emphasis.*)

SAM: I don't.

JOSH: Like I am a dog. A dog. So I get—I get . . .

SUE: Mad—defiant?—Maybe it's like—"I will show him. I will say No—you can't make me"? [Interpretation/conjecture in proxy voice—clarifying reactive surface emotion.]

JOSH: *Yes.* Yes. Yes.

SAM: Well, we are changing this. I do back off and you do hear me more . . . but . . .

JOSH: You back off just a little . . . ?

SAM: I try.

JOSH: If you say, "Can you do this today," I do it. Like, "Can you mow the lawn today?" Treat me like an equal.

SUE: Hm—that is a bit tricky, Josh, 'cause this guy here is your dad, and you are 11. So he is responsible for bringing you up. That is his job—showing you the ropes. So maybe "equal" isn't quite right. Sometimes he needs to be in charge.

JOSH: Well then—treat me like a person.

SUE: Treat you with "respect"? (*Josh nods.*)

SAM: I am trying to do that. But I am the parent, and I am responsible for things getting done.

JOSH: You forget stuff. You are old. I have more brain cells. Yours are dying. I read it in a book.

SAM: (*Flushes red.*) That is rude, Josh. I have experience.

SUE: Heh, Josh—I am old, too, older than your dad. Wonder how many brain cells I have left? About 10, I guess. (*I laugh, and Josh laughs.*) Even if he has less brain cells, your dad has learned lots over the years, and his job is to sometimes take charge here and to ask you to do things. Are you mad at your dad right now? (*Josh calmly shakes his head.*) What happens to you when dad tells you what to do, and you hear his drill sergeant voice? [Contain potential escalation with humor. Ask evocative question to elicit softer emotions—Tango Move 2.]

JOSH: (*Soft voice, looking down.*) Like a dog.

SUE: (*Matching soft voice.*) Like a dog? Like your feelings don't matter? Small. Like you are bad?

JOSH: That voice—I hear that he doesn't think I can do much. Small like a dog. He doesn't think much of me.

SUE: Oh wow, that hurts, yes? (*Josh nods.*) That really hurts. So you get really mad then (*He nods.*), because it hurts.

JOSH: I have to go to the bathroom. (*He leaps up, and Sam goes with him to show him the way to the washroom. I understand that this is Josh's way of regulating his emotions. Sam and Josh return.*)

SUE: Are you okay? We were talking about how your dad and I don't have many brain cells left (*Josh laughs.*) and about how when Dad tells you what to do, this hurts. You feel criticized—kind of put down? (*Josh sits very still, but he keeps eye contact with me.*) Can you help Josh with this feeling, Sam? (*I judge that if I am there to help, Sam can begin to see and respond to his son's vulnerability.*) [Tango Move 3—shape an enactment, but focus on the parent helping the son rather than on mutual risk taking.]

SAM: In fact, I think very highly of your ability. Look how you helped me mow the lawn, look how you help me with other things. (*Josh turns toward Sam.*) I am proud of you—all of the things you do, all the sports you play. (*Josh looks down and is silent.*)

SUE: What is happening, Josh? Can you hear your dad? Maybe you are still caught up in that feeling of being "put down," is that it? [Tango Move 4—processing an enactment.]

JOSH: He doesn't think I can do it. But if he just asks me—I will do it.

SUE: Can you tell him that?

JOSH: (*Turning to Sam.*) I will do stuff—if you talk to me like you trust me.

SUE: Yes. It's like you are saying to your dad, "I do so want you to see me as a good kid."

SAM: (*Leaning toward Josh.*) I'll try my best, Josh. I do see you as a good kid. And if you don't do it—what should I do then? [Therapist resists the urge to problem solve—say, "Simply and calmly give consequences," which we have spoken about in the sessions with Sam and Emma, because Emma can do this and can help Sam do it.]

JOSH: I will try, Dad. Yes, I will try to do this.

SUE: Right. And there will be times when you guys get stuck in this dance that looks like a power struggle, 'cause that is what happens to dads and sons. It's part of your dad's job to give you direction, and if you feel put down or criticized 'cause you are a sensitive kid, then you refuse, and then you both get stuck in this dreadful dance that has you feeling like a bad kid and your dad feeling like a bad dad (*Sam nods.*), a dad who can't get his kid to do anything without a big blowup. But right here, you can sort out how to help each other hear—how to talk so that the other person still feels respected—so you can cooperate. You can do this, guys. [Summarize the authority issue, normalize, pinpoint the emotional hurt/need driving the negative interaction pattern and the present positive exception—Tango Move 5.]

Josh and Sam both nod and smile at each other. I now go back to the second issue that Sam brought up at the beginning of the session—the fact that he cannot reach for his son to offer connection and comfort and have Josh let him in. Once the negative cycle of giving orders and angry refusal has begun to be contained, the creation of the beginnings of a positive cycle of secure connection between dad and son is the priority.

SUE: So I would like to go back to what you brought up at the beginning, Sam. There was this issue of being able to ask Josh to do things and Josh responding, but there was also the issue of times when you are reaching for your son, especially recently, and feel like you can't connect with him. My sense is that this is very painful for you? [Back to Tango Move 3—assembling emotion and encouraging Sam to be emotionally present to his son.]

SAM: Yes, it is. (*Purses his lips and looks sad, turns to Josh.*) Like the other day, I came and I reached out for you but you don't . . . you won't let me in. I get this wall.

JOSH: (*Looking down and away.*) I am uncomfortable with some topics.

SAM: (*More urgency in his voice.*) I can hear that it's hard to talk sometimes, but you say things like "Shut up," and "Get out," and that hurts, Josh.

SUE: Yes. Can I guess a little here as to what is happening? (*Josh nods at me.*) Josh, my sense is that you kind of get overwhelmed by feelings sometimes—they seem confusing and too much to deal with. (*Josh smiles at me and nods vigorously.*) Feeling angry at someone and needing to know they think you are a good kid, worrying that they don't feel that way, that is hard, and it is happening all at once. (*Josh nods again.*) So maybe you are still mad or needing to keep your distance from your dad—kind of keep your wall up. So then it's hard to shift gears and really see when he is reaching for you. (*Josh looks at Sam.*) He is trying to connect, which I think is what you want. At those times, he is reaching for you and trying to show that he sees you're hurting. He is trying to be there for you—to show he cares and you are special to him. Is that okay, Sam? [Interpretation/conjecture, normalizing Josh's difficulty in regulating his emotion and highlighting the positive signal coming from his dad. Tango Move 4—processing new emotions through enactments.]

SAM: Yes, yes, yes. I know I haven't been good at this in the past.

SUE: You end up feeling kind of rejected—shut out—like you have failed as a dad. You said at the beginning of the session, it's like "I am losing him." In that moment, you feel like you are losing your son. (*Sam looks tearful.*) And that hurts very much—to lose that connection—to be shut out by Josh. (*Sam nods. I turn to Josh.*) What is it like, Josh, to hear that in these moments when it is hard for you to let him in, that your dad feels all these things—hurt, rejected, like he is losing you? [evocative questions.]

JOSH: It feels weird. Do dads feel that? He is tough—he is a man.

SUE: Oh, yes. Your dad has these softer feelings—he doesn't want lose you—to lose his Josh—his precious son, so when he can't reach you . . . can't connect . . . Can you tell him, Sam? (*Gesturing with my hand from Sam to Josh.*) [Structure enactment with deepened emotional cues—Tango Move 3.]

SAM: (*Softly, leaning forward.*) Josh, our relationship is precious to me. It really, really bothers me when you push me away. I don't want to lose my connection with you.

SUE: Can you hear him, Josh? What is happening to you as your dad says this?

JOSH: Wow—sucker punch, sucker punch, and another sucker punch! This is like . . . surprising . . . surprising. He cares! (*He smiles, but it is obvious he is moved, but shy of showing his feelings.*)

SUE: Can you take that in—that he cares? This is not the way you have seen your dad. Can you let yourself feel it? (*Turning to Sam.*) Can you tell him again, Sam?

SAM: I don't want you to shut me out. I am so sorry that you didn't think I cared for you, Josh. (*Josh begins to twist all his tissues into a small ball.*)

SUE: (*To Sam.*) Yeah. I remember Josh telling you in the first session at the hospital that he wasn't going to listen to you because he didn't think you cared about him. It's hard to take all this in—that the dad who he sees as so in charge can feel these soft feelings. That Josh doesn't need to be so afraid that he isn't important to you. All dads and sons fight about things like chores and schedules, but if you guys can reach for each other after the fights then . . . you can have your togetherness too. I think that is what you want isn't it, Josh?

JOSH: Yes. It's weird. It's weird, (*Turns to Sam, talks in a soft voice.*) 'cause you are not around much. You are always working. Not around to talk to or to play with. You are not there. (*He is twisting more tissues into balls—a sign to me that his window of tolerance for this emotionally charged conversation is closing. It is so often the case that a sense of abandonment is the impetus behind a kid's rage.*)

SAM: Yes. I know. I feel so bad. Everyone hurts because of this. I have talked to my boss and it is a little better, but it seems like it's the way it is in my field. I have no one to delegate to. I try my best to be home as much as I can. The job demands so much of me. It's hard on your mom too. I want to be with you guys. I want to be with you. I am not always sure how to do it right. (*Josh looks up and smiles at Sam.*)

SUE: (*Making the decision that this is enough. It is all Josh can tolerate and we have done a good piece of work that we can integrate next time.*) Sam, I want you to know that it is amazing that you can be so open and so honest and share so much with your son. And Josh is such a clever, honest kid. It takes courage to come into these sessions because he is sensitive too, and these sessions can be hard—lots of difficult feelings come up. But here, with just a little help, he hangs in and opens up. He lets you in because he wants the connection with you. And it is wonderful, Sam, that you are reaching for him the way you did here. Do you know how special that is, Josh, how rare and wonderful to have a dad who can do that? How many dads do you think can do that? [Tango Move 5—validate and integrate.]

JOSH: (*Smiling broadly.*) Oh, I don't know. About 75% maybe.

SUE: Nope—nowhere close. You have a very special dad. He works very hard to protect and support his family. And he is learning to reach out—maybe he never saw his dad do that when he was a kid!!

JOSH: (*Yelling.*) He is a provider. Dads are supposed to do that.

SUE: Yes. Your dad is a strong man. He takes care of his family by working hard; he tries to give you all he can when he comes home; he is struggling to be a good dad to you and your brothers, and to be a good husband to your mom. He is strong. And it's very hard because it means that he has to spend so much time away from his family whom he loves. But your Dad does more than that. Do you know many dads who can take care of the family in all the practical ways *and* come in here and open up and show their softer feelings and reach for their kid? That takes a really strong man, a man who can show his softer feelings to those he loves—can invite them in—try to take care of them emotionally. That is special. (*Sam murmurs, "Thank you," and tears up.*) He must love you very much, Josh—very much. (*I am aware of offering Josh a model of masculinity, and also validating Sam and the changes he has made. I am also talking to Josh's amygdala, his longing for connection and reassurance, expanding his model of who his dad is.*)

JOSH: (*Grinning at me.*) Okay then, so he is like—it's like—25% who can do that—will do that.

SUE: Dads who really love their son and see that their son needs them to come close, even when things are going wrong and there are lots of angry times in the family, do that. Special dads risk reaching out—like your dad did in this session—to the kid he doesn't want to lose. (*Josh smiles and looks out the window.*)

SAM: (*To me.*) Thank you for that.

SUE: You are welcome. I think we should stop now. Josh, you did so well to come to the session and to share the way you did—you are good at this. Just like you open up and share with your friend—the little disabled kid—the one your mom told me about. It must be all those extra brain cells you have—that must be it. (*He grins some more.*)

But I think we are done. We should stop now. And, Sam, next time I would like to see you and Emma, if that is okay. (*He nods.*) So let's stop for now. You guys were brilliant. I so enjoy working with you. We explored how you are managing those stuck demand–refuse places where anger comes up, and we explored how you both can connect and come close so you don't lose each other. Well done. [Summarize process of the session in terms of disconnection and connection moments and validate.]

After the session I reflect that Sam now seems much more engaged and open with his family. He is a withdrawer who is now attempting to re-engage, so he can begin to be more present and responsive to his son. He will need to work with his wife, though, to really change their negative interaction patterns, and future couple therapy would seem to be indicated here. With Josh I am aware of the need to monitor the emotional intensity of the session carefully so as not to overwhelm him. Part of the time, I play and joke and exit into little chats where Josh can relax (a couple of which I have omitted here). He is precocious for his age, but is also very sensitive.

WORKING WITH SAM AND EMMA

This session with Sam and Emma is a session with the couple, but is focused on the family context.

We begin the session by reviewing the "demon" dance that has emerged in previous sessions and taken over Sam and Emma's family. I paint the picture I have and ask them to please correct me. I suggest that Josh feels cutoff from and unimportant to Sam, and he protests with tantrums and refusals; Emma also feels shut out from Sam, and is then alone and overwhelmed with anxiety in her role of mother, finding herself angry with Josh and in constant conflict encounters with Sam; Sam feels lost and "incompetent" (his words) as a father and husband, and tries to reason with Emma and tell Josh what to do—when this does not work, he retreats to his office and numbs out with work. The more Sam directs and withdraws, the more desperate Emma and Josh become, and the more they yell and complain, the more Sam wants to flee into his work. The cycle spins uncontrollably. Emma adds in a panicky voice that she just cannot parent her children "alone," that she is losing her balance at work, and that she is permanently "freaked out." Sam agrees with my summary, and adds that their difficulties get to the point where he just wants to "run away."

I focus on Josh as a highly intelligent, sensitive kid who, in this dance, does not have a safe place to feel accepted, calmed, and reassured. He does not have a good connection with his dad, cannot really feel held by his mom (even though she really tries her best), who is busy dealing with her own anxiety and stress. I validate how hard it is to parent sensitively, to attune to a child and respond congruently when we do not have our own emotional balance. Josh is also unsure of the safety in the family, because he sees his parents fight, his mother's panic, and his dad's apparent distance and unavailability.

Emma tells me that she sees Josh as just a "sad little boy," and that she feels lost in struggling with her own emotions about her marriage—her sense of abandonment and her fears for her son. She tells Sam, "You just lecture Josh, and you don't give me or him the connection we need." I focus on the fact that they both see the other as failing with Josh and feel unsupported in their parenting roles.

SAM: (*To Emma.*) You take Josh's side and undermine me—that is what happens! You resent my job and . . .

EMMA: I just try to comfort him.

SUE: Can I stop you just for a minute? You guys get stuck here around how to parent Josh. It's hard to be a team when you are struggling with your own relationship, yes? Emma, I believe you when you say you tune in to Josh's need for comfort from you *and* from Sam, because you feel that need for Sam's comfort too—yes? (*Emma nods.*) And we did talk about your relationship in a previous session, and how you guys need to repair it, but let's stay with what blocks you from helping each other as parents. I think you both have the same goals here. You both want Josh to become more stable, calmer, less distressed, and easier to talk to and be with. (*They both nod.*) Emma, you are trying to tell your husband that the way you see him talking to his kid isn't working—isn't meeting Josh where he lives, and Sam, you are defending yourself. I guess if this was at home it would end up with you getting exasperated and leaving, Sam? [Reflect present process of interaction—Tango Step 1.]

SAM: Yes. I would just go back to the office. Her and the kid, it's a roller coaster. I never do it right. She gets angry at Josh too— not just me. She lashed out and smacked him the other day. (*To Emma.*) You are angry too.

EMMA: I did, I did. I felt terrible about it. (*Cries. Emma has talked about this before and the therapist is clear that this is a momentary loss of temper.*) But I can't do this alone.

SUE: [Tango Step 1—reflecting the inner emotional loops now.] Yes—you both lose your balance with Josh—both feel overwhelmed and can't seem to reach out and support each other. Sam, what happens to you when you hear from Emma that she sees you lecturing and staying distant from your kid? You said it's a "roller coaster" where you never "get it right"? So you shut down.

SAM: Yes. I don't know how to parent Josh. I try. But he doesn't listen and his anger actually scares me. I know that sounds silly. She is angry at me for working so hard. He is angry at me. So I run.

SUE: It's overwhelming—and you don't feel safe enough to go and talk about this place where you don't feel sure of yourself as a parent with Emma because you think you will hear that it's all your fault. (*Sam nods and tears up.*) And Emma, is this one of those times where you are trying to poke Sam, to get him to listen, hear your concerns, and be there more—respond emotionally more to Josh?

EMMA: Yes—I know he feels criticized by me. But I don't know how to get him to see that we need him. I am losing it with Josh and him. [This response makes sense from an attachment point of view. Separation distress turns into angry desperation in the face of stonewalling or nonresponsiveness.]

SUE: So you get overwhelmed too—lose it. And you get desperate and try to explain, call to Sam to come close and help. But it doesn't work and . . .

EMMA: We are going down the tubes and Sam just walks out the door!

SUE: Right. So you are left bouncing between anger and feeling abandoned and afraid—overwhelmed just like Sam. Alone. But all Sam sees is your anger and that even comes out with Josh now and then you feel terrible about that.

SAM: I see we are both struggling—alone. I see that. But her anger scares the hell out of me! She is unreasonable! My family were very cool and calm. This scares the hell out of me.

SUE: [Tango Move 2—assemble and deepen emotion.] Let's stay with that. Sounds like your "running" seems like the only option when this fear hits you? And you really don't see the "reason" in her rage? Both Josh and Emma get so mad that it feels literally dangerous to you—

SAM: Yes—yes. There was the time that Josh was making threats about knives with me, and then a time when Emma tried to hit me—and she is mad at me all the time. So . . . if I try to explain that I have to work till late at night, she just dismisses that. (*He stares blankly at the floor.*)

SUE: What is happening to you right now, Sam, as you talk about this. Your face looks blank. You are very still. Where are you?

SAM: I am . . . I am . . . lost.

SUE: Lost—there is no way out here. If you stay, you hear people want to hurt you or, what . . . ?

SAM: That I am no good at anything. Useless. Useless.

SUE: And if you run—leave—then everyone is so enraged with you. . . . There is no way out. It's hopeless—you are helpless? (*Sam nods and nods.*) Is there anything that brings you a sense of comfort, stability?

SAM: I keep to my schedule—I keep my lists of tasks. She says all I care about is my schedule.

EMMA: It's your priority. . . .

SUE: (*To Sam.*) But that is your way of staying sane—keeping the helplessness at bay. Can you tell her . . . [Tango Step 3—choreographing engaged encounters. I could have helped him more by distilling the message.]

SAM: (*In a quiet voice.*) I do run off. One thing I can do is provide—earn money. I do lean on my schedule. All this emotional stuff—it's so hard for me. But when you get so angry . . . I just . . . I don't know what the word is—big fear . . . just hopelessness.

SUE: Panic maybe? (*Sam nods, then tears up.*)

SUE: [Tango Step 4—processing the encounter.] How does it feel to say this to her right now?

SAM: It feels strange. I am worried that she will be mad. (*Looking up at Emma.*) Are you mad?

EMMA: (*Softly.*) No. No, I am not mad, Sam. I know I get extreme—I don't like myself for that. It feels like a relief to hear what is happening with you. I never think I am having any impact at all. It's like you don't care. Then I get to feel so so . . . deserted by you. I guess we both feel useless in all this, and that hurts.

SUE: Yes. Your anger is you calling and calling to try to get him to respond. (*Emma weeps and agrees.*) You don't want to be angry all the time. Right now, he is risking and coming out to be with you, and that is reassuring. [Tango Step 5—validating.] Look at what you guys just did right here. Sam, you did not lecture or explain or run—you found another way. You told Emma what your commitment to tasks and schedules was all about—about your feeling of being useless—out of your depth—hopeless. And, Emma, you then stepped past your franticness—your anger at being left alone in all this and responded to him, saw his pain. That is amazing. (*They smile at me, even though their smiles are a little weepy.*) You guys are caught in your own dance as a couple, and sometimes it looks like the other is the enemy, but you are both in the same boat as parents, with Josh.

EMMA: Yes. (*To Sam.*) If I could come to you and tell you about my day with Josh and my . . . my fears, get some comfort, I think things would be different. But (*Now she really weeps.*) I think if I can't get Josh to behave, tone down, then you will leave us, leave me. I can't find you now, and if those bad times happen again . . .

SUE: Ah hm—And you are carrying all this weight of trying to manage this crisis, deal with Josh, and find a way to keep Sam from moving further away. No wonder you break under all this pressure—the franticness has to find a way out. But you are telling Sam, "If you can share with me and I see your fears, not just you walking away from me, and if I can tell you my fears and about the pressure on me to hold everything together in the family, with us, and just get comfort, this could make a real difference."

EMMA: (*To me—I motion to her to tell Sam.*) It would calm me down. Just to feel we were in the same boat. I know I show you anger when I get agitated. I send mixed messages.

SUE: What could Sam do for you at those moments, Emma? I remember in an earlier session we mentioned that we sometimes send angry signals when we are afraid—and I noted that some couples can use a code word that means "I am drowning . . . just need to know you are by my side even if you don't have any solution." In a way, being able to do this *is* the solution because it grounds folks—they are a team when the stress rolls in. When you are both off balance and stressed, that is when Josh really goes wild—yes? There is no stronger, wiser parent for him to use as a touchstone. He can't handle his emotions, and then he can't count on you to help him handle them either. [The EFT style of coaching parenting skills from the bottom up.]

SAM: Yes, *yes, yes.* (*To Emma.*) The other day Josh was revving up and you turned and said, "This is the storm," and then something different happened.

EMMA: Right. You didn't turn away. You came and stood beside me and you were calm even though I was losing it with Josh. You touched my arm, said something like, "We can all calm down now. We are all getting confused." And then Josh went off with you into the garage to find his fishing gear and . . . it kind of defused everything.

SUE: Hm. So you guys both get overwhelmed and hopeless, feel "useless," and scared, but you *can* find another way. You can use the code "storm" to tell each other when the tsunami is hitting and ground each other. No one is blamed here. It's just that a storm is coming in. Everything is changed just by being there for each other. Just helping each other get your balance. Josh has to take that in too: Nothing is more frightening for a kid than seeing that when he is melting down his parents can't hold him—catch him. And then the kid often decides that it must be that he is a bad kid, instead of seeing how off balance his "stronger" parents are. This is brilliant, guys. Just helping each other with these softer feelings makes such a difference. Does this make sense to you, Sam?

SAM: Yes, it does. Kind of different. I get it. I want to be there for her.

EMMA: I don't want to be so angry or make physical threats to you, Sam. It feels terrible. And Josh told me the other day that I had said to him that it was his "obnoxiousness" that was destroying the family. That felt terrible. Makes me feel so bad about myself. Adds to the tension in the house. I get that my anger scares you. But I can't do this alone, Sam.

SAM: Okay. Hear that. Maybe we can use the "tsunami" word then—help make things less scary. I could use this too to tell you when I am getting lost, cornered with Josh. Think it would help. It helps for me just to feel like you are hearing me here. (*Emma reaches over and touches Sam's arm softly.*)

I do not give parenting advice or techniques per se, but focus on shaping a new corrective emotional experience of parenting support for this couple and a way that they can help regulate each other's difficult emotions around the dilemmas of parenting and so provide a more secure base for their son. When the family sessions are over, they accept my suggestion that they go into couple therapy and work on their relationship.

At a follow-up inquiry, the family reports that Josh is generally calmer and there are now no more "storms" or threats of violence or suicide. Josh is doing better in school, and Sam and Emma are better at cooperating as parents and are also working on their relationship. Emma suggested that she really appreciated that Sam now seemed to understand that discipline and rules, in and of themselves, did not work with Josh unless he also "reached" for his son and connected with him. The couple agreed that with Josh's level of anxiety and his other diagnosed problems (such as ADHD), there would be other crises in the future, but they felt better able to handle them. Emma suggested that the "bonding piece really worked here. It was critical. Without it we weren't going anywhere. It hit the nail on the head." Josh and Sam began to do activities like playing pool together, and Sam was more tolerant when Josh did "creative" things like decide to replaster the walls in his room or make his older brother a huge birthday cake that took over the kitchen for 2 days.

This was a perfect "storm" in that a highly sensitive child with significant special needs for secure connection began the transition to adolescence at a time when the parent's marriage hit a low point. Both parents are challenged as a couple in their parental role and as individuals facing rejection, abandonment, and loss of control. Therapy consisted of an initial family session, sessions with the parents, sessions with Sam and Josh, and a session with Emma and Josh, then a final session with both parents and Josh.

EXERCISES

1. Identify at least two places in the transcripts where your first inclination would have been to do something different in terms of intervention. Can you formulate a rationale for why I intervened as I did?

2. How does this above treatment process differ from traditional models of systemic family therapy, both in terms of overall structure and specific interventions?

3. What specific positive effects on each person and on the family as a system can you imagine arising from each of the two sessions I discuss?

4. If you had seen this family for a consultation session, what do you think you would have found most difficult about working with them?

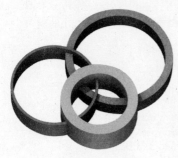

Chapter 10

A Postscript

The Promise of Attachment Science

An algorithm is a methodical set of steps that can be used to
... reach decisions ... the method followed when making the
calculation. . . . Even Nobel Laureates in economics make only a
tiny fraction of their decisions using pen, paper and calculator:
99 percent of our decisions, including the most important life
choices . . . are made by the highly refined algorithms we call
sensations, emotions and desires. . . . However, one core emotion
is apparently shared by all mammals: the mother–infant bond.
                              —YUVAL NOAH HARARI (2017, p. 97)

Trying to understand mental illness without accounting for the
power of social connection . . . is like studying planet motion
without accounting for gravity.
                              —DAVID DOBBS (July 2017, p. 83)

The argument presented in this book is that a focus on the core universal elements of our species—on our social bonding nature and on the
key place of emotions in connecting physiology, mental states, and patterns of interpersonal engagement—offers an elegant, eminently practical, and unifying way forward for the field of psychotherapy. This path
steers away from fragmentation toward integration and from compartmentalization toward wholeness. In attachment terms, it gives practitioners a secure base on which to stand in the growing chaos of our field.

On the most general level, attachment science suggests that the "between" part of a person's life should always be made an active part of therapy. Self and system and within and between are two sides of the same coin. It makes no sense to view or treat them separately. Compartmentalization distorts. Seeing individuals as constantly defining themselves in attachment contexts and in a way that reflects their attachment history is not only more accurate and holistic, it is empowering for the therapist, opening up possibilities for change that *use* the built-in power of the attachment system. For example, once we tap into the power of attachment bonds, seeing decades of debilitating shame simply dissolve in a client with PTSD becomes a regular event. Such a client tells me he has "failed" in numerous individual therapies, so real change is just not possible. However, in couple therapy, when he speaks his shame, and his wife tells him how she not only accepts him, but sees him as her chosen one—the one she needs—a seismic cascade of changes occur. There are shifts in his sense of self, in the nature of his connection with his wife, and in his sense of how to deal with the dragons we all face as just part of being human. Asserting oneself with an attachment figure in an imagined encounter also has a potent charge that is missing from a coaching process in which individuals learn general assertiveness skills. Helping clients deal with relationship loss will be more effective when the therapist understands that such loss involves the restructuring of self-concept and that lack of self-concept clarity plays a unique role in post-breakup emotional distress (Slotter et al., 2010).

UNITING SCIENCE AND PRACTICE

When the attachment perspective and the rich integrative science associated with it is merged with the experiential model of therapy, we have an effective intervention that honors and prioritizes the following:

- Psychotherapy as an essentially relational, attachment-oriented endeavor. This dictates the specific nature of the optimal therapeutic alliance. Emotional connection with a therapist is not simply a basis for coaching specific new behaviors, but a genuine encounter wherein the therapist is a surrogate attachment figure who offers clients a safe haven and a secure base. This safe connection expands their intrapsychic and interpersonal horizons. Feeling safe, sensitively attuned to, and securely connected with someone who helps regulate vulnerability is inherently growth producing for human beings.

- The significance of emotion and emotional experience in psychotherapy, both as a focus and an agent of change. Attachment is a developmental theory of personality, and it is also a theory of affect regulation. Emotional balance and flexibility are part of constructive dependency, and emotion is the most potent mover and motivator in the change process. The unique momentum created by evoking emotion and the indelible imprint of corrective emotional experiences may well be the touchstone of all effective psychotherapy—one that still seems to be drastically underutilized. To be truly used as a change agent, emotion has to be outlined as a process, clearly identified, put into an enlightening explanatory frame, and the momentum of its motivational force needs to be awakened.

• The integration of the inner and the between. Therapy has to address the reciprocal processes in which the self and the context in which the self plays out—a client's key relational systems—constantly define each other. Understanding causality as a circular, patterned process is crucial. The self is expressed in open or constricted ways that shape patterns of response from others; these patterns then feed back into a person's sense of self and response repertoire. Lasting change is always an intrapsychic and interpersonal phenomena. The view of human beings suggested here is essentially relational, and so mental health problems and solutions to these problems must be placed in this context. So teaching my client individual self-soothing or coping skills for her moments of panic is likely to be of very limited value unless I actively address her inability to trust others and reach out to them for help. As Bowlby notes, the capacity to make intimate connections in both careseeking and caregiving roles is the "principal feature of effective personality functioning and mental health" (1988, p. 121).

• A focus on core existential realities and meanings. These realities naturally arise when the therapist evokes a client's deeper emotional fears and longings in session. Optimally, therapy is a chance to struggle with the core dilemmas of life, such as how to deal with universal threats including emotional isolation, emotional and physical vulnerability, and the inevitability of loss and the finiteness of life, as well issues of personal significance (i.e., finding meaning in one's life journey and one's relationships). The attachment perspective suggests that in the end, it is connection with others that allows us to stare down life's impossible unsolvable dilemmas, and therefore isolation is the ultimate existential trauma.

• Interventions that do not narrowly focus solely on symptoms or problem alleviation but see the whole person in an interpersonal context and the possibilities that are hidden within each person and in each relational dance. Dysfunction is seen in terms of stuck patterns that once served a somewhat positive function, but now constrict optimal functioning. It is the therapist's job to validate the client's so-called defenses and self-limiting responses as protective strategies that have now become prisons, and to respectfully lead clients out of these prisons, much as a good parent does with a child.

- A basic orientation to empiricism. In the microcosm of therapy, this involves the attuned observation of present process, the ongoing identification of core variables that lead to the prediction of pattern, and a clear explanatory framework. This orientation offers a secure base to therapist and client, making sense of life dilemmas and difficulties. On a broader level, therapy must be based on a clear theory of personality and how personality develops and changes over time.

The Practitioner: Present and Attuned

To take a different perspective, the adoption of attachment science as the basis for psychotherapy helps us to avoid potential pitfalls. If we stay consistent with the arguments presented here, then a renewed focus on therapists' relational authenticity, that is, the ability to be really present with and attuned to our clients, may counter the movement toward reductionistic and mechanical interventions that seem to be growing more common in our field. These interventions, supported by claims that CBT is the gold standard for psychotherapy in terms of outcome research, a claim that has been effectively challenged (Leichsenring & Steinert, 2017), seem to be creating a psychotherapy discipline that is becoming more and more, to use the words of Irvin Yalom (2002), "impoverished." Coaching in coping techniques and mental health tips may have their own place, lending themselves to online interventions in which the involvement of a therapist is minimal, but in order to help a client move beyond simply managing symptoms, we have no better approach than in-person therapy with an attuned, fully present practitioner, especially a practitioner who has an integrated and empirically sound map of how we as human beings are constituted. Symptom management is also an endlessly expanding task when the underlying needs and dilemmas inherent in just being human are not being acknowledged or met.

An attachment orientation highlights the dangers inherent in a world that is becoming more and more deprived of personal connection and makes sense of the evidence that increasing emotional isolation, sometimes termed a modern plague, is an active threat to mental and physical health (Hawkley & Cacioppo, 2010). It would be a supreme irony if therapy, designed to help with the impact of stressors such as isolation, also became, at the same time, less and less relational; that is, if, even in therapy, human connection was downgraded from, as Cacioppo and Patrick (2008) frame it, an "essential to an incidental." Attachment science offers us a unique opportunity to take the therapeutic endeavor back to its roots—that of understanding the organizing principles that make us who we are and of leading us out into optimal aliveness and growth.

HONORING EMOTION

But attachment is not the only organizing principle that has, until recently, been missed or minimized in the world of psychotherapy. In general, empirically based therapies too often avoid or minimize emotion, and certainly do not think of emotion as a key resource in the creation of change. In the last two decades, we have seen the field devote a huge amount of attention to correcting cognitions, under that assumption that a focus on reason would shift affect and behavior. Indeed, other texts have presented more cognitive, insight-oriented interventions as the natural expression of attachment science (Wallin, 2007). Our field also seems enamored recently with the brain as an organ; authors speak of "brain-based" therapy. Allen Frances, one of the fathers of the DSM-IV, recently criticized the idea of considering psychiatric problems as primarily brain disorders, the resulting overuse of drugs (antidepressant use nearly quadrupled from 1988 to 2008), and the increasing medicalization of normal distress. He suggests that neuroscience advances have not in any way increased effective intervention (Frances, 2013). This viewpoint now seems to be shared even by Tom Insel, the former head of the National Institute of Mental Health, who previously (for over a decade) had channeled funding into research focused myopically on physiological variables or anything beginning with the prefix "neuro" (Dobbs, 2017). Pharmacological solutions are generally oversold, and evidence suggests that findings of benefit are more dependent on interpersonal factors, for example, an empathic, caring person dispensing the drugs, than is commonly believed (Greenberg, 2016). Even in disorders such as schizophrenia, effect sizes tend to be larger for interventions aimed at social variables, such as expressed hostility and criticism, than for new medications (Hooley, 2007). As a species we have strong self-healing capacities; mostly they involve supportive connection with others. However, the reductive biological model generally ignores the overwhelming evidence that social isolation and factors like perceived rejection prime and aggravate stress and mental health issues, while social support ameliorates them and shapes resilience.

This book presents the integration of experiential and systemic perspectives on intervention, concentrating on emotion as a natural outgrowth of the attachment perspective. However, as stated previously, while Bowlby always stressed the primacy of affect, he never found a unique or specific way of using affect to shape the change process. Nevertheless, all the clinical examples that he included in his writing echo a focus on following, validating, and expanding ongoing emotional experience in a manner that Carl Rogers would have applauded. Continuing to sideline emotion as an active change agent can be seen as a core pitfall in modern psychotherapy. Even as more behavioral approaches attempt to become nominally more inclusive of emotion, they tend to deal with it simply from a coping perspective; for example, reappraisal, acceptance, and suppression are offered as alternative strategies for affect control (Hoffman et al., 2009), with reappraisal always winning the empirical sweepstakes. The term "reappraisal" mostly refers to examining unreasonable dysfunctional thoughts or trying to adopt an "unemotional detached attitude" to emotions in order to decrease them (Gross, 1998b). Alternatively, emotional exposure may be used with the belief that habituation will occur. What is missing from this picture is any recognition that emotions are regulated and maintained through others. Also missing is a sense of the logic and adaptive nature of emotion and the active processing of emotion, including concepts such as increasing granularity, that are presented here. We need to reinforce the view of psychotherapy as necessarily a journey into and through emotion, while using emotion to direct and gain momentum in the change process.

Approaches that minimize the impact of emotion and active ways of discovering and working with it, that rely increasingly on drugs or on fast behavioral interventions, or that discount interpersonal relationships as a key resource in healing drastically limit our strategies for effective psychotherapy in the 21st century.

The adoption of an attachment frame that focuses on universal human factors does not imply that there is no need to match treatment to client—to give different strokes for different folks. Any good therapist takes the personal differences of clients into account and adapts the scope, focus, pace, and intensity of intervention to their specific needs. This is especially true in an experiential approach, wherein respect for and attunement to each client is the sine qua non of therapy. The overall principle in any helping relationship is, as Kierkegaard suggested in 1948, that "one first has to make sure one finds where the other is and start there."

In fact, from both attachment and experiential therapy perspectives attunement is the beginning and end of effective psychotherapy. It is then fascinating to realize that so often the ability to create this attunement is entirely omitted from psychotherapy training. As client disorders and change techniques have multiplied, the focus has been on instilling knowledge about this plethora of information. Older ideas, such as the principle that a therapist needs to actively cultivate the self-awareness that is a prerequisite for flexibly responding to many different kinds of clients, and that this self-awareness often requires some kind of personal therapy as part of training, seem to have gone' out of style. Genuine empathy, being able to put yourself in the shoes of another, requires open curiosity and a leap of imagination. Such leaps are difficult if one is mired in one's own reactive responses. Lack of self-awareness also closes down one of the main pathways to connecting with clients: An openness to and faith in one's own emotional signals and intuitions. Working with the emotions, especially the core longings and fears of others, requires an ability to look at these things in oneself. The training and supervision of therapists should then offer a safe haven and secure base where this kind of openness and attunement can be cultivated.

THE VALUE OF RELATIONSHIPS

The attachment orientation also takes us into an area that is filled with confusion and conflict—that of values. Psychotherapy is a value laden-enterprise, even if the values underlying interventions often are left unstated. We constantly decide that people are better off if they're one way or another. As Aristotle also noted, "What is honored will be cultivated." The values implicit in attachment theory and science echo the values demonstrated in experiential models of therapy. The most overriding value, it seems to me, is the sacredness of connection—of relationships as the primary source of meaning and growth in human life. There are many ways to prioritize human connection as a value. Some may see human connection as a spiritual matter and find support for it in religious teachings and belief in a great cosmic plan. Others simply look at the science that recognizes connection with others as the overriding given of human evolution, survival, and well-being. Jean-Jacques Rousseau, one of the great founders of humanism, states in his novel *Emile* that rules of conduct can be found "in the depths of my heart, traced by nature in characters which nothing can efface." What attachment science does, together with complementary lines of enquiry into areas such as the inherent nature of empathy (de Waal, 2009), is take this kind of statement, which can be dismissed as fluffy sentimentality, and give it grounding in empiricism. It is our job in the 21st century to build a discipline based on human beings' most fundamental needs, on the nature of deprivation and human pain, and on who we are at our most functional and at our best. We are Homo sapiens, and we are *Homo vinculum*—the one who bond—that is, the one who is truly safe and sound only when infused with a felt sense of secure connection to a valued other.

Promoting such a discipline presents quite a challenge in a context where many novel, enormous social experiments are under way that threaten to take us in a different direction. For example, more people now live alone and have no one to confide in (nearly 40% of Americans now identify as lonely, up from just 1 in 10 in the 1970s). Greater numbers of us spend much more time staring at a screen than looking into another's face. Concentrated attention that lasts for more than a few seconds is becoming a luxury. Everything is for sale, whether it is drugs that provide an escape from tangible life or sex dolls that make contact with real sex partners unnecessary. Depression is rampant. In 2011, 3.5 million children in the United States were taking medication for ADHD (Centers for Disease Control and Prevention, 2016). Clearly, human misery is not waning; in fact, it's being actively created by the way we structure our societies. The job of mental health professionals then is not simply to heal distress in individuals, couples, and families whenever possible, but to study, advocate, and educate, and to take a leadership role in crafting a healthier society, in which human beings can thrive. To do this, we need a vision to unify psychotherapy and make this discipline into a coherent force for good in the world. We cannot do this if we remain a collection of diverse cults all haggling over territory and over who has the lead in the psychotherapy competition.

Philosopher Kwame Anthony Appiah of New York University makes the following point: "In life, the challenge is not so much to figure out how best to play the game; the challenge is to figure out what game you are playing." As I have stated previously (Johnson, 2013), anchoring our models and techniques in the science of attachment and placing emotion at the center of what we do have the potential to change our game in psychotherapy. Ultimately, the only game that is worth playing is to build a more humane society—one that is attuned to who we are as social bonding animals. For example, evidence tells us that the more securely attached we are, the more tolerant of differences, the more empathic and altruistic we can be (Mikulincer et al., 2005). Attachment science is a blueprint, not just for the optimal development of psychotherapy, but also for a better, more essentially, human society.

Appendix 1

Measuring Attachment

Before turning to formal measures of attachment, it is useful to hone the ability to grasp and assess levels of security and the responses associated with these levels from simply observing clients in session. Developing this skill helps the clinicians tune in to clients' emotional realities. It also helps the clinician grasp when and how clients are making progress and when they have arrived at a more secure bond. It is worth remembering that both secure and more insecure attachment responses are on a continuum. The point is not to label clients with an attachment style but to tune in to current response patterns and processes.

LOOKING THROUGH THE ATTACHMENT LENS: LEARNING TO OBSERVE THE ATTACHMENT DRAMA

In the beginning of therapy Harry admits that he did, some months ago, send one email to his former lover. He did this after he had formally ended this very brief relationship to repair his relationship with his wife. He explains that this is the only contact he has had with this former lover, and that he felt guilty about his affair but needed to email her to be sure that she was coping. His wife, Zoe, tells the therapist that she believes Harry, and that they have made great progress in therapy. Then she explodes. Let us look at some of ways she responds that cue the therapist that Zoe is not simply distressed in her relationship, but insecurely attached in her orientation to relationships generally, and in her relationship to Harry as it has evolved over many years.

1. She is still extremely distraught at the news about the email, and her emotional response seems chaotic. She flips between virulent anger and intense sadness and expressions of hurt. She has trouble organizing her thoughts and threatens to leave the session and the relationship. Her high reactivity suggests that she is experiencing a very high level of threat.

2. Her messages to Harry are confused and confusing. She demands that he agree to show her his email every night, and then that he again write to his ex-lover stating that he regretted the relationship. When he agrees to the first demand but balks at writing the letter, she begins catastrophizing about how

their relationship was never meant to be and can never be healed. She tells him tearfully that she needs him to prove his love and gives him a list of specific actions that might achieve this.

3. When Harry takes responsibility for sending the email and not telling her about it, she seems not to hear him. He attempts to empathize, reach out, and offer her reassurance, but his efforts do not seem to make even a small dent in Zoe's distress. She cannot seem to take in his reassurances and expressions of love. She mostly dismisses his comments and returns to complaining about his behavior in their negative cycle that existed before the injury of the affair.

4. Even after this incident is dealt with in the session and the emotional music is calmer, Zoe seems hypervigilant and reluctant to give Harry the benefit of the doubt, to the point of downplaying even positive suggestions Harry brings up about spending time together, saying that she doesn't trust he will really come through.

This is a picture of significant anxious attachment played out from a pursuing position in a moment of stress and uncertainty. Zoe's preoccupation with a sense of threat (anxious attachment is often also termed preoccupied), her ambivalence about trust, and her difficulty with regulating her emotions are clear.

Ten weeks later, how does the therapist know if Zoe's attachment orientation has begun to shift toward security in her relationship with Harry? If it has, this is a shift that could then be generalized to apply to her general orientation toward depending on others.

Zoe finds a picture of Harry and his friends that includes his former lover (which she had asked him to throw away) in his desk. She brings the picture to therapy and takes it from her handbag. Harry seems surprised and apologizes, saying he did throw away one picture, but did not know that this picture was there. She asks him to simply put it in the therapist's garbage, and Harry agrees. How do Zoe's responses differ from the first session described here?

1. Zoe is angry as she confronts Harry, but her anger is much more ordered and coherent than it was previously. She then goes on to express her fear that this injury will continue to turn up in and haunt their relationship, and that Harry is still attached to his former lover. She is distressed, but her emotions are much clearer and less intense. She is able to explore exactly what it was about the affair that made it such a "freak out," which was that she had, for various reasons, become much more trusting and felt safer and closer with Harry just before its disclosure.

2. Zoe's improved affect regulation shows up in her signals to Harry. She can focus on the fear that this incident with the picture brought up in her and links this pain back to other betrayals in her early life. She is more balanced in her narrative. She can explore her responses rather than obsessing about Harry's motives, and is able to link the affair itself to the negative cycle created by them both in her relationship with Harry in the years before the affair. She also does not become caught in catastrophizing and is able to send clear messages about her hurt and how Harry can help her with that hurt.

3. When Harry offers understanding, regret, and care, she seems to tune in and respond to his comfort. She can reiterate her need for reassurance, ask him for a specific kind of physical contact, and tell him the words he uses that she finds most comforting.

4. Zoe can then move on to exploring with Harry how he is sometimes triggered by her tone of voice and wants to withdraw, and how she can help him become less sensitive and stay connected with her.

This is a picture of growing secure connection and the maintenance of emotional balance in the face of vulnerability. Zoe cannot hold onto this felt sense of security all the time, but even when she does exhibit more insecure responses, they are less intense and she can dial them down more easily.

In individual therapy, clients' attachment orientations are displayed in narratives about their lives and relationships and in interactions with the therapist. It is important here, though, to be aware of the expectations we as therapists create, and the responses we evoke. Most clients, no matter what their dominant attachment style, tend to display avoidant behaviors when confronted with therapist responses that appear detached, judgmental, and lacking in empathy.

MORE FORMAL MEASURES OF ATTACHMENT

Two examples of questionnaires of adult attachment are presented in this appendix. These are offered, first, because these measures are used in research, and reviewing them may make this research more meaningful for clinicians; second, because knowing how a phenomenon is measured brings it to life and makes it concrete; and third, because in using the first measure, readers can assess the attachment style or main strategy that is front and center for them in their current life.

It is good to remember that if you choose to complete the Relationship Scales Questionnaire, the questions are stated in terms of a person's general attachment. A person's style with a specific relationship partner may differ from this general orientation. The second measure, the Experiences in Close Relationships Scale—Revised, is framed specifically in terms of one's current partner.

All styles are useful and functional at different times and circumstances and, although they are often stable, they can also change with new experiences. Most individuals also have a main dominant style and then a backup alternative. I may generally rate as secure on these scales, but at times of high stress might rate as more anxiously attached.

Relationship Scales Questionnaire (RSQ)

Please read each of the following statements and rate the extent to which you believe each statement best describes your feelings about *close relationships,* using the following rating scale:

1	2	3	4	5
Not at all		Somewhat like me		Very much like me

1. I find it difficult to depend on other people.
2. It is very important to me to feel independent.
3. I find it easy to get emotionally close to others.
4. I want to merge completely with another person.
5. I worry that I will be hurt if I allow myself to become too close to others.
6. I am comfortable without close emotional relationships.
7. I am not sure that I can always depend on others to be there when I need them.
8. I want to be completely emotionally intimate with others.
9. I worry about being alone.
10. I am comfortable depending on other people.
11. I often worry that romantic partners don't really love me.
12. I find it difficult to trust others completely.
13. I worry about others getting too close to me.
14. I want emotionally close relationships.
15. I am comfortable having other people depend on me.
16. I worry that others don't value me as much as I value them.
17. People are never there when you need them.
18. My desire to merge completely sometimes scares people away.
19. It is very important to me to feel self-sufficient.
20. I am nervous when anyone gets too close to me.
21. I often worry that romantic partners won't want to stay with me.
22. I prefer not to have other people depend on me.
23. I worry about being abandoned.
24. I am somewhat uncomfortable being close to others.
25. I find that others are reluctant to get as close as I would like.
26. I prefer not to depend on others.
27. I know that others will be there when I need them.
28. I worry about having others not accept me.

Source: Griffin, D. W., & Bartholomew, K. (1994). The metaphysics of measurement: The case of adult attachment. In K. Bartholomew & D. Perlman (Eds.), *Advances in personal relationships: Attachment processes in adulthood* (Vol. 5, pp. 17–52). London: Jessica Kingsley.

29. Romantic partners often want me to be closer than I feel comfortable being.
30. I find it relatively easy to get close to others.

Note. Items 6, 9, and 28 must be reverse-keyed prior to computing the following four attachment style scores:

    1. The *Secure Style* score is computed by averaging items 3, 9, 10, 15, and 28. Higher scores reflect more secure attachment.

    2. The *Preoccupied (Anxious) Style* score is computed by averaging items 6, 8, 16, and 25. Higher scores reflect more preoccupied attachment.

    3. The *Dismissing Avoidant Style* score is computed by averaging items 2, 6, 19, 22, and 26. Higher scores reflect more dismissing avoidance.

    4. The *Fearful Avoidant Style* score is computed by averaging items 1, 5, 12, and 24. Higher scores reflect more fearful avoidance.

The fearful avoidant style is less well known by health professionals. In a sense, this style combines both anxious and avoidant tendencies. This style is associated with parenting by attachment figures who were both desperately needed and also seemed dangerous, and so had to be avoided. Connection is anxiously longed for and, when offered, imbued with threat. Others are a source of fear and a solution to fear.

Experiences in Close Relationships Scale—Revised (ECR-R)

The following statements concern how you generally feel in close relationships (e.g., with romantic partners, close friends, or family members). Respond to each statement by indicating how much you agree or disagree with it, using the following rating scale:

1	2	3	4	5	6	7
Disagree strongly	Disagree	Disagree slightly	Neutral/ mixed	Agree slightly	Agree	Agree strongly

Secure attachment consists of low scores on both avoidance and anxiety items. This version is stated in terms of romantic partners.

Avoidance Items

1. I prefer not to show a partner how I feel deep down.
2. I feel comfortable sharing my private thoughts and feelings with my partner.*

Source: Fraley, R. C., Waller, N. G., & Brennan, K. A. (2000). An item response theory analysis of self-report measures of adult attachment. *Journal of Personality and Social Psychology, 78,* 350–365.

3. I find it difficult to allow myself to depend on romantic partners.
4. I am very comfortable being close to romantic partners.*
5. I don't feel comfortable opening up to romantic partners.
6. I prefer not to be too close to romantic partners.
7. I get uncomfortable when a romantic partner wants to be very close.
8. I find it relatively easy to get close to my partner.*
9. It's not difficult for me to get close to my partner.*
10. I usually discuss my problems and concerns with my partner.*
11. It helps to turn to my romantic partner in times of need.*
12. I tell my partner just about everything.*
13. I talk things over with my partner.*
14. I am nervous when partners get too close to me.
15. I feel comfortable depending on romantic partners.*
16. I find it easy to depend on romantic partners.*
17. It's easy for me to be affectionate with my partner.*
18. My partner really understands me and my needs.*

Anxiety Items

1. I'm afraid that I will lose my partner's love.
2. I often worry that my partner will not want to stay with me.
3. I often worry that my partner doesn't really love me.
4. I worry that romantic partners won't care about me as much as I care about them.
5. I often wish that my partner's feelings for me were as strong as my feelings for him or her.
6. I worry a lot about my relationships.
7. When my partner is out of sight, I worry that he or she might become interested in someone else.
8. When I show my feelings for romantic partners, I'm afraid they will not feel the same about me.
9. I rarely worry about my partner leaving me.*
10. My romantic partner makes me doubt myself.
11. I do not often worry about being abandoned.*
12. I find that my partner(s) don't want to get as close as I would like.
13. Sometimes romantic partners change their feelings about me for no apparent reason.
14. My desire to be very close sometimes scares people away.
15. I'm afraid that once a romantic partner gets to know me, he or she won't like who I really am.
16. It makes me mad that I don't get the affection and support I need from my partner.
17. I worry that I won't measure up to other people.
18. My partner only seems to notice me when I'm angry.

Note. *Denotes items that are reverse-keyed.

Appendix 2

General Factors and Principles in Therapy

Many general factors bring about change in therapy. For sure, client factors, relationship factors, and therapist and technique factors all seem to play a role.

The American Psychological Association Division 12 Task Force on the promotion and dissemination of psychological procedures (Chambless et al., 1998) identified these factors in the following terms:

- Client factors, such as gender, attachment style, and level of motivation and engagement, and expectations and readiness for change.
- Therapeutic relationship factors, such as alliance quality and empathy, and therapist factors, such as warmth, positive regard for the client, and authenticity.
- General technique factors include the level of therapist directiveness, a focus on symptom change versus a focus on growth and development, treatment intensity, an interpersonal versus an intrapsychic focus of intervention, the prominence of the role emotion plays in therapy, and a focus on intensive versus short-term procedures.

CLIENT FACTORS

Focusing on these factors raises the issue of matching client to intervention: The most sensible concept of matching that this writer has noted is that overly emotional clients may require more emotionally containing interventions, while detached clients need techniques that facilitate emotional engagement and expression (Stiles, Agnew-Davies, Hardy, Barkham, & Shapiro, 1998). Attempting to integrate all the research in this field and relate all these factors to everyday therapy practice can be confusing. Keeping the main findings in mind is a good place to start. Here are the most pertinent findings concerning client factors.

1. Comorbid personality disorders seem to make the treatment of disorders like depression more difficult.

2. There is less-documented dropout if patients and therapists come from the same ethnic backgrounds.

3. Some research suggests that clients who tend to impulsivity and external blame, often called externalizers, may benefit from therapies for depression that focus on symptom reduction, skill building, and managing impulses, rather than on self-awareness, while the opposite may be true for more introspective clients (Beutler, Blatt, Alimohamed, Levy, & Antuaco, 2006).

4. The attachment style of clients seems to predict both alliance and outcome; clients who exhibit a more avoidant attachment style seem to have more difficulty making a positive alliance with their therapist and often have poorer outcomes (Byrd, Patterson, & Turchik, 2010; Marmarosh et al., 2009; Bachelor, Meunier, Lavadiere, & Gamache, 2010).

5. In treating anxiety, the severity and duration of symptoms appear to negatively impact treatment; likewise, a client's level of social support has been found to predict treatment effectiveness (Newman, Crits-Christoph, Connelly Gibbons, & Erickson, 2006).

6. As with so many other indicators of coping, being married has been found to predict sustained improvement in anxiety, but being *unhappily* married seems to diminish positive change (Durham, Allan, & Hackett, 1997). As always, the quality of relationships shows up as a potent source of health or, if those relationships are negative, as a source of susceptibility to problems. In studies of PTSD, relationship distress predicts symptom severity (Riggs, Byrne, Weathers, & Litz, 2005). In fact, perceived hostility from significant others has been generally found to trigger relapses in both anxiety and depression (Hooley & Teasdale, 1989).

7. Single diagnoses and good interpersonal contacts seem to be typical of those who are most likely to benefit from therapy for anxiety; negative parenting and attachment relationships in childhood make the effective treatment of anxiety more difficult (Beutler, Harwood, Alimohamed, & Malik, 2002).

THERAPIST FACTORS

In terms of therapeutic alliance and therapist factors, there is general agreement that the relationship with the therapist, especially the empathy and the authenticity offered in this relationship, influences outcome and, when positive, fosters client collaboration and engagement in therapy. For example, Zuroff and Blatt (2006) found that across therapy models and accounting for patient characteristics and symptom severity, clients' early rating of the alliance impacted outcome and follow-up in the NIMH study on depression (Elkin et al., 1989). It is important to note, however, that, in general, the association of alliance quality and therapy outcome is relatively small. Studies imply that around 10% of the variance in outcome is accounted for by the alliance (Castonguay et al., 2006; Beutler, 2002). This finding confirms our general understanding in EFT that *alliance is a necessary but not sufficient element* for creating positive change.

And yet, in one study of EFT for couples (Johnson & Talitman, 1996), alliance was found to account for as much as 20% of the variance in outcome.

It is also important to note that alliance may not be quite such a "general" factor as we thought. It seems to differ substantially across models of therapy in nature, quality, and impact, and also seems to play a different role in different therapies. Also, technique and alliance can be hard to separate, as they constantly interact with and influence one another.

The concept of therapeutic alliance can be differentiated into three elements: Bond, goal agreement, and task (Bordin, 1994). Perhaps the most interesting result in EFT research was found in the Johnson and Talitman (1986) study. In that study, it was the *task* element of the alliance, rather than the bond with the therapist or agreement about goals, that predicted better outcomes. This task element as measured by Bordin, captures the client's experience that the therapist is on target—that interventions are relevant for the client and are critical to setting the stage for change. The result of this EFT study was surprising to us given that EFT emphasizes the presence of the therapist and his or her availability, responsiveness, and engagement. One way of understanding this finding is that the task element translates into a felt sense that the therapist is tuned in to and aligned with the client in a way that is relevant to the client's concerns and goals.

In terms of therapist characteristics, some evidence shows that therapists with an anxious preoccupied attachment style tend to respond less empathically with clients, and secure attachment in the therapist seems to contribute to session depth and better outcome (Rubino, Barker, Roth, & Fearon, 2000; Levy, Ellison, Scott, & Bernecker, 2011). Qualities such as flexibility, persuasiveness, affect modulation and expressiveness, warmth and acceptance, and the ability to communicate hope have also been found to impact the alliance and treatment outcome.

GENERAL TECHNIQUES

As already discussed, it is impossible for practitioners to learn even a significant portion of the interventions outlined in lists of empirically supported treatments, since they are so numerous (Follette & Greenberg, 2006). The impact of specific techniques is also extremely difficult to isolate and research, embedded as they are in a rich set of intermingled interventions in the ongoing drama of a therapy session. There is also the issue that, even in manualized and empirically validated therapies, it is often hard to determine what the active component of change really is. When CBT works, is it because of the intervention called challenging the negative beliefs of the client? There is growing evidence that targeting negative thinking is not necessary to achieve positive outcomes in CBT (Tang & DeRubeis, 1999; Dimidjian et al., 2006). In fact, as stated previously in Chapter 3, in CBT, it seems to be the quality of the alliance and the depth of emotional experiencing that predict treatment success for depressed clients (Castonguay et al., 1996).

The labels of interventions and techniques themselves can also confuse as well as clarify. Mindfulness, for example, which comes from the Pali word *sati,* meaning "awareness or attention," can be used to refer to many different elements. Germer, Siegel, and Fulton (2003) point out that the classic version of mindfulness, in which a person turns toward his or her present experience without judgment, paying attention to the "unfolding of experience moment to moment" (p. 145), is "strikingly similar" to humanistic experiential approaches, such as Gendlin's focusing interventions (1996). Indeed the parallel with EFT is obvious here, and the links between EFT and Buddhist thought have been outlined in the literature (Furrow, Johnson, Bradley, & Amodeo, 2011). However mindfulness can also be used as a way into detachment from experience or even as stress management or relaxation training. Many clinicians now view mindfulness as part of CBT treatment, without recognizing that experiential therapies have been using this technique in its classic form for many decades, albeit without the specific practice of sitting cross-legged by yourself in silence. In the classic form described by Germer, and as implemented in EFT, the process of focusing on experience "mindfully," as it occurs, also changes people's relationship to their experience in that they recognize that they are actively *constructing* their experience, rather than having it simply happen to them. This awareness may indeed include, as suggested in Buddhist thought (Olendzki, 2005), a new sense of the self as a *process* that is actively and constantly reconstructed in a particular context, rather than being a fixed entity. It is also interesting to note that ways into this new level of awareness can vary, whether we call it mindfulness or attunement into the experiential unfolding of experience. One study (Pinniger, Brown, Thorsteinsson, & McKinley, 2012) compared the impact of Argentine tango and mindfulness practice on depression. It found that both interventions were more effective than a wait control in reducing symptoms, but that only the tango reduced stress and made people more mindful!

It is also hard to compare the effectiveness of specific techniques or interventions. With all the variables that are involved in a therapy model, the differing impact of the implementation of a model with different clients, and the bluntness of our measures, it would be surprising if outcome differences resulting from different specific techniques were not lost, especially when many studies lack the statistical power to find these differences (Kazdin & Bass, 1989). We also rely on meta-analyses in psychotherapy studies, which mix high- and low-quality studies and studies of very different phenomena, and are notoriously subject to distortion. When methodological problems are taken into account, effect sizes from meta-analyses can drop dramatically. A review of trials for depression found an unadjusted effect size of 0.74, but this dropped to 0.22 after controlling for methodological quality (Cuijpers, van Straten, Bohlmeijer, Hollon, & Andersson, 2010). The famous NIMH study on depression (Elkin et al., 1989), which compared interpersonal and cognitive behavioral interventions, is often used to argue the so-called Dodo bird hypothesis—that is, that there are really no differences in outcome across any models of psychotherapy. Since studies with widely differing methodologies are grouped together in meta-analyses, labeling often obscures what is actually done in treatment (so that one CBT intervention may not resemble another). The practice of averaging averages as these analyses do almost certainly masks considerable variability in outcome. I suggest, as do others (Tolin, 2014), that we dispense with this misleading metaphor.

Comparative studies also suffer from confounding issues, such as that many clients terminate therapy prematurely or relapse, or that across models, some therapists appear to be unusually effective while others are not (Wampold, 2006). Perhaps the most pertinent question for the practicing therapist is, are there general techniques for the treatment of anxiety and depression that almost any model should include in one way or another?

GOALS OF THERAPY

There seems to be some consensus (Follette & Greenberg, 2006; Woody & Ollendick, 2006) that, considering the data on therapies that have been shown to be effective, any effective treatment should include techniques focused on a few key general goals.

- The challenging of cognitive appraisals with new experience.
- An increase in positive reinforcement.
- An active addressing of avoidance behaviors.
- Gradated exposure to feared or difficult situations.
- Improving a client's interpersonal functioning.
- Improving marital and family environments.
- Improving the awareness and regulation of emotion.

Treatments for anxiety, in particular, seem to vary regarding issues, such as how much focus to place on coaching coping skills versus how much the processing of emotion should be directly addressed. In CBT approaches, the evocation of emotion is seen as simply a by-product of challenging cognitions (Woody & Ollendick, 2006, p. 180), and the focus is solely intrapsychic rather than interpersonal. However, luminaries like David Barlow challenge both of these trends. In a 1984 study, Barlow, O'Brien, and Last found that 86% of women whose partners accompanied them to exposure treatments for agoraphobia improved, compared to only 43% of women who completed the treatment without their partner, and this gap in efficacy continued to rise at follow-up. Barlow, in his seminal book *Anxiety and Its Disorders* (2002), also advocates more attentiveness to emotion and emotion theory. He points out that emotion *is* behavior, it *is* cognition, and it *is* biology. As Woody and Ollendick point out, "Many clients speak of the experience of anxiety and fear: The sense of dread, danger and drama that leads to the fight and flight response. As clients describe this experience, it is more than cognitions, more than avoidance and more than physiological arousal. This felt experience seems to be lacking in our current depiction of these core emotions and their treatment" (2006, p. 181).

What does this metafocus on common factors and the correlates of change and general principles of intervention mean for the practicing therapist? This knowledge can help us adapt our therapeutic relationship to and interventions with particular clients to refine treatment and enhance outcome. It can help us look critically at any model and ask whether the techniques that are considered core to the model include the key elements of effective treatment, whether the interventions are clear and labeled appropriately, and how unique the interventions are to particular models. But the common-factors perspective does not offer a model of intervention. Predictors of treatment success and principles of therapy can be abstracted in general terms, but therapy is not conducted on this general level. The practicing therapist wants to know what element to focus on and what specific kind of intervention to use at a particular moment, so that the model he or she uses becomes a source of confidence and competence. Suffice it to say that the literature on general factors in many ways supports the premises of an experiential attachment model of therapy. For example, EFT stresses the importance of alliance in outcome, and EFT seems to align with the general goals laid out for effective therapy previously outlined. However, the literature on general factors can also be very confusing, and is sometimes used to dismiss the need for coherent models of intervention or to imply that the nature of interventions does not matter since one is as effective as another. Obviously this book does not subscribe to this view. In fact, it states the opposite. It argues that many models of therapy lack a solid empirical understanding of human beings from a developmental and personality standpoint, and that such an understanding is necessary for the development of the field of psychotherapy and future improvements in therapy outcome.

Appendix 3

Emotionally Focused Individual Therapy and Other Empirically Tested Models That Include the Attachment Perspective

It is first important to note that psychodynamic approaches to the treatment of anxiety and depression (which gave rise to and are close cousins of experiential approaches) have been shown to be effective (Shedler, 2010; Abbass, Hancock, Henderson, & Kisley, 2006; Leichsenring, Rabung, & Leibing, 2004), and consistent trends show that effect sizes for these interventions become larger at follow-up. These results suggest that these interventions, which are often somewhat longer than behavioral therapies, are successful in creating ongoing change. Many studies include patients with a range of conditions, which, since comorbidity is the norm, would seem to be more representative of real-world practice than the discrete patient groups often used in the more numerous efficacy studies that examine effects in CBT. When considering outcomes, it is also important to note that CBT interventions tend to be more didactic and skill based, while the essence of nonbehavioral interventions is a focus on helping the client gain an awareness of previously implicit feelings and meanings. This kind of change does not always fit easily into the framework of randomized control studies, the accepted barometer of empiricism in psychotherapy. Such studies tend to stress the alleviation of acute symptoms (the focus of behavioral approaches) rather than the more growth-oriented generation of "inner capacities and resources focused on in dynamic and experiential therapies that allow people to live life with a greater sense of freedom and possibility" (Shedler, 2010, p. 105). It seems that symptom-oriented outcome measures do not, in fact, do justice to the possible changes psychotherapy can engender.

INTERPERSONAL PSYCHOTHERAPY (IPT)

One empirically tested approach that does refer to attachment theory is the IPT model. This model is known best as an intervention for depression (Klerman, Weissman, Rounsaville, & Chevron, 1984; Cuijpers et al., 2010). In a recent study, using a large sample size (237 clients) which allows for rigorous conclusions of "non-inferiority" or true equivalence between treatments, IPT was shown to be as effective at treating depression as cognitive therapy (Connolly Gibbons et al., 2016). However, in spite of their improvement, some 80% of clients continued to have some depressive symptoms at the end of treatment. Interestingly, the authors of this study note that the sample size, which determines the power of analyses of outcome, is most often insufficient in psychotherapy studies to demonstrate real equivalence between treatments.

There are similarities between the IPT and EFIT models presented in this book. The IPT model focuses on social stressors and loss as potent triggers for depression and uses attachment theory as part of its theoretical base. Interpersonal encounters are discussed, communication patterns are analyzed to find problematic patterns of relating, and future interactions are planned. Loss, grief, disputes, and role transitions are particularly attended to. A client's history, especially trauma, is framed as creating a vulnerability to present problems, and education is offered that normalizes depressive mood. Empathic questions and reflections are used to explore relationships that are chronologically and emotionally linked to symptoms. New ways of communicating are practiced in role plays. This approach somewhat parallels the use of imaginal encounters and enactments with others in EFIT. The normalizing and framing of emotions as powerful but not dangerous, the focus on working in the here and now, and the optimistic stance that clients can and will handle difficulties and grow seem particularly consonant with EFIT.

There are also significant differences between IPT and EFIT; for example, IPT emphasizes renegotiation in role disputes similar to more behavioral interventions. Also "catharsis" is referred to as an intervention, implying that ventilation of emotion in and of itself is useful—a view that is not espoused in EFT in general or in EFIT. Although in both IPT and EFIT approaches emotion is identified, there is no reference in IPT to actively processing or deepening emotion, or to using newly processed emotion as a pathway into more adaptive behaviors. In fact, John Markowitz suggests (in his notes in his seminars) that IPT is a nonexposure treatment, and therefore practitioners should use CBT or EMDR first when dealing with trauma. Attachment seems to be more of a backdrop in this approach, rather than an active existential frame that distills the "hot" cognitions and meanings that are the music of attachment relationships. From this point of view, IPT as practiced seems to be closer to a coaching behavioral model aimed at building interpersonal skills than is EFIT. Since there is also little process-of-change research on the IPT model, the mechanism of change is unclear.

PROCESS EXPERIENTIAL/EMOTION-FOCUSED THERAPY (PE/EF)

The PE/EF model (process experiential therapy, now most often called emotion-focused therapy, outlined by Elliott, Watson, et al., 2004) is grouped with EFIT under the general rubric of an emotion-focused therapy, as used by Greenberg (2011). This term seems now to be used in a generic way to refer to all therapies, be they cognitive-behavioral, or systemic or humanistic, that attempt in any way to include emotion. However, there is an enormous difference between a behavioral therapy, in which emotion is simply identified, and a therapy such as EFIT, so using this generic term seems to create confusion rather than clarity. PE/EF also subscribes to attachment theory, at least on a general theoretical level, and is derived from the same root, Rogerian experiential psychotherapy, as is the EFIT model. This model of individual psychotherapy has good empirical validation (Elliott et al., 2013), showing large effect sizes (as defined by Cohen, 1988), especially for depression. These results are equivalent to those found in more behavioral therapies, especially when researcher allegiance is accounted for. This is less true of effects for anxiety disorders, however, particularly for GAD, where effects were often smaller and results favor CBT, although substantial pre–post effects have been found for PE/EF in most studies. This approach targets specific therapeutic tasks, such as the resolving of unfinished business from the past or the resolution of splits (where parts of the self are in conflict). A small study found that this resolution of splits focus resulted in more self-compassion and less self-criticism, depression, and anxiety in clients (Sharar et al., 2011). In terms of the change process, studies find that the higher the experiencing level in session, the better the outcome that can be expected (Elliott, Watson, et al., 2004). Watson and Bedard (2006) found that good-outcome clients in both PE/EF and CBT for depression began and ended therapy at higher levels of experiencing. For both these models, good-outcome clients referred to their emotions more frequently, were more internally focused, and were more capable of reflecting on experience, as well as also being more willing to create new meanings. It seems to be the case that emotional arousal is necessary for the reorganization of "hot" cognitions—the main goal of CBT (Goldfried, 2003). However, as might be expected, CBT clients in this study were still generally more distant and disengaged with their emotions in session than were PE/EF clients. Research on the PE/EF model consistently shows that the therapist's depth of experiential focus, which brings the client in contact with deeper experiencing, predicts good outcomes.

In terms of similarities between EFIT and PE/EF, the relationship with the therapist in both models is collaborative and authentic, rather than role bound; indeed, a genuine alliance is viewed as essential to the process of change. Clients are also viewed holistically, not just in terms of presenting symptomatology, and in both models, the manner in which the client constructs his or her immediate ongoing experiencing is the focus of intervention. The therapist guides the client's experiencing, with interventions such as empathic reflection and evocative questioning, in the direction of integration and positive agency. Both EFT and PE/EF are experiential models, so it makes sense that research on models shows that deepening experience in session and opening up in a more affiliative way with others predicts positive outcomes. The similarities in these models may be summarized as follows: *The goal in EFT and PE/EF is to move into blocked, undifferentiated emotion and change how this emotion is processed and regulated in a way that leads to new meanings and new agency.*

There are also a significant number of differences between EFIT and PE/EF.

• EFIT is considerably more intertwined with and saturated by attachment theory and science as a guide to both inner and interpersonal dramas. This fact reflects its beginnings as an interpersonally focused couple modality oriented to shaping constructive dependency and secure attachment. The portrayal of attachment theory in EFIT also appears to be more accurate. For example, the addition of a focus on identity as a necessary part of attachment in PE/EFT is misplaced, since working models of self are a core feature of attachment theory. The EFIT model and attachment theorists' interactional patterns with others form crucial self-perpetuating feedback loops that actively shape working models of self (Mikulincer, 1995). In EFIT, attachment is also used in a more all-encompassing existential manner, in that connection and disconnection with others is framed as a life-and-death process. As in PE/EF, dysfunctional behavior is often described by the EFIT therapist, but it is also routinely validated as a desperate attempt to maintain some kind of belonging or dull the agony of isolation. So I may say to a client, "Staying with self-criticism seems comfortable, familiar, and less difficult than really feeling how impossibly alone, how 'left behind' and helpless you feel when you think of your father and how he treated you."

• EFIT was developed outside the intrapsychic frame characteristic of PE/EF, and is more explicitly interpersonal and systemic in nature, emphasizing circular-process patterns of causality and reciprocal constraining feedback loops in emotional processing within individuals and in responses between significant others. For example, the family version of PE/EF focuses on meeting parents separately and coaching them as individuals to be better parents, whereas EFFT focuses on de-escalating dances of disconnection as they occur in the session. EFFT then guides family members into safe haven dialogues that expand both the concept of self in individuals and the nature of their dance. The EFFT goal is to guide adolescents into interactions that build effective constructive dependency. This in turn fosters individuation and autonomy.

• The theoretical formulations of EFIT and PE/EF have developed differently in terms of emotion. In EFIT, for example, emotion is not formulated as maladaptive, as is presented in PE/EF. The EFIT therapist focuses on stuck and self-defeating ways of *regulating* emotion. All primary emotions, anger, fear, shame, sadness, joy, and surprise, are considered adaptive when they suit a particular context and when they are used in a balanced and flexible way. We also do not speak of "emotion schemes," preferring the clearer and more-substantiated attachment concept of working models of self and other that are infused with emotion, resulting in a "felt sense" that guides perception, attribution, and action.

• The EFIT therapist is much less focused on the specific tasks as mapped out in PE/EF, such as resolving splits or unfinished business. Coaching people through set steps in a set task does not capture the process of EFIT, wherein therapists tend to concentrate instead on how people process threat and pain and the resulting problems in attaining emotional balance and attachment security with others. In contrast to the formulations of PE/EF, the EFIT therapist does not speak of changing one emotion for another emotion as a core part of change, but rather of assembling, distilling, and disclosing emotion to create constructive coregulation with others and to bring new action tendencies to light. For instance, Mary's anger is modified by her awareness of the desperation underneath her rage, but change really occurs when she is able to allow this desperateness to move her toward new expressions of longing for her attachment figure.

- In many ways, the EFIT process appears to be considerably more parsimonious; the map for EFIT is laid out in this book in terms of three stages; a core process (the EFT Tango) and a set of generic, experiential microinterventions. PE/EF offers a plethora of complicated categorizations, for example, four types of processing difficulties, with 11 different markers for four types of therapy tasks. In terms of techniques, EFIT therapists tend to use basic Gestalt techniques, such as imaginal encounters with emotional realities, parts of self, and attachment figures less frequently and in a more fluid, organic way than is common in PE/EF. When these techniques are used, we prefer to simply ask clients to close their eyes and concentrate on a particular aspect of their experience, rather than actually change chairs to represent different parts of self or to represent other people as in traditional Gestalt therapy. When PE/EF is used with couples, steps have also been added that teach people to regulate their emotions themselves before engaging with others. Research on EFT suggests that this step is unnecessary; the EFT therapist prefers to first foster effective coregulation given the limitations of the self-regulation process (noted in Chapter 2). In brief, EFIT appears to more directly reflect the elegance and simplicity of attachment theory and science than do the IPT or PE/EF models.

Resources

LEARNING RESOURCES

Information on training events; becoming a certified EFT therapist; EFIT, EFT, and EFFT publications; and training DVDs of EFT for couples, EFIT, and EFFT are available at *www.iceeft.com*.

RELATIONSHIP EDUCATION PROGRAMS

For Professionals

The following group educational programs are available for professionals to offer to the public:

1. Hold Me Tight®: Conversations for Connection
2. Created for Connection: The Hold Me Tight® Program for Christian Couples
3. Healing Hearts Together: The Hold Me Tight® Program for Couples Facing Heart Disease
4. Hold Me Tight®—Let Me Go: For Families with Teens

Go to *www.iceeft.com* for more information.

For the Public

The Hold Me Tight® online program with Dr. Susan M. Johnson presents 8–12 hours of online and on-target relationship education, including video clips of couples, expert comments, cartoons, teaching, and exercises.

Go to *www.holdmetightonline.com* for more information.

References

Abbass, A. A., Hancock, J. T., Henderson, J., & Kisley, S. (2006). Short term psychodynamic therapies for common mental disorders. *Cochrane Database of Systematic Reviews, 4,* Art. No. CD004687.

Acevedo, B., & Aron, A. (2009). Does a long term relationship kill romantic love? *Review of General Psychology, 13,* 59–65.

Aikin, N., & Aikin, P. (2017). *The Hold Me Tight®—Let Me Go program: Conversations for connection: A relationship education and enhancement program for families with teens.* Ottawa, Ontario, Canada: International Centre for Excellence in Emotionally Focused Therapy.

Ainsworth, M. D., Blehar, M. C., Waters, E., & Wall, S. (1978). *Patterns of attachment: A study of the Strange Situation.* Hillsdale, NJ: Erlbaum.

Aldao, A., Nolen Hoeksema, S., & Schweiser, S. (2010). Emotion regulation across psychopathology: A meta-analytic review. *Clinical Psychology Review, 30,* 217–237.

Alexander, F., & French, T. (1946). *Psychoanalytic therapy: Principles and application.* New York: Ronald Press.

Alexander, P. C. (1993). Application of attachment theory to the study of sexual abuse. *Journal of Consulting and Clinical Psychology, 60,* 185–195.

Allan, R., & Johnson, S. M. (2016). Conceptual and application issues: Emotionally focused therapy with gay male couples. *Journal of Couple and Relationship Therapy: Innovations in Clinical and Educational Interventions, 16,* 286–305.

Allen, J. P. (2008). The attachment system in adolescence. In J. Cassidy & P. Shaver (Eds.), *Handbook of attachment: Theory, research, and clinical applications* (2nd ed., pp. 419–435). New York: Guilford Press.

Allen, J. P., & Land, D. J. (1999). Attachment in adolescence. In J. Cassidy & P. R. Shaver (Eds.), *Handbook of attachment: Theory, research, and clinical applications* (pp. 319–335). New York: Guilford Press.

Anders, S. L., & Tucker, J. S. (2000). Adult attachment style, interpersonal communication competence and social support. *Personal Relationships, 7,* 379–389.

Armsden, G. C., & Greenberg, M. T. (1987). The inventory of parent and peer attachment: Relationships to well-being in adolescence. *Journal of Youth and Adolescence, 16,* 427–454.

Arnold, M. B. (1960). *Emotion and personality*. New York: Columbia University Press.

Asarnow, J. R., Goldstein, M. J., Tompson, M., & Guthrie, D. (1993). One year outcomes of depressive disorders in child psychiatric in-patients: Evaluation of the prognostic power of a brief measure of expressed emotion. *Journal of Child Psychology and Psychiatry, 34,* 129–137.

Bachelor, A., Meunier, G., Lavadiere, O., & Gamache, D. (2010). Client attachment to therapist: Relation to client personality and symptomatology, and their contributions to the therapeutic alliance. *Psychotherapy, Theory, Research, Practice and Training, 47,* 454–468.

Barlow, D. H. (2002). *Anxiety and its disorders: The nature and treatment of anxiety and panic* (2nd ed.). New York: Guilford Press.

Barlow, D. H., Allen, L. B., & Choate, M. L. (2004). Toward a unified treatment for emotional disorders. *Behavioral Therapy, 35,* 205–230.

Barlow, D. H., Farshione, T., Fairholme, C., Ellard, K., Boisseau, C., Allen, L., et al. (2011). *Unified protocol for transdiagnostic treatment of emotional disorders.* New York: Oxford University Press.

Barlow, D. H., O'Brien, G., & Last, C. (1984). Couples treatment of agoraphobia. *Behavior Therapy, 15,* 41–58.

Barlow, D. H., Sauer-Zavala, C. J., Bullis, J., & Ellard, K. (2014). The nature, diagnosis and treatment of neuroticism: Back to the future. *Clinical Psychological Science, 2,* 344–365.

Barrett, L. F. (2004). Feelings or words?: Understanding the content in self-reported ratings of experienced emotion. *Journal of Personality and Social Psychology, 87,* 266–281.

Bartholomew, K., & Horowitz, L. (1991). Attachment styles among young adults: A test of a four category model. *Journal of Personality and Social Psychology, 61,* 226–244.

Basson, R. (2000). The female sexual response: A different model. *Journal of Sex and Marital Therapy, 26,* 51–65.

Baucom, D. H., Porter, L. S., Kirby, J. S., & Hudepohl, J. (2012). Couple-based interventions for medical problems. *Behavior Therapy, 43,* 61–76.

Baum, K. M., & Nowicki, S. (1998). Perception of emotion: Measuring decoding accuracy of adult prosaic cues varying in intensity. *Journal of Nonverbal Behavior, 22,* 89–107.

Beck, A. T., & Steer, R. A. (1993). *Beck Anxiety Inventory Manual*. San Antonio, TX: Psychological Corp.

Beck, A. T., Steer, R. A., & Brown, G. K. (1996). *Manual for the Beck Depression Inventory–II.* San Antonio, TX: Psychological Corp.

Beckes, L., Coan, J., & Hasselmo, K. (2013). Familiarity promotes the blurring of self and other in the neural representation of threat. *Social Cognitive and Affective Neuroscience, 8,* 670–677.

Benjamin, L. (1974). The structural analysis of social behavior. *Psychological Review, 81,* 392–425.

Bertalanffy, L. von. (1968). *General system theory*. New York: George Braziller.

Beutler, L. E. (2002). The dodo bird is extinct. *Clinical Psychology: Science and Practice, 9,* 30–34.

Beutler, L. E., Blatt, S. J., Alimohamed, S., Levy, K., & Antuaco, L. (2006). Participant factors in treating dysphoric disorders. In L. Castonguay & L. Beutler

(Eds.), *Principles of therapeutic change that work* (pp. 13–63). New York: Oxford University Press.

Beutler, L. E., Harwood, T. M., Alimohamed, S., & Malik, M. (2002). Functional impairment and coping style. In J. Norcross (Ed.), *Psychotherapy relationships that work* (pp. 145–170). New York: Oxford University Press.

Bhatia, V., & Davila, J. (2017). Mental health disorders in couple relationships. In J. Fitzgerald (Ed.), *Foundations for couples therapy: Research for the real world* (pp. 268–278). New York: Brunner-Routledge.

Birmaher, B., Brent, D. A., Kolko, D., Baugher, M., Bridge, J., Holder, D., et al. (2000). Clinical outcome after short-term psychotherapy for adolescents with major depressive disorder. *Archives of General Psychiatry, 57,* 29–36.

Birnbaum, G. E. (2007). Attachment orientations, sexual functioning, and relationship satisfaction in a community sample of women. *Journal of Social and Personal Relationships, 24,* 21–35.

Birnbaum, G. E., Reis, H. T., Mikulincer, M., Gillath, O., & Orpaz, A. (2006). When sex is more than just sex: Attachment orientations, sexual experience, and relationship quality. *Journal of Personality and Social Psychology, 91,* 929–943.

Bloch, L., & Guillory, P. T. (2011). The attachment frame is the thing: Emotion-focused family therapy in adolescence. *Journal of Couple and Relationship Therapy, 10,* 229–245.

Bograd, M., & Mederos, F. (1999). Battering and couples therapy: Universal screening and selection of treatment modality. *Journal of Marital and Family Therapy, 25,* 291–312.

Bordin, E. (1994). Theory and research on the therapeutic working alliance. In A. O. Horvath & L. S. Greenberg (Eds.), *The working alliance: Theory research and practice* (pp. 13–37). New York: Wiley.

Bouaziz, A. R., Lafontaine, M. F., Gabbay, N., & Caron, A. (2013). Investigating the validity and reliability of the caregiving questionnaire with individuals in same-sex relationships. *Journal of Relationships Research, 4*(e2), 1–11.

Bowen, M. (1978). *Family therapy in clinical practice.* New York: Jason Aronson

Bowlby, J. (1944). Forty-four juvenile thieves: Their characters and home life. *International Journal of Psychoanalysis, 25,* 19–52.

Bowlby, J. (1969). *Attachment and loss: Vol. 1. Attachment.* New York: Basic Books.

Bowlby, J. (1973). *Attachment and loss: Vol. 2. Separation: Anxiety and anger.* New York: Basic Books.

Bowlby, J. (1979). *The making and breaking of affectional bonds.* London: Tavistock.

Bowlby, J. (1980). *Attachment and Loss: Vol. 3. Loss.* New York: Penguin Books.

Bowlby, J. (1988). *A secure base.* New York: Basic Books.

Bowlby, J. (1991). *Postscript.* In C. M. Parkes, J. Stevenson-Hinde, & P. Marris (Eds.), *Attachment across the lifespan* (pp. 293–297). New York: Routledge.

Brennen, K. A., Clark, C. L., & Shaver, P. R. (1998). Self-report measurement of adult attachment: An integrative overview. In J. A. Simpson & W. S. Rholes (Eds.), *Attachment theory and close relationships* (pp. 46–76). New York: Guilford Press.

Brown, T. A., Campbell, L. A., Lehman, C. L., Grisham, J. R., & Mancill, R. B. (2001). Current and lifetime comorbidity of the DSM-IV anxiety and mood disorders in a large clinical sample. *Journal of Abnormal Psychology, 110,* 49–58.

Budd, R., & Hughes, I. (2009). The Dodo bird verdict—Controversial, inevitable and important: A commentary on 30 years of meta-analyses. *Clinical Psychology and Psychotherapy, 16,* 510–522.

Burgess Moser, M., Johnson, S. M., Dalgleish, T. L., Wiebe, S. A., & Tasca, G. A. (2018) The impact of blamer-softening on romantic attachment in emotionally focused couples therapy. *Journal of Marital and Family Therapy, 44,* 640–654.

Burgess Moser, M., Johnson, S. M., Tasca, G., & Wiebe, S. (2015). Changes in relationship specific romantic attachment in emotionally focused couple therapy. *Journal of Marital and Family Therapy, 42,* 231–245.

Byrd, K., & Bea, A. (2001). The correspondence between attachment dimensions and prayer in college students. *International Journal for the Psychology of Religion, 11,* 9–24.

Byrd, K. R., Patterson, C. L., & Turchik, J. A. (2010). Working alliance as a mediator of client attachment dimensions and psychotherapy outcome. *Psychotherapy: Theory, Research, Practice, Training, 47,* 631–636.

Cacioppo, J. T., & Patrick, W. (2008). *Loneliness: Human nature and the need for social connection.* New York: Norton.

Cano, A., & O'Leary, D. K. (2000). Infidelity and separations precipitate major depressive episodes and symptoms of nonspecific depression and anxiety. *Journal of Consulting and Clinical Psychology, 68,* 774–781.

Cassidy, J., & Shaver, P. R. (Eds.). (2008). *Handbook of attachment: Theory, research, and clinical applications* (2nd ed.). New York: Guilford Press.

Castonguay, L. G., Goldfried, M. R., Wiser, S., Raue, P., & Hayes, A. (1996). Predicting the effect of cognitive therapy for depression: A study of unique and common factors. *Journal of Consulting and Clinical Psychology, 64,* 497–504.

Castonguay, L. G., Grosse Holtforth, M., Coombs, M., Beberman, R., Kakouros, A., Boswell, J., et al. (2006). Relationship factors in treating dysphoric disorders. In L. Castonguay & L. Beutler (Eds.), *Principles of therapeutic change that work* (pp. 65–81). New York: Oxford University Press.

Chambless, D. L., Baker, M. J., Baucom, D. H., Beutler, L. E. Calhoun, K. S., Crits-Christoph, P., et al. (1998). Update on empirically validated therapies: II. *Clinical Psychologist, 51,* 3–16.

Chambless, D. L., & Ollendick, T. H. (2001). Empirically supported psychological interventions: Controversy and evidence. *Annual Review of Psychology, 52,* 685–716.

Chango, J., McElhaney, K., Allen, J., Schad, M., & Marston, E. (2012). Relational stressors and depressive symptoms in late adolescence: Rejection sensitivity as a vulnerability. *Journal of Abnormal Child Psychology, 40,* 369–379.

Coan, J. A. (2016). Towards a neuroscience of attachment. In J. Cassidy & P. Shaver (Eds.), *Handbook of attachment: Theory, research, and clinical applications* (3rd ed., pp. 242–269). New York: Guilford Press.

Coan, J. A., & Sbarra, D. A. (2015). Social baseline theory: The social regulation of risk and effort. *Current Opinion in Psychology, 1,* 87–91.

Coan, J. A., Schaefer, H. S., & Davidson, R. J. (2006). Lending a hand: Social regulation of the neural response to threat. *Psychological Science, 17,* 1032–1039.

Cobb, R., & Bradbury, T. (2003). Implications of adult attachment for preventing adverse marital outcomes. In S. M. Johnson & V. Whiffen (Eds.), *Attachment processes in couple and family therapy* (pp. 258–280). New York: Guilford Press.

Cohen, D. A., Silver, D. H., Cowan, C. P., Cowan, P. A., & Pearson, J. (1992). Working models of childhood attachment and couple relationships. *Journal of Family Issues, 13,* 432–449.

Cohen, J. (1988). *Statistical power analyses for the behavioral sciences* (2nd ed.). Hillsdale, NJ: Erlbaum.

Cohen, S., O'Leary, K., & Foran, H. (2010). A randomized trial of a brief, problem-focused couple for depression. *Behavior Therapy, 41,* 433–446.

Collins, N. L., & Read, S. J. (1994). Cognitive representations of attachment: The structure and functioning of working models. In K. Bartholomew & D. Perlman (Eds.), *Advances in personal relationships: Vol. 5. Attachment processes in adulthood* (pp. 53–92). London: Jessica Kingsley.

Connolly Gibbons, M. B., Gallop, R., Thompson, D., Luther, D., Crits-Christoph, K., Jacobs, J., et al. (2016). Comparative effectiveness of cognitive therapy and dynamic psychotherapy for major depressive disorders in community mental health settings: A randomized clinical non-inferiority trial. *JAMA Psychiatry, 73,* 904–912.

Conradi, H. J., Dingemanse, P., Noordhof, A., Finkenauer, C., & Kamphuis, J. H. (2017, September 4). Effectiveness of the "Hold Me Tight" relationship enhancement program in a self-referred and a clinician referred sample: An emotionally focused couples therapy-based approach. *Family Process.* [Epub ahead of print]

Coombs, M., Coleman, D., & Jones, E. (2002). Working with feelings: The importance of emotion in both cognitive-behavioral and interpersonal therapy in the NIMH treatment of depression collaborative research program. *Psychotherapy, Theory, Research, Practice, Training, 39,* 233–244.

Corsini, R. J., & Wedding, D. (2008). *Current psychotherapies* (8th ed.). Belmont, CA: Thomson/Brooks Cole.

Costello, P. C. (2013). *Attachment-based psychotherapy: Helping clients develop adaptive capacities.* Washington, DC: American Psychological Association.

Cowan, P. A., Cowan, C. P., Cohn D. A., & Pearson, J. L. (1996). Parents attachment histories and childrens' externalizing and internalizing behaviors: Exploring family systems models of linkage. *Journal of Consulting and Clinical Psychology, 64,* 53–63.

Cozolino, L., & Davis, V. (2017). How people change. In M. Solomon & D. J. Siegel (Eds.), *How people change: Relationship and neuroplasticity in psychotherapy* (pp. 53–72). New York: Norton.

Creasey, G., & Ladd, A. (2005). Generalized and specific attachment representations: Unique and interactive roles in predicting conflict behaviors in close relationships. *Personality and Social Psychology Bulletin, 31,* 1026–1038.

Crowell, J. A., Treboux, D., Gao, Y., Fyffe, C., Pan, H., & Waters, E. (2002). Assessing secure base behavior in adulthood: Development of a measure, links to adult attachment relations and relations to couples communication and reports of relationships. *Developmental Psychology, 38,* 679–693.

Csikszentmihalyi, M. (1990). *Flow: The psychology of optimal experience.* New York: Harper & Row.

Cuijpers, P., van Straten, A., Bohlmeijer, E., Hollon, S., & Andersson, G. (2010). The effects of psychotherapy for depression are overestimated: A meta-analysis of study quality and effect size. *Psychological Medicine: A Journal of Research in Psychiatry and the Allied Sciences, 40,* 211–223.

Dalton, J., Greenman, P., Classen, C., & Johnson, S. M. (2013). Nurturing connections in the aftermath of childhood trauma: A randomized control trial of emotionally focused couple therapy for female survivors of childhood abuse. *Couple and Family Psychology, Research and Practice, 2*(3), 209–221.

Damasio, A. R. (1994). *Decartes' error: Emotion, reason and the human brain.* New York: Putnam.

Daniel, S. I. F. (2006). Adult attachment patterns and individual psychotherapy: A review. *Clinical Psychological Review, 26,* 968–984.

Davila, J., Karney, B. R., & Bradbury, T. N. (1999). Attachment change processes in the early years of marriage. *Journal of Personality and Social Psychology, 76*(5), 783–802.

De Oliveira, C., Moran, G., & Pederson, D. (2005). Understanding the link between maternal adult attachment classifications and thoughts and feelings about emotions. *Attachment and Human Development, 7,* 153–170.

De Waal, F. (2009). *The age of empathy.* New York: McClelland Stewart.

Dekel, R., Solomon, Z., Ginzburg, K., & Neria, Y. (2004). Long-term adjustment among Israeli war veterans: The role of attachment style. *Journal of Stress, Anxiety and Coping, 17,* 141–152.

Denton, W., Wittenborn, A. K., & Golden, R. N. (2012). A randomized trial of emotionally focused therapy for couples. *Journal of Marital and Family Therapy, 26,* 65–78.

Diamond, D., Stovall-McCloush, C., Clarkin, J., & Levy, K. (2003). Patient therapist attachment in the treatment of borderline personality disorder. *Bulletin of the Menninger Clinic, 67,* 227–260.

Diamond, G. (2005). Attachment-based family therapy for depressed an anxious adolescents. In J. Lebow (Ed.), *Handbook of clinical family therapy* (pp. 17–41). Hoboken, NJ: Wiley.

Diamond, G., Russon, J., & Levy, S. (2016). Attachment-based family therapy: A review of empirical support. *Family Process, 55,* 595–610.

Dimidjian, S., Hollon, S. D., Dobson, K. S., Schmaling, K. B., Kohlenberg, R. J., Addis, M. E., et al. (2006). Randomized trial of behavior activation, cognitive therapy, and antidepressant medication in the acute treatment of adults with major depression. *Journal of Consulting and Clinical Psychology, 74,* 658–670.

Dobbs, D. (2017, July/August). The smartphone psychiatrist. *The Atlantic.*

Dozier, M., Stovall-McClough, C., & Albus, K. (2008). Attachment and psychopathology in adulthood. In J. Cassidy & P. R. Shaver (Eds.), *Handbook of attachment: Theory, research, and clinical applications* (2nd ed., pp. 718–744). New York: Guilford Press.

Drach-Zahavy, A. (2004). Toward a multidimensional construct of social support: Implications of providers self-reliance and request characteristics. *Journal of Applied Social Psychology, 34,* 1395–1420.

Duggal, S., Carlson, E. A., Sroufe, L. A., & Egland, B. (2001). Depressive symptomatology in childhood and adolescence. *Development and Psychopathology, 13,* 143–164.

Durham, R. C., Allan, T., & Hackett, C. (1997). On predicting improvement and relapse in generalized anxiety disorder following psychotherapy. *British Journal of Clinical Psychology, 36,* 101–119.

Ein-Dor, T., & Doron, G. (2015). Psychopathology and attachment. In J. Simpson & S. Rholes (Eds.), *Attachment theory and research: New directions and emerging themes* (pp. 346–373). New York: Guilford Press.

Ekman, P. (2003). *Emotions revealed*. New York: Henry Holt.

Elkin, I., Shea, M. T., Watkins, J. T., Imber, S. T., Sotsky, S. M., Collins, J. F., et al. (1989). National Institute of Mental Health Treatment of Depression Collaborative Research Program: General effectiveness of treatments. *Archives of General Psychiatry, 46,* 971–982.

Elliott, R., Greenberg, L. S., & Lietaer, G. (2004). Research on experiential therapies. In M. J. Lambert (Ed.), *Bergin and Garfield's handbook of psychotherapy and behavior change* (5th ed., pp. 493–540). Hoboken, NJ: Wiley.

Elliott, R., Greenberg, L. S., Watson, J., Timulak, L., & Friere, E. (2013). Research on humanistic–experiential psychotherapies. In M. J. Lambert (Ed.), *Bergin and Garfield's handbook of psychotherapy and behavioral change* (6th ed., pp. 495–538). Hoboken, NJ: Wiley.

Elliott, R., Watson, J., Goldman, R., & Greenberg, L. (2004). *Learning emotion-focused therapy: The process experiential approach to change*. Washington, DC: American Psychological Association.

Epstein, N. B., Baldwin, L., & Bishop, D. (1983). The McMaster Family Assessment Device. *Journal of Martial and Family Therapy, 9,* 171–180.

Erickson, E. H. (1968). *Identity: Youth and crisis*. New York: Norton.

Fairbairn, W. R. D. (1952). *An object relations theory of the personality*. New York: Basic Books.

Feeney, B. C. (2007). The dependency paradox in close relationships: Accepting dependence promotes independence. *Journal of Personality and Social Psychology, 92,* 268–285.

Feeney, B. C., & Collins, N. L. (2001). Predictors of caregiving in adult intimate relationships: An attachment theoretical perspective. *Journal of Personality and Social Psychology, 80,* 972–994.

Feeney, J. (2005). Hurt feelings in couple relationships. *Personal Relationships, 12,* 253–271.

Felitti, V. J., Anda, R. F., Nordenberg, D., Williamson, D. F., Sptiz, A. M., Edwards, V., et al. (1998). The relationship of adult health status to childhood abuse and household dysfunction. *American Journal of Preventative Medicine, 14,* 245–258.

Fillo, J., Simpson, J. A., Rholes, W. S., & Kohn, J. L. (2015). Dads doing diapers: Individual and relational outcomes associated with the division of childcare across the transition to parenthood. *Journal of Personality and Social Psycholgy, 108,* 298–316.

Finzi-Dottan, R., Cohen, O., Iwaniec, D., Sapir, Y., & Weisman, A. (2003). The drug-user husband and his wife: Attachment styles, family cohesion and adaptability. *Substance Use and Misuse, 38,* 271–292.

Follette, W., & Greenberg, L. (2006). Technique factors in treating dysphoric disorders. In L. Castonguay & L. Beutler (Eds.), *Principles of therapeutic change that work* (pp. 83–109). New York: Oxford University Press.

Fonagy, P., Steele, M., Steele, H., Leigh, T., Kennedy, R., Matton, G., et al. (1995). Attachment, the reflective self and borderline states. In S. Goldberg, R. Muir, & J. Kerr (Eds.), *Attachment theory: Social, developmental and clinical perspectives* (pp. 233–279). Hillsdale, NJ: Analytic Press.

Fonagy, P., Steele, M., Steele, H., Moran, G. S., & Higgit, M. (1991). The capacity for understanding mental states: The reflective self in parent and child and its significance for security of attachment. *Infant Mental Health Journal, 12,* 201–218.

Fosha, D. (2000). *The transforming power of affect: A model for accelerated change.* New York: Basic Books.

Fraley, R. C., Fazzari, D. A., Bonanno G. A., & Dekel, S. (2006). Attachment and psychological adaptation in high exposure survivors of the 9/11 attack on the World Trade Center. *Journal of Personality and Social Psychology, 32,* 538–551.

Fraley, R. C., & Shaver, P. R. (1998). Airport separations: A naturalistic study of adult attachment dynamics in separating couples. *Journal of Personality and Social Psychology, 75,* 1198–1212.

Fraley, R. C., Waller, N. G., & Brennan, K. A. (2000). An item response theory analysis of self report measures of adult attachment. *Journal of Personality and Social Psychology, 78,* 350–365.

Frances, A. (2013). *Saving normal.* New York: William Morrow.

Frederickson, B. L., & Branigan, C. (2005). Positive emotions broaden the scope of attention and thought-action repertoires. *Cognition and Emotion, 19,* 315–322.

Frijda, N. H. (1986). *The emotions.* Cambridge, UK: Cambridge University Press.

Funk, J. L., & Rogge, R. D. (2007). Testing the ruler with item response theory: Increasing precision of measurement for relationship satisfaction with the Couples Satisfaction Index. *Journal of Family Psychology, 21,* 572–583.

Furrow, J., Johnson, S. M., Bradley, B., & Amodeo, J. (2011). Spirituality and emotionally focused therapy: Exploring common ground. In J. Furrow, S. M. Johnson, & B. Bradley (Eds.), *The emotionally focused casebook: New directions in treating couples* (pp. 343–372). New York: Routledge.

Furrow, J., & Palmer, G. (2007). EFFT and blended families: Building bonds from the inside out. *Journal of Systemic Therapies, 26,* 44–58.

Furrow, J., Palmer, G., Johnson, S. M., Faller, G., & Palmer-Olsen, L. (in press). *Emotionally focused family therapy: Restoring connection and promoting resilience.* New York: Routledge.

Garfield, S. (2006). The therapist as a neglected variable in psychotherapy research. *Clinical Psychology: Science and Practice.*

Gendlin, E. T. (1996). *Focusing oriented psychotherapy: A manual of the experiential method.* New York: Guilford Press.

Germer, C. K. (2005). Mindfulness: What is it and what does it matter? In C. Germer, R. Siegel, & P. Fulton (Eds.), *Mindfulness and psychotherapy* (pp. 3–27). New York: Guilford Press.

Germer, C. K., Siegel, R. D., & Fulton, P. R. (2003). *Mindfulness and psychotherapy.* New York: Guilford Press.

Gillath, O., & Canterbury, M. (2012). Neural correlates of exposure to subliminal and supraliminal sex cues. *Social Cognitive and Affective Neuroscience, 7,* 924–936.

Gillath, O., Mikulincer, M., Birnbaum, G., & Shaver, P. R. (2008). When sex primes love: Subliminal sexual priming motivates relationship goal pursuit. *Personality and Social Psychology Bulletin, 34,* 1057–1069.

Goldfried, M. R. (2003). Cognitive-behavioral therapy: Reflections on the evolution of a therapeutic orientation. *Cognitive Therapy and Research, 27,* 53–69.

Goleman, D. (1995). *Emotional intelligence.* New York: Bantam Books.

Gordon, K. M., & Toukmanian, S. G. (2002). Is how it is said important?: The association between quality of therapist interventions and client processing. *Counselling and Psychotherapy Research, 2,* 88–98.

Gotta, G., Green, R. J., Rothblum, E., Solomon, S., Balsam, K., & Schwartz, P. (2011). Heterosexual, lesbian and gay male relationships: A comparison of couples in 1975 and 2000. *Family Process, 50,* 354–376.

Gottman, J. M. (1999). *The seven principles for making marriage work.* New York: Crown Publishing Group.

Gottman, J. M., Coan, J., Carrier, S., & Swanson, C. (1998). Predicting marital happiness and stability from newly-wed interactions. *Journal of Marriage and the Family, 60,* 5–22.

Gottman, J. M., Katz, L., & Hooven, C. (1997). *Meta-emotion: How families communicate emotionally.* Hillsdale, NJ: Erlbaum.

Granquist, P., Mikulincer, M., Gewirtz, V., & Shaver, P. R. (2012). Experimental findings on God as an attachment figure: Normative processes and moderating effects of internal working models. *Journal of Personality and Social Psychology, 103,* 804–818.

Greenberg, R. P. (2016). The rebirth of psychosocial importance in a drug-filled world. *American Psychologist, 71,* 781–791.

Greenman, P. S., & Johnson, S. M. (2012). United we stand: Emotionally focused therapy (EFT) for couples in the treatment of post-traumatic stress disorder. *Journal of Clinical Psychology: In Session, 68,* 561–569.

Greenman, P. S., & Johnson, S. M. (2013). Process research on emotionally focused therapy (EFT) for couples: Linking theory to practice. *Family Process, 52,* 46–61.

Greenman, P. S., Wiebe, S., & Johnson, S. M. (2017). Neurophysiological processes in couple relationships: Emotions, attachment bonds and the brain. In J. Fitzgerald (Ed.), *Foundations for couples therapy: Research for the real world* (pp. 291–301). New York: Routledge.

Gross, J. J. (1998a). Antecedent and response-focused emotion regulation: Divergent consequences for experience, expression and physiology. *Journal of Personality and Social Psychology, 74,* 224–237.

Gross, J. J. (1998b). The emerging field of emotion regulation: An integrative review. *Review of General Psychology, 2,* 271–299.

Gross, J. J., & Profitt, D. (2013). The economy of social resources and its influence on spatial perceptions. *Frontiers in Human Neurosience, 7,* 772.

Gump, B. B., Polk, D. E., Karmarck, T. W., & Shiffman, S. M. (2001). Partner interactions are associated with reduced blood pressure in the natural environment: Ambulatory monitoring evidence from a healthy multiethnic adult sample. *Psychsomatic Medicine, 63,* 423–433.

Hammen, C. (1995). The social context of risk for depression. In K. Craig & K. Dobson (Eds.), *Anxiety and depression in adults and children* (pp. 82–96). Los Angeles: SAGE.

Harari, Y. N. (2017). *Homo deus: A brief history of tomorrow.* New York: Harper.

Hawkley, L. C., & Cacioppo, J. T. (2010). Loneliness matters: A theoretical and empirical review of consequences and mechanisms. *Annals of Behavioral Medicine, 40,* 218–227.

Hawton, K., Catalan, J., & Fagg, J. (1991). Sex therapy for erectile dysfunction: Characteristics of couples, treatment outcome and prognostic factors. *Archives of Sexual Behavior, 21,* 161–175.

Hayes, S. C., Levin, M. E., Plumb-Vilardaga, J., Villstte, J., & Pistorello, J. (2013). Acceptance and commitment therapy: Examining the progress of a distinctive model of behavioral and cognitive therapy. *Behavior Therapy, 44,* 180–198.

Hazan, C., & Zeifman, D. (1994). Sex and the psychological tether. In K. Bartholomew & D. Perlman (Eds.), *Advances in personal relationships: Attachment relationships in adulthood* (Vol. 5, pp. 151–177). London: Jessica Kingsley.

Herman, J. L. (1992). *Trauma and recovery.* New York: Basic Books.

Hesse, E. (2008). The Adult Attachment Interview. In J. Cassidy & P. R. Shaver (Eds.), *Handbook of attachment: Theory, research, and clinical applications* (2nd ed., pp. 552–598). New York: Guilford Press.

Hoffman, K., Cooper, G., & Powell, B. (2017). *Raising a secure child.* New York: Guilford Press.

Hofmann, S. G., Heering, S., Sawyer, A. T., & Asnaani, A. (2009). How to handle anxiety: The effects of reappraisal, acceptance, and suppression strategies on anxious arousal. *Behaviour Research and Therapy, 47,* 389–394.

Holmes, J. (1996). *Attachment, intimacy and autonomy: Using attachment theory in adult psychotherapy.* Northdale, NJ: Jason Aronson.

Holmes, J. (2001). *The search for the secure base: Attachment theory and psychotherapy.* New York: Brunner/Routledge.

Holt-Lunstad, J., Uchino, B. N., Smith, T. W., Olson-Cerny, C., & Nealey-Moore, J. B. (2003). Social relationships and ambulatory blood pressure: Structural and qualitative predictors of cardiovascular function during everyday social interactions. *Health Psychology, 22,* 388–397.

Hooley, J. M. (2007). Expressed emotion and relapse of psychopathology. *Annual Review of Clinical Psychology, 3,* 329–352.

Hooley, J. M., & Teasdale, J. D. (1989). Predictors of relapse in unipolar depressives: Expressed emotion, marital distress and perceived criticism. *Journal of Abnormal Psychology, 98,* 229–235.

Horvath, A. O., & Bedi, R. P. (2002). The alliance. In J. Norcross (Ed.), *Psychotherapy relationships that work* (pp. 37–69). New York: Oxford University Press.

Horvath, A. O., & Symonds, B. D. (1991). Relationship between working alliance and outcome in psychotherapy: A meta-analysis. *Journal of Counselling Psychology, 38,* 139–149.

House, J. S., Landis, K. R., & Umberson, D. (1988). Social relationships and health. *Science, 241,* 540–545.

Hughes, D. (2004). An attachment-based treatment of maltreated children and young people. *Attachment and Human Development, 6,* 263–278.

Hughes, D. (2006). *Building the bonds of attachment* (2nd ed.). New York: Jason Aronson.

Hughes, D. (2007). *Attachment focused family therapy.* New York: Norton.

Huston, T. L., Caughlin, J. P., Houts, R. M., Smith, S., & George, L. J. (2001). The connubial crucible: Newlywed years as predictors of marital delight, distress and divorce. *Journal of Personality and Social Psychology, 80,* 237–252.

Iacoboni, M. (2008). *Mirroring people: The new science of how we connect with others.* New York: Farrar, Straus & Giroux.

Immardino Yeng, M. H. (2016). *Emotions, learning and the brain: Exploring the educational implications of affective neuroscience.* New York: Norton.

Izard, C. E. (1990). Facial expressions and the regulation of emotion. *Journal of Personality and Social Psychology, 58,* 487–498.

Izard, C. E. (1992). Basic emotions, relations among emotions and emotion cognition relations. *Psychological Review, 99,* 561–564.

James, P. (1991). Effects of a communication training component added to an emotionally focused couples therapy. *Journal of Marital and Family Therapy, 17,* 263–276.

Johnson, S. M. (2002). *Emotionally focused couple therapy with trauma survivors: Strengthening attachment bonds.* New York: Guilford Press.

Johnson, S. M. (2003). Emotionally focused couples therapy: Empiricism and art. In T. Sexton, G. Weeks, & M. Robbins (Eds.), *Handbook of family therapy* (pp. 263–280). New York: Brunner-Routledge.

Johnson, S. M. (2004). *The practice of emotionally focused couple therapy: Creating connection* (2nd ed.). New York: Brunner-Routledge.

Johnson, S. M. (2005). Broken bonds: An emotionally focused approach to infidelity. *Journal of Couple and Relationship Therapy, 4,* 17–29.

Johnson, S. M. (2008a). *Hold Me Tight: Seven conversations for a lifetime of love.* New York: Little, Brown.

Johnson, S. M. (2008b). Couple and family therapy: An attachment perspective. In J. Cassidy & P. R. Shaver (Eds.), *Handbook of attachment: Theory, research, and clinical applications* (2nd ed., pp. 811–829). New York: Guilford Press.

Johnson, S. M. (2009). Extravagant emotion: Understanding and transforming love relationships in emotionally focused therapy. In D. Fosha, D. Siegel, & M. Solomon (Eds.), *The healing power of emotion: Affective neuroscience, development and clinical practice* (pp. 257–279). New York: Norton.

Johnson, S. M. (2010). *The Hold Me Tight program: Conversations for connection* (Facilitator's guide). Ottawa, Ontario, Canada: International Centre for Excellence in Emotionally Focused Therapy.

Johnson, S. M. (2011). The attachment perspective on the bonds of love: A prototype for relationship change. In J. Furrow, S. M. Johnson, & B. Bradley (Eds.), *The emotionally focused casebook: New directions in treating couples* (pp. 31–58). New York: Routledge.

Johnson, S. M. (2013). *Love sense: The revolutionary new science of romantic relationships.* New York: Little, Brown.

Johnson, S. M. (2017). An emotionally focused approach to sex therapy. In Z. Peterson (Ed.), *The Wiley handbook of sex therapy* (pp. 250–266). New York: Wiley.

Johnson, S. M., & Best, M. (2003). A systematic approach to restructuring adult attachment: The EFT model of couples therapy. In P. Erdman & T. Caffery (Eds.), *Attachment and family systems: Conceptual, empirical and therapeutic relatedness* (pp. 165–192). New York: Brunner-Routledge.

Johnson, S. M., Bradley, B., Furrow, J., Lee, A., Palmer, G., Tilley, D., et al. (2005). *Becoming an emotionally focused couple therapist: The workbook.* New York: Brunner-Routledge.

Johnson, S. M., Burgess Moser, M., Beckes, L., Smith, A., Dalgleish, T., Halchuk, R., et al. (2013). Soothing the threatened brain: Leveraging contact comfort with emotionally focused therapy. *PLOS ONE, 8*(11), e79314.

Johnson, S. M., & Greenberg, L. S. (1985). The differential effects of experiential and problem solving interventions in resolving marital conflict. *Journal of Consulting and Clinical Psychology, 53,* 175–184.

Johnson, S. M., Lafontaine, M., & Dalgleish, T. (2015). Attachment: A guide to a new era of couple interventions. In J. Simpson & W. S. Rholes (Eds.), *Attachment theory and research: New directions and emerging themes* (pp. 393–421). New York: Guilford Press.

260   References

Johnson, S. M., Maddeaux, C., & Blouin, J. (1998). Emotionally focused family therapy for bulimia: Changing attachment patterns. *Psychotherapy, 35,* 238–247.

Johnson, S. M., & Sanderfer, K. (2016). *Created for connection: The "Hold Me Tight" guide for Christian couples.* New York: Little, Brown.

Johnson, S. M., & Sanderfer, K. (2017). *Created for connection: The "Hold Me Tight" program for Christian couples: Facilitator's guide for small groups.* Ottawa, Ontario, Canada: International Centre for Excellence in Emotionally Focused Therapy.

Johnson, S. M., & Talitman, E. (1987). Predictors of success in couple and family therapy. *Journal of Marital and Family Therapy, 23,* 135–152.

Johnson, S. M., & Whiffen, V. (Eds.). (2003). *Attachment processes in couple and family therapy.* New York: Guilford Press.

Johnson, S. M., & Williams-Keeler, L. (1998). Creating healing relationships for couples dealing with trauma: The use of emotionally focused marital therapy. *Journal of Marital and Family Therapy, 24,* 25–40.

Johnson, S. M., & Zuccarini, D. (2010). Integrating sex and attachment in emotionally focused couple therapy. *Journal of Marital and Family Therapy, 36,* 431–445.

Jones, E. E., & Pulos, S. M. (1993). Comparing the process in psychodynamic and cognitive-behavioral therapies. *Journal of Consulting and Clinical Psychology, 16,* 306–316.

Jones, J. D., Cassidy, J., & Shaver, P. R. (2015). Parents self-reported attachment styles: A review of the link with parenting behaviors, emotions and cognitions. *Personality and Social Psychological Review, 19,* 44–76.

Jurist, E. L., & Meehan, K. B. (2009). Attachment, mentalizing and reflective functioning. In J. H. Obegi & E. Berant (Eds.), *Attachment theory and research in clinical work with adults* (pp. 71–73). New York: Guilford Press.

Kashdan, T. B., Feldman Barrett, L., & McKnight, P. E. (2015). Unpacking emotion differentiaton: Transforming unpleasant experience by perceiving distinctions in negativity. *Current Directions in Psychological Science, 24,* 10–19.

Kazdin, A., & Bass, D. (1989). Power to detect differences between alternative treatments in comparative psychotherapy outcome research. *Journal of Consulting and Clinical Psychology, 57,* 138–147.

Kennedy, N., Johnson, S. M., Wiebe, S., & Tasca, G. (in press). Conversations for connection: An outcome assessment of the Hold Me Tight relationship education program for couples. *Journal of Marital and Family Therapy.*

Kirkpatrick, L. A. (2005). *Attachment, evolution and the psychology of religion.* New York: Guilford Press.

Klein, M. H., Mathieu, P. L., Gendlin, E. T., & Kiesler, D. J. (1969). *The Experiencing Scale: A research and training manual* (Vol. 1). Madison: Wisconsin Psychiatric Institute.

Klerman, G., Weissman, M. M., Rounsaville, B. J., & Chevron, E. S. (1984). *Interpersonal psychotherapy for depression.* New York: Jason Aronson.

Kobak, R. (1999). The emotional dynamics of disruptions in attachment relationships: Implications for theory, research and clinical intervention. In J. Cassidy & P. R. Shaver (Eds.), *Handbook of attachment: Theory, research, and applications* (pp. 21–43). New York: Guilford Press.

Kobak, R. R., Cole, H. E., Ferenz-Gilles, R., Fleming, W., & Gamble, W. (1993).

Attachment and emotion regulation during mother–teen problem solving: A control theory analysis. *Child Development, 64,* 231–245.

Krueger, R. F., & Markon, K. E. (2011). A dimensional-spectrum model of psychopathology: Progress and opportunities. *Archives of General Psychiatry, 68,* 10–11.

Landau-North, M., Johnson, S. M., & Dalgleish, T. (2011). Emotionally focused couple therapy and addiction. In J. Furrow, S. M. Johnson, & B. Bradley (Eds.), *The emotionally focused casebook: New directions in treating couples* (pp. 193–218). New York: Routledge.

Leichsenring, F., Rabung, S., & Leibing, E. (2004). The efficacy of short-term psychodynamic psychotherapy in specific psychiatric disorders: A meta-analysis. *Archives of General Psychiatry, 61,* 1208–1216.

Leichsenring, F., & Steinert, C. (2017). Is cognitive behavioral therapy the gold standard for psychotherapy?: The need for plurality in treatment and research. *Journal of the American Medical Association.*

Levy, K. N., Ellison, W. D., Scott, L. N., & Bernecker, S. L. (2011). Attachment style. *Journal of Clinical Psychology: In Session, 67,* 193–203.

Luhrmann, T. M., Nusbaum, H., & Thisted, R. (2012). Lord, teach us to pray: Prayer practice affects cognitive processing. *Journal of Cognition and Culture, 13,* 159–177.

Lutkenhaus, P., Grossman, K. E., & Grossman, K. (1985). Infant mother attachment at twelve months and style of interaction with a stranger at the age of three years. *Child Development, 56,* 1538–1542.

MacIntosh, H. B., Hall, J., & Johnson, S. M. (2007). Forgive and forget: A comparison of emotionally focused and cognitive-behavioral models of forgiveness and intervention in the context of couples infidelity. In P. R. Peluso (Ed.), *Infidelity: A practitioners guide to working with couples in crisis* (pp. 127–147). New York: Routledge.

MacIntosh, H. B., & Johnson, S. M. (2008). Emotionally focused therapy for couples and childhood sexual abuse survivors. *Journal of Marital and Family Therapy, 34,* 298–315.

Magnavita, J., & Anchin, J. (2014). *Unifying psychotherapy: Principles, methods and evidence from clinical science.* New York: Springer.

Main, M., Kaplan, N., & Cassidy, J. (1985). Security, in infancy, childhood and adulthood. A move to the level of representation. In I. Bretherton & E. Waters (Eds.), Growing points in attachment theory and research. *Monographs of the Society for Research in Child Development, 50*(1–2, Serial No. 209), 66–104.

Makinen, J., & Johnson, S. M. (2006). Resolving attachment injuries in couples using EFT: Steps towards forgiveness and reconciliation. *Journal of Consulting and Clinical Psychology, 74,* 1055–1064.

Manos, R. C., Kanter, J. W., & Busch, A. M. (2010). A critical review of assessment strategies to measure the behavioral activation model of depression. *Clinical Psychology Review, 30,* 547–561.

Marcus, D. K., O'Connell, D., Norris, A. L., & Sawaqdeh, A. (2014). Is the Dodo bird endangered in the 21st century?: A meta-analysis of treatment comparison studies. *Clinical Psychology Review, 34,* 519–530.

Marmarosh, C. L., Gelso, C., Markin, R., Majors, R., Mallery, C., & Choi, J. (2009). The real relationship in psychotherapy: Relationships to adult attachments, working alliance, transference and therapy outcome. *Journal of Counselling Psychology, 53,* 337–350.

McBride, C., & Atkinson, L. (2009). Attachment theory and cognitive behavioral therapy. In J. Obegi & E. Berant (Eds.), *Attachment theory and research in clinical work with adults* (pp. 434–458). New York: Guilford Press.

McCoy, K. P., Cummings, E. M., & Davis, P. T. (2009). Constructive and destructive marital conflict, emotional security and childrens' prosocial behavior. *Journal of Child Psychology and Psychiatry, 50,* 270–279.

McEwen, B., & Morrison, J. (2013). Brain on stress: Vulnerability and plasticity of the prefrontal cortex over the life course. *Neuron, 79,* 16–29.

McWilliams, L., & Bailey, S. J. (2010). Associations between adult attachment ratings and health conditions: Evidence from the National Comorbidity Survey Replication. *Health Psychology, 29,* 446–453.

Mennin, D. S., & Farach, F. (2007). Emotion and evolving treatments for adult psychopathology. *Clinical Psychology: Science and Practice, 14,* 329–352.

Merkel, W. T., & Searight, H. R. (1992). Why families are not like swamps, solar systems or thermostats: Some limits of systems theory as applied to family therapy. *Contemporary Family Therapy, 14,* 33–50.

Mikulincer, M. (1995). Attachment style and the mental representation of the self. *Journal of Personality and Social Psychology, 69,* 1203–1215.

Mikulincer, M. (1997) Adult attachment style and information processing: Individual differences in curiosity and cognitive closure. *Journal of Personality and Social Psychology, 69,* 1203–1215.

Mikulincer, M. (1998). Adult attachment style and individual differences in functional versus dysfunctional experiences of anger. *Journal of Personality and Social Psychology, 74,* 513–524.

Mikulincer, M., Birnbaum, G., Woodis, D., & Nachmias, O. (2000). Stress and accessibility of proximity-related thoughts: Exploring normative and intraindividual components of attachment theory. *Journal of Personality and Social Psychology, 78,* 509–523.

Mikulincer, M., Ein-Dor, T., Solomon, Z., & Shaver, P. R. (2011). Trajectory of attachment insecurities over a 17-year period: A latent curve analysis of war captivity and posttraumatic stress disorder. *Journal of Social and Clinical Psychology, 30,* 960–984.

Mikulincer, M., & Florian, V. (2000). Exploring individual differences in reactions to mortality salience: Does attachment style regulate terror management mechanisms? *Journal of Personality and Social Psychology, 79,* 260–273.

Mikulincer, M., Florian, V., & Weller, A. (1993). Attachment styles, coping strategies and posttraumatic psychological stress: The impact of the Gulf War in Israel. *Journal of Personality and Social Psychology, 64,* 817–826.

Mikulincer, M., Gillath, O., Halvey, V., Avihou, N., Avidan, S., & Eshkoli, N. (2001). Attachment theory and reaction to other's needs: Evidence that the activation of the sense of attachment security promotes empathic responses. *Journal of Personality and Social Psychology, 81,* 1205–1224.

Mikulincer, M., & Shaver, P. R. (2016). *Attachment in adulthood: Structure, dynamics, and change* (2nd ed.). New York: Guilford Press.

Mikulincer, M., Shaver, P. R., Gillath, O., & Nitzberg, R. A. (2005). Attachment, caregiving and altruism: Boosting attachment security increases compassion and helping. *Journal of Personality and Social Psychology, 89,* 817–839.

Mikulincer, M., Shaver, P. R., & Horesh, N. (2006). Attachment bases of emotion regulation and posttraumatic adjustment. In D. K. Snyder, J. A. Simpson, & J. N. Hughes (Eds.), *Emotion regulation in families: Pathways to dysfunction and health* (pp. 77–99). Washington, DC: American Psychological Association.

Mikulincer, M., Shaver, P. R., & Pereg, D. (2003). Attachment theory and affect regulation: The dynamics, development and cognitive consequences of attachment strategies. *Motivation and Emotion, 27,* 77–102.

Mikulincer, M., & Sheffi, E. (2000). Adult attachment style and reactions to positive affect: A test of mental categorization and creative problem solving. *Motivation and Emotion, 24,* 149–174.

Minka, S., & Vrshek-Schallhorn, S. (2014). Co-morbidity of unipolar depressive and anxiety disorders. In I. Gotlieb & C. Hammen (Eds.), *Handbook of depression* (3rd ed., pp. 84–102). New York: Guilford Press.

Minuchin, S., & Fishman, H. C. (1981). *Techniques of family therapy.* Cambridge, MA: Harvard University Press.

Mitchell, S. (2000). *Relationality: From attachment to intersubjectivity.* New York: Analytic Press.

Moretti, M. M., & Holland, R. (2003). The journey of adolescence: Transitions in self within the context of attachment relationships. In S. M. Johnson & V. Whiffen (Eds.), *Attachment processes in couple and family therapy* (pp. 234–257). New York: Guilford Press.

Morris, A., Steinberg, L., & Silk, J. (2007). The role of family context in the development of emotion regulation. *Social Development, 16,* 361–388.

Morris, C., Miklowitz, D. J., & Waxmonsky, J. A. (2007). Family-focused treatment for bipolar disorder in adults and youth. *Journal of Clinical Psychology, 63,* 433–445.

Naaman, S. (2008). *Evaluation of the clinical efficacy of emotionally focused couples therapy on psychological adjustment and natural killer cell cytotoxicity in early breast cancer.* Doctoral dissertation, University of Ottawa, Ottawa, Ontario, Canada.

Newman, M. G., Crits-Christoph, L. P., Connelly Gibbons, M. B., & Erikson, T. M. (2006). Participant factors in treating anxiety disorders. In L. G. Castonguay & L. E. Beutler (Eds.), *Principles of therapeutic change that work* (pp. 121–154). New York: Oxford University Press.

Niedenthal, P., Halberstadt, J. B., & Setterlund, M. B. (1999). Emotional response categorization. *Psychological Review, 106,* 337–361.

Nolen-Hoeksema, S., & Watkins, E. R. (2011). A heuristic for developing transdiagnostic models of psychpathology: Explaining multifinality and divergent trajectories. *Perspectives on Psychological Science, 6,* 589–609.

Norwicki, S., & Duke, M. (1994). Individual differences in the non-verbal communication of affect. *Journal of Nonverbal Behavior, 18,* 9–35.

O'Leary, D., Acevedo, B., Aron, A., Huddy, L., & Mashek, D. (2012). Is long-term love more than a rare phenomenon?: If so, what are its correlates? *Social Psychology and Personality Science, 3,* 241–249.

Olendzki, A. (2005). The roots of mindfulness. In C. Germer, R. Siegel, & P. Fulton (Eds.), *Mindfulness and psychotherapy* (pp. 241–261). New York: Guilford Press.

Ortigo, K., Westen, D., DeFife, J., & Bradley, B. (2013). Attachment, social cognition and posttraumatic stress symptoms in a traumatized urban population:

Evidence for the mediating role of object relations. *Journal of Traumatic Stress, 26,* 361–368.

Paivio, S. C., & Pascual-Leone, A. (2010). *Emotion-focused therapy for complex trauma.* Washington, DC: American Psychological Association.

Palmer, G., & Efron, D. (2007). Emotionally focused family therapy: Developing the model. *Journal of Systemic Therapies, 26,* 17–24.

Panksepp, J. (1998). *Affective neuroscience: The foundations of human and animal emotions.* New York: Oxford University Press.

Panksepp, J. (2009). Brain emotional systems and qualities of mental life: From animal models of affect to implications for psychotherapeutics. In D. Fosha, D. J. Siegel, & M. Solomon (Eds.), *The healing power of emotion: Affective neuroscience, development and clinical practice* (pp. 1–26). New York: Norton.

Parmigiani, G., Tarsitami, L., De Santis, V., Mistretta, M., Zampetti, G., Roselli, V., et al. (2013). Attachment style and posttraumatic stress disorder after cardiac surgery. *European Psychiatry, 28*(Suppl. 1), 1.

Pasual-Leone, A., & Yeryomenko, N. (2016). The client "experiencing" scale as a predictor of treatment outcomes: A meta-analysis on psychotherapy process. *Journal of Psychotherapy Research, 27,* 653–665.

Peloquin, K., Brassard, A., Delisle, G., & Bedard, M. (2013). Integrating the attachment, caregiving and sexual systems into the understanding of sexual satisfaction. *Canadian Journal of Behavioral Science, 45,* 185–195.

Peloquin, K., Brassard, A., Lafontaine, M., & Shaver, P. R. (2014). Sexuality examined through the lens of attachment theory: Attachment, caregiving and sexual satisfaction. *Journal of Sex Research, 51,* 561–576.

Pennebaker, J. W. (1990). *Opening up: The healing power of confiding in others.* New York: Morrow.

Pietromonaco, P. R., & Collins, N. L. (2017). Interpersonal mechanisms linking close relationships to health. *American Psychologist, 72,* 531–542.

Pinniger, R., Brown, R., Thorsteinsson, E., & McKinley, P. (2012). Argentine tango dance compared to mindfulness meditation and a waiting list control: A randomized trial for treating depression. *Complementary Therapies in Medicine, 20,* 377–384.

Pinsof, W. M., & Wynne, L. C. (2000). The effectiveness and efficacy of marital and family therapy: Introduction to the special issue. *Journal of Marital and Family Therapy, 21,* 341–343.

Porges, S. W. (2011). *The polyvagal theory: Neurophysiological foundations of emotion, attachment, communication and self-regulation.* New York: Norton.

Powell, B., Cooper, G., Hoffman, K., & Marvin, B. (2014). *The circle of security intervention: Enhancing attachment in early parent–child relationships.* New York: Guilford Press.

Rholes, S., & Simpson, J. (2015). Introduction: New directions and emerging themes. In S. Rholes & J. Simpson (Eds.), *Attachment theory and research* (pp. 1–8). New York: Guilford Press.

Rice, L. N. (1974). The evocative function of the therapist. In L. N. Rice & D. A. Wexler (Eds.), *Innovations in client centered therapy* (pp. 289–311). New York: Wiley.

Riggs, D. S., Byrne, C. A., Weathers, F. W., & Litz, B. T. (2005). The quality of the intimate relationships of male Vietnam veterans: Problems associated with posttraumatic stress. *Journal of Traumatic Stress, 11,* 87–101.

Roberts, B. W., & Robins, R. (2000). Board dispositions, broad aspirations: The intersection of personality traits and major life goals. *Journal of Personality and Social Psychology Bulletin, 26,* 1284–1296.

Rogers, C. (1961). *On becoming a person.* Boston: Houghton Mifflin.

Rubino, G., Barker, C., Roth, T., & Fearon, P. (2000). Therapist empathy and depth of interpretation in response to potential alliance ruptures—The role of therapist and patient attachment styles. *Psychotherapy Research, 10,* 408–420.

Salovey, P., Hsee, C., & Mayer, J. D. (1993). Emotional intelligence and the self regulation of affect. In D. Wegner & J. W. Pennebaker (Eds.), *Handbook of mental control* (pp. 258–277). Englewood Cliffs, NJ: Prentice-Hall.

Salovey, P., Mayer, J., Golman, L., Turvey, C., & Palfai, T. (1995). Emotional, attention clarity and repair: Exploring emotional intelligence using the trait meta-mood scale. In J. Pennebaker (Ed.), *Emotion, disclosure and health* (pp. 125–154). Washington, DC: American Psychological Association.

Satir, V. (1967). *Conjoint family therapy.* Palo Alto, CA: Science & Behavior Books.

Sbarra, D. (2006). Predicting the onset of emotional recovery following nonmarital relationship dissolution: Survival analysis of sadness and anger. *Personality and Social Psychology Bulletin, 32,* 298–312.

Scharf, M., Mayseless, O., & Kivenson-Baron, I. (2004). Adolescents attachment representations and developmental tasks in emerging adulthood. *Developmental Psychology, 40,* 430–444.

Schiller, D., Monfils, M., Raio, C., Johnson, D., LeDoux, J., & Phelps, E. (2010). Preventing the return of fear in humans using reconsolidation update mechanisms. *Nature, 463,* 49–53.

Schmidt, N. B., Keough, M. E., Timpano, K., & Richey, J. (2008). Anxiety sensitivity profile: Predictive and incremental validity. *Journal of Anxiety Disorders, 22,* 1180–1189.

Schnall, S., Harber, K., Stefanucci, J., & Proffitt, D. (2008). Social support and the perception of geographical slant. *Journal of Experimental Social Psychology, 44,* 1246–1255.

Scott, R. L., & Cordova, J. V. (2002). The influence of adult attachment styles on the association between marital adjustment and depressive symptoms. *Journal of Marriage and the Family, 62,* 1247–1268.

Selchuk, E., Zayas, V., Gunaydin, G., Hazan, C., & Kross, E. (2012). Mental representations of attachment figures facilitate recovery following upsetting autobiographical memory recall. *Journal of Personality and Social Psychology, 103,* 362–378.

Senchak, M., & Leonard, K. E. (1992). Attachment styles and marital adjustment among newlywed couples. *Journal of Social and Personal Relationships, 9,* 51–64.

Sexton, T., Gordon, K., Gurman, A., Lebow, J., Holtzworth-Munroe, A., & Johnson, S. M. (2011). Guidelines for classifying evidence-based treatments in couple and family therapy. *Family Process, 50,* 377–392.

Sharar, B., Carlin, E., Engle, D., Hegde, J., Szepsenwol, A., & Arkowitz, H. (2011). A pilot investigation of emotion focused two chair dialogue intervention for self-criticism. *Clinical Psychology and Psychotherapy, 19,* 496–507.

Shaver, P. R., & Clarke, C. L. (1994). The psychodynamics of adult romantic attachment. In J. Masling & R. Bornstein (Eds.), *Empirical perspectives on object relations theory* (pp. 105–156). Washington, DC: American Psychological Association.

Shaver, P. R., Collins, N., & Clarke, C. L. (1996). Attachment styles and internal working models of self and relationship partners. In G. O. Fletcher & J. Fitness (Eds.), *Knowledge structures in close relationships: A social psychological approach* (pp. 25–61). Mahwah, NJ: Erlbaum.

Shaver, P. R., & Hazan, C. (1993). Adult romantic attachment: Theory and evidence. In D. Perlman & W. Jones (Eds.), *Advances in personal relationships* (Vol. 4, pp. 29–70). London: Jessica Kingsley.

Shaver, P. R., & Mikulincer, M. (2002). Attachment-related psychodynamics. *Attachment and Human Development, 4,* 133–161.

Shaver, P. R., & Mikulincer, M. (2007). Attachment and emotional regulation. In J. J. Gross (Ed.), *Handbook of emotion regulation* (pp. 446–465). New York: Guilford Press.

Shedler, J. (2010). The efficacy of psychodynamic psychotherapy. *American Psychologist, 65,* 98–109.

Siegel, D. (2013). *Brainstorm: The power and purpose of the teenage brain.* New York: Tarcher/Penguin.

Simpson, J. A., Collins, A., Tran, S., & Haydon, K. (2007). Attachment and the experience and expression of emotions in romantic relationships: A developmental perspective. *Journal of Personality and Social Psychology, 92,* 355–367.

Simpson, J. A., & Overall, N. (2014). Partner buffering of attachment insecurity. *Current Directions in Psychological Science, 23,* 54–59.

Simpson, J. A., Rholes, W. S., & Nelligan, J. S. (1992). Support seeking and support giving within couples in an anxiety provoking situation: The role of attachment styles. *Journal of Personality and Social Psychology, 62,* 434–446.

Simpson, J. A., Rholes, W. S., & Phillips, D. (1996). Conflict in close relationships: An attachment perspective. *Journal of Personality and Social Psychology, 71,* 899–914.

Slade, A. (2008). The implications of attachment theory and research for adult psychotherapy. In J. Cassidy & P. R. Shaver (Eds.), *Handbook of attachment: Theory, research, and clinical applications* (2nd ed., pp. 762–782). New York: Guilford Press.

Slotter, E. B., Gardner, W. C., & Finkel, E. J. (2010). Who am I without you?: The influence of romantic breakup on the self-concept. *Personality and Social Psychology Bulletin, 36,* 147–160.

Spanier, G. (1976). Measuring dyadic adjustment. *Journal of Marriage and Family, 13,* 113–126.

Sroufe, L. A., Egeland, B., Carlson, E. A., & Collins, A. (2005). *The development of the person: The Minnesota Study of Risk and Adaptation from Birth to Adulthood.* New York: Guilford Press.

Stegge, H., & Meerum Terwogt, M. (2007). Awareness and regulation of emotion in typical and atypical development. In J. J. Gross (Ed.), *Handbook of emotion regulation* (pp. 269–286). New York: Guilford Press.

Steill, K., & Hailey, G. (2011). Emotionally focused therapy for couples living with aphasia. In J. Furrow, S. M. Johnson, & B. Bradley (Eds.), *The emotionally focused casebook: New directions in treating couples* (pp. 113–140). New York: Routledge.

Stern, D. N. (2004). *The present moment in psychotherapy and everyday life.* New York: Norton.

Stiles, W. B., Agnew-Davies, R., Hardy, G. E., Barkham, M., & Shapiro, D. A. (1998). Relations of the alliance with psychotherapy outcome: Findings in the Second Sheffield Psychotherapy Project. *Journal of Consulting and Clinical Psychology, 66*, 791–802.

Suchy, Y. (2011). *Clinical neuropsychology of emotion.* New York: Guilford Press.

Sullivan, H. S. (1953). *Conceptions of modern psychiatry.* New York: Norton.

Sullivan, K. T., Pasch, L. A., Johnson, M. D., & Bradbury, T. N. (2010). Social supoport, problem-solving, and the longitudinal course of newlywed marriage. *Journal of Personality and Social Psychology, 98*, 631–644.

Szalavitz, M. (2017). Dopamine: The currency of desire. *Scientific American Mind, 28*, 48–53.

Tang, T. Z., & DeRubeis, R. J. (1999). Sudden gains and critical sessions in cognitive behavioral therapy for depression. *Journal of Consulting and Clinical Psychology, 67*, 894–904.

Tolin, D. F. (2014). Beating a dead dodo bird: Looking for signal vs nose in cognitive behavioral therapy for anxiety disorders. *Clinical Psychology: Practice and Science, 21*, 351–362.

Tomkins, S. (1986). *Affect, imagery and consciousness.* New York: Springer.

Tottenham, N. (2014). The importance of early experiences for neuro-affective development. *Current Topics in Behavioral Neuroscience, 16*, 109–129.

Tronick, E. (1989). Emotions and emotional communication in infants. *American Psychologist, 44*, 112–119.

Tronick, E. (2007). *The neurobehavioral and social–emotional development of infants and children.* New York: Norton.

Tulloch, H., Greenman, P., Demidenko, N., & Johnson, S. M. (2017). *Healing Hearts Together Relationship Education Program: Facilitators guide for small groups.* Ottawa, Ontario, Canada: International Centre for Excellence in Emotionally Focused Therapy.

Tulloch, H., Johnson, S. M., Greenman, P., Demidenko, N., & Clyde, M. (2016). *Healing Hearts Together: A pilot intervention program for cardiac patients and their partners.* Presentation at the Canadian Association of Cardiac Prevention and Rehabilitation National Conference, Montreal, Quebec, Canada.

Uchino, B. N., Smith, T. W., & Berg, C. A. (2014). Spousal relationship quality and cardiovascular risk: Dyadic perceptions of relationship ambivalence are associated with coronary-artery calcification. *Psychological Science, 25*, 1037–1042.

van der Kolk, B. (2014). *The body keeps the score: Brain, mind and body in the healing of trauma.* New York: Penguin Books.

Wade, T. D., & Kendler, K. S. (2000). The relationship between social support and major depression: Cross-sectional, longitudinal and genetic perspectives. *Journal of Nervous and Mental Disease, 188*, 251–258.

Wallin, D. J. (2007). *Attachment in psychotherapy.* New York: Guilford Press.

Wampold, B. (2006). What should be validated: The psychotherapist. In J. C. Norcross, L. E. Beutler, & R. E. Levant (Eds.), *Evidence-based practices in mental health: Debate and dialogue* (pp. 200–208). Washington, DC: American Psychological Association.

Warren, S., Huston, L., Egeland, B., & Sroufe, L. A. (1997). Childhood anxiety disorders and attachment. *Journal of the American Academy of Child and Adolescent Psychiatry, 36*, 637–644.

Watson, J. C., & Bedard, D. L. (2006). Client's emotional processing in psychotherapy: A comparison between cognitive behavioral and process–experiential therapies. *Journal of Consulting and Clinical Psychology, 74,* 152–159.

Weissman, M. M., Markowitz, J. C., & Klerman, G. L. (2007). *Clinican's quick guide to interpersonal psychotherapy.* New York: Oxford University Press.

Whisman, M. A., & Baucom, D. H. (2012). Intimate relationships and psychopathology. *Clinical Child and Family Psychology Review, 15,* 4–13.

Wiebe, S. A., Elliott, C., Johnson, S. M., Burgess Moser, M., Dalgleish, T. L., Lafontaine, M., & Tasca, G. A. (2018). Attachment change in emotionally focused couple therapy and sexual satisfaction outcomes in a two-year follow-up study. *Journal of Couple and Relationship Therapy, 18,* 1-21.

Wiebe, S. A., Johnson, S. M., Lafontaine, M. F., Burgess Moser, M., Dalgleish, T., & Tasca, G. A. (2016). Two-year follow-up outcomes in emotionally focused couple therapy: An investigation of relationship satisfaction and attachment trajectories. *Journal of Marital and Family Therapy, 43,* 227–244.

Wilson, E. O. (1998). *Consilience: The unity of knowledge.* New York: Vintage Books.

Winnicott, D. W. (1965). *The maturational process and the facilitating environment.* London: Hogarth Press.

Woody, S., & Ollendick, T. (2006). Technique factors in treating anxiety disorders. In L. Castonguay & L. Beutler (Eds.), *Principles of therapeutic change that work* (pp. 167–186). New York: Oxford University Press.

Yalom, I. (1980). *Existential psychotherapy.* New York: Basic Books.

Yalom, I. (1989). *Love's executioner.* New York: Basic Books.

Yalom, I. D. (2000). *The gift of therapy.* New York: Harper Perennial.

Young, M., Riggs, S., & Kaminski, P. (2017). Role of marital adjustment in associations between romantic attachment and coparenting. *Family Relations, 66,* 331–345.

Zajonc, R. B. (1980). Feeling and thinking: Preferences need no inferences. *American Psychologist, 35,* 151–175.

Zemp, M., Bodenmann, G., & Cummings, E. M. (2016). The significance of interparental conflict for children. *European Psychologist, 21,* 99–108.

Zucccarini, D., Johnson, S. M., Dalgleish, T., & Makinen, J. (2013). Forgiveness and reconciliation in emotionally focused therapy for couples: The client change process and therapy interventions. *Journal of Marital and Family Therapy, 39,* 148–162.

Zuroff, D. C., & Blatt, S. J. (2006). The therapeutic relationship in the brief treatment of depression: Contributions to clinical improvement and enhanced adaptive capacities. *Journal of Consulting and Clinical Psychology, 74,* 130–140.

Index